2006
YEAR BOOK OF
SURGERY®

The 2006 Year Book Series

Year Book of Allergy, Asthma, and Clinical Immunology™: Drs Rosenwasser, Boguniewicz, Milgrom, Routes, and Weber

Year Book of Anesthesiology and Pain Management™: Drs Chestnut, Abram, Black, Gravlee, Lee, Mathru, and Roizen

Year Book of Cardiology®: Drs Gersh, Cheitlin, Elliott, Graham, Sundt, and Waldo

Year Book of Critical Care Medicine®: Drs Dellinger, Parrillo, Balk, Bekes, Dorman, and Dries

Year Book of Dentistry®: Drs McIntyre, Belvedere, Buhite, Davis, Henderson, Johnson, Jureyda, Ohrbach, Olin, Scott, Spencer, and Zakariasen

Year Book of Dermatology and Dermatologic Surgery™: Drs Thiers and Lang

Year Book of Diagnostic Radiology®: Drs Osborn, Birdwell, Dalinka, Gardiner, Levy, Maynard, Oestreich, and Rosado de Christenson

Year Book of Emergency Medicine®: Drs Burdick, Hamilton, Handly, Quintana, and Werner

Year Book of Endocrinology®: Drs Mazzaferri, Bessesen, Clarke, Howard, Kennedy, Leahy, Meikle, Molitch, Rogol, and Schteingart

Year Book of Family Practice®: Drs Bowman, Apgar, Dexter, Miser, Neill, and Scherger

Year Book of Gastroenterology™: Drs Lichtenstein, Burke, Campbell, Dempsey, Drebin, Ginsberg, Katzka, Kochman, Morris, Rombeau, Shah, and Stein

Year Book of Hand and Upper Limb Surgery®: Drs Chang and Steinmann

Year Book of Medicine®: Drs Barkin, Frishman, Garrick, Loehrer, Phillips, Pillinger, and Snydman

Year Book of Neonatal and Perinatal Medicine®: Drs Fanaroff, Maisels, and Stevenson

Year Book of Neurology and Neurosurgery®: Drs Gibbs and Verma

Year Book of Nuclear Medicine®: Drs Coleman, Blaufox, Royal, Strauss, and Zubal

Year Book of Obstetrics, Gynecology, and Women's Health®: Dr Shulman

Year Book of Oncology®: Drs Loehrer, Arceci, Glatstein, Gordon, Hanna, Morrow, and Thigpen

Year Book of Ophthalmology®: Drs Rapuano, Cohen, Eagle, Flanders, Hammersmith, Myers, Nelson, Penne, Sergott, Shields, Tipperman, and Vander

Year Book of Orthopedics®: Drs Morrey, Beauchamp, Peterson, Swiontkowski, Trigg, and Yaszemski

Year Book of Otolaryngology-Head and Neck Surgery®: Drs Paparella, Gapany, and Keefe

Year Book of Pathology and Laboratory Medicine®: Drs Raab, Parwani, Bejarano, and Bissell

Year Book of Pediatrics®: Dr Stockman

Year Book of Plastic and Aesthetic Surgery™: Drs Miller, Bartlett, Garner, McKinney, Ruberg, Salisbury, and Smith

Year Book of Psychiatry and Applied Mental Health®: Drs Talbott, Ballenger, Buckley, Frances, Jensen, and Markowitz

Year Book of Pulmonary Disease®: Drs Phillips, Barker, Lewis, Maurer, Tanoue, and Willsie

Year Book of Rheumatology, Arthritis, and Musculoskeletal Disease™: Drs Panush, Furst, Hadler, Hochberg, Lahita, and Paget

Year Book of Sports Medicine®: Drs Shephard, Alexander, Cantu, Feldman, McCrory, Nieman, Rowland, Sanborn, and Shrier

Year Book of Surgery®: Drs Copeland, Bland, Cerfolio, Daly, Eberlein, Fahey, Mozingo, Pruett, and Seeger

Year Book of Urology®: Drs Andriole and Coplen

Year Book of Vascular Surgery®: Dr Moneta

2006
The Year Book of SURGERY®

Editor-in-Chief
Edward M. Copeland III, MD
The Edward R. Woodward Distinguished Professor of Surgery, Department of Surgery, University of Florida, Gainesville, Florida

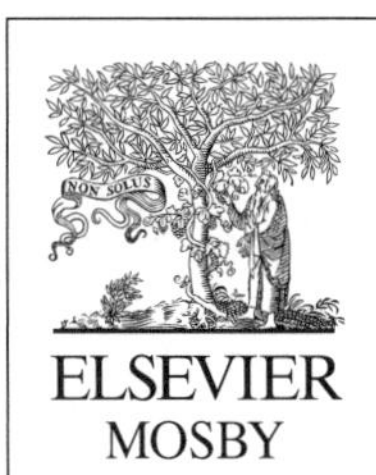

ELSEVIER
MOSBY

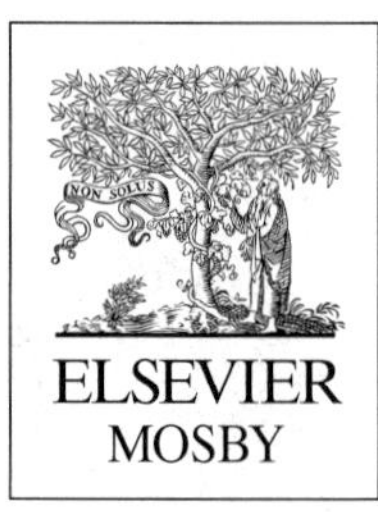

Vice President, Continuity: John A. Schrefer
Associate Developmental Editor: Ruth Malwitz
Senior Manager, Continuity Production: Idelle L. Winer
Senior Issue Manager: Jason Gonulsen
Illustrations and Permissions Coordinator: Dawn Vohsen

2006 EDITION

Printed in the United States of America
Composition by Thomas Technology Solutions, Inc.
Printing/binding by Sheridan Books, Inc.

Editorial Office:
Elsevier
1600 John F. Kennedy Blvd.
Suite 1800
Philadelphia, PA 19103-2899

International Standard Serial Number: 0090-3671
International Standard Book Number: 1-4160-3300-9
978-1-4160-3300-4

Editorial Board

Table of Contents

Journals Represented

Journals represented in this YEAR BOOK are listed below.

American Journal of Infection Control
American Journal of Kidney Diseases
American Journal of Medicine
American Journal of Pathology
American Journal of Physiology Heart and Circulation Physiology
American Journal of Physiology, Endocrinology and Metabolism
American Journal of Physiology-Lung Cellular and Molecular Physiology
American Journal of Surgery
American Journal of Transplantation
American Surgeon
Anesthesia and Analgesia
Annals of Plastic Surgery
Annals of Surgery
Annals of Thoracic Surgery
Archives of Dermatology
Archives of Disease in Childhood. Fetal and Neonatal Edition
Archives of Physical Medicine and Rehabilitation
Archives of Surgery
British Journal of Cancer
British Journal of Surgery
Burns
Canadian Journal of Surgery
Chest
Circulation
Clinical Cancer Research
Clinical Chemistry
Critical Care Medicine
Diabetes
Diabetes Care
Digestive Diseases and Sciences
Diseases of the Colon and Rectum
European Journal of Endocrinology
Gastroenterology
Gastrointestinal Endoscopy
Health Technology Assessment
Intensive Care Medicine
Journal of Burn Care and Rehabilitation
Journal of Clinical Endocrinology and Metabolism
Journal of Clinical Investigation
Journal of Clinical Oncology
Journal of Gastrointestinal Surgery
Journal of Immunology
Journal of Investigative Dermatology
Journal of Microbiology, Immunology and Infection
Journal of Pediatric Surgery
Journal of Pediatrics
Journal of Pharmacology and Experimental Therapeutics
Journal of Surgical Research
Journal of Thoracic and Cardiovascular Surgery

Journal of Trauma: Injury, Infection, and Critical Care
Journal of Vascular Surgery
Journal of the American College of Surgeons
Journal of the American Geriatrics Society
Journal of the American Medical Association
Journal of the National Cancer Institute
Lancet
New England Journal of Medicine
Pediatrics
Radiology
Surgery
Transplantation
Transplantation Proceedings
Virchows Archiv: An International Journal of Pathology
World Journal of Surgery

STANDARD ABBREVIATIONS

The following terms are abbreviated in this edition: acquired immunodeficiency syndrome (AIDS), cardiopulmonary resuscitation (CPR), central nervous system (CNS), cerebrospinal fluid (CSF), computed tomography (CT), deoxyribonucleic acid (DNA), electrocardiography (ECG), health maintenance organization (HMO), human immunodeficiency virus (HIV), intensive care unit (ICU), intramuscular (IM), intravenous (IV), magnetic resonance (MR) imaging (MRI), ribonucleic acid (RNA), and ultrasound (US).

NOTE

The YEAR BOOK OF SURGERY is a literature survey service providing abstracts of articles published in the professional literature. Every effort is made to assure the accuracy of the information presented in these pages. Neither the editor nor the publisher of the YEAR BOOK OF SURGERY can be responsible for errors in the original materials. The editors' comments are their own opinions. Mention of specific products within this publication does not constitute endorsement.

To facilitate the use of the YEAR BOOK OF SURGERY as a reference tool, all illustrations and tables included in this publication are now identified as they appear in the original article. This change is meant to help the reader recognize that any illustration or table appearing in the YEAR BOOK OF SURGERY may be only one of many in the original article. For this reason, figure and table numbers appear to be out of sequence within the YEAR BOOK OF SURGERY.

1 General Considerations

Introduction

Much has been written in 2005 about the impact of the 80-hour workweek imposed on surgical training programs by various governmental agencies and the Accreditation Council for Graduate Medical Education. Residency Review Committees now police training programs to ensure that the 80-hour mandate is followed. In some states, a financial penalty is imposed upon the teaching hospital if the mandate is violated. I have included several articles that address the safety of the new training paradigm. I admit that a bit of my prejudice against the 80-hour mandate has probably slipped into my selection of articles and in my commentaries on them.

The National Surgical Quality Improvement Program (NSQIP) developed in the Veterans Administration System is the best method available to determine the reasons for surgical morbidity and mortality and the cost associated with both. The 80-hour workweek was instituted to ensure *better* care for the surgical patient. A recent VA study concluded that patient outcome was the same as before implementation and without a significant increase in the involvement by the attending surgeon. Often, interns are required to be up all night caring for patients, and there is evidence that motor vehicle accidents involving interns were reduced after implementation of work-hour limitations. This assumes that interns do not stay up late on nights off!! Maybe interns are different from the "old days." Students at Ohio State Medical School found that residents who were working 100 hours per week before work-hour implementation thought that surgery was a rewarding career, had big egos, and were demanding of hospital personnel. Are these bad traits? Almost all the studies agree that contact with patients in the outpatient setting has suffered in the new paradigm. Most show that operative volume has not been affected. Now we might know how to operate, but not when!

There has been a repopulation of the empty surgical residency spots of a few years ago. The work-hour restrictions get the credit and, no doubt, deservedly so. Are the people now attracted to surgery different with different goals and aspirations? Time will tell! One study found that there was a fall-off in interest in surgery between the first and fourth years of medical school. It is hard to totally blame lifestyle and debt on this decreased interest. Possibly motivation of students by surgical faculty members might have been lacking. Much of student and resident contact in the past came in the more relaxed environment of pre- and postoperative patient care either as an inpatient or outpatient. It is not surprising that motivation toward a surgical career by surgical faculty has declined as contact time has declined. A survey showed that male and female students select the same reasons for becoming surgeons. So, we do not have to change our motivational techniques entirely because of gender. The disturbing aspect to this study is that 25% of both male and female surgeons would not recommend the surgical profession to medical students. The chance of a medical student encountering a disgruntled surgeon during the critical formative years is almost 100% if the dissatisfaction rate of 25% is accurate. One solution to the problem of surgeon work hours and, possibly, surgeon dissatisfaction has been to limit surgical practice to a narrow focus such as breast surgery. This, of course, begs the question of who is going to do the "general" surgery? There is mounting evidence that patients requiring complex operative procedures such as pancreatectomies and hepatectomies for cancer have better survival and lower complication rates when operated upon in high-volume hospitals. The increased interests in narrowing the scope of surgical practice will soon result in patients with more complex surgical problems having no choice but to search out high-volume hospitals regardless of the inconvenience to the patient. The malpractice environment is, likewise, limiting patient access to specialty care as some of these surgeons eliminate from their practice patients with diseases with high litigation potential or leave areas of high liability risk.

The surgeons' contribution to the hospital bottom line is outlined in an excellent article from the University of Pennsylvania where the authors were allowed access to hospital collection data (not a universal trait of most hospitals). The answers to why some of the favoritism shown to certain surgical services by hospital administrators are contained therein. In some training institutions, residents are still required (or allowed) to dictate the operative records. The money lost by inaccurate documentation leading to inaccurate procedure coding is staggering (assuming you are interested in making a living). NSQIP has determined that preoperative risk factors and surgical complexity are more predictive of hospital costs than are postoperative complications, once again indicating the importance of direct involvement of the attending surgeon in the pre- and intraoperative period. So there are areas that those surgeons, who by definition of their specialty may not add greatly to the hospital bottom line, can improve on what they do contribute.

Because of many of the ever-mounting issues with surgical education described in the preceding paragraphs, The American Surgical Association convened a "Blue Ribbon Committee" to address the issues and make recommendations for solutions to the problems. The description and identification of the problems are excellent. Many of the solutions require "new" money into the educational system that is not identified because the group had no means of doing so. Additional methods of addressing the changing practice paradigm is to take a lesson from the airline industry that the captain of the ship is not all powerful and must work within the boundaries of multiple individuals with different but important components leading to a safe flight. Patient safety is now more diffused within the team atmosphere. This diffusion will increase as those trained in the 80-hour workweek graduate into practice and carry the style of teamwork, "hand offs," and seamless communication with them. This style, of course, dictates that everyone dealing with a patient has the same skills and motivation to ensure patient safety. It has the added benefit of multiple individuals thinking about the same patient problem. It does, however, put more of a burden on the medical professions to ensure that all graduating physicians are responsible and have the ability for self-improvement. Characteristics of unprofessional behavior can be detected while in medical school, and when uncorrected, can lead to disaster in the team approach to patient care. Since the inability for self-improvement means that irresponsible behavior cannot be corrected, these individuals must be identified and removed from the medical profession as early as possible.

I have chosen to write this introduction in narrative fashion. The articles selected follow the narrative and the commentaries include more in-depth discussion. If the narrative has stimulated your interest, you will enjoy the commentaries—they are entirely my thoughts on the various subjects, many derived from personal observations (a few may even be controversial).

Edward M. Copeland III, MD

Does Resident Hours Reduction Have an Impact on Surgical Outcomes?

Kaafarani HMA, Itani KMF, Petersen LA, et al (Baylor College of Medicine, Houston)

J Surg Res 126:167-171, 2005 1–1

Background.—We assessed the impact of restricting surgical resident work hours as required by the Accreditation Council for Graduate Medical Education (ACGME), on postoperative outcomes.

Materials and Methods.—The divisions of General and Vascular Surgery at the Michael E. DeBakey Houston Veteran Affairs Medical Center implemented a limited work hours schedule effective October 1, 2002. We compared the rate of postoperative morbidity and mortality before and after the new schedule. Clinical data were collected by the VA National Surgical Quality Improvement Program (NSQIP) for the periods of October 1, 2001 to September 30, 2002 (preintervention), and October 1, 2002 to September 30, 2003 (postintervention). We assessed risk-adjusted observed to expected (O/E) ratios of mortality and prespecified postoperative morbidity for each study period.

Results.—In the preintervention period, there were 405 general surgery and 202 vascular surgery cases as compared to 382 and 208 cases, respectively in the postintervention period. There were no significant differences in mortality O/E ratios between the pre- and postintervention periods (0.63 versus 0.60 in general surgery; 0.78 versus 0.81 in vascular surgery; $P = 0.90$ and 0.94, respectively) or in morbidity O/E ratios (1.06 versus 1.27 in general surgery; 1.47 versus 1.50 in vascular surgery; $P = 0.20$ and 0.90, respectively).

Conclusion.—The restricted resident work hour schedule in general and vascular surgery in our facility did not significantly affect postoperative outcomes.

▶ This study comes from the Veterans Affairs system, in which the NSQIP has been implemented and, in my opinion, represents the best analysis of outcomes available to us today. Therefore, the results of this study have been as strictly controlled as possible. Likewise the Veterans Affairs system has an excellent method of determining the involvement of the attending surgeon in the operative procedure. The authors' conclusion is that patient outcomes after implementation of the 80-hour workweek is the same as before its implementation and without a significant increase in the involvement of the attending surgeon in the operative procedure. One of the prevailing reasons to implement the 80-hour workweek was to improve patient outcomes because the prediction was that tired residents made more medical and surgical errors. I would argue that this study dispels that theory, at least in this hospital.

E. M. Copeland III, MD

Extended Work Shifts and the Risk of Motor Vehicle Crashes Among Interns

Barger LK, for the Harvard Work Hours, Health, and Safety Group (Brigham and Women's Hosp, Boston; Harvard Med School, Boston)

N Engl J Med 352:125-134, 2005 1–2

Background.—Long work hours and work shifts of an extended duration (≥24 hours) remain a hallmark of medical education in the United States. Yet their effect on health and safety has not been evaluated with the use of validated measures.

Methods.—We conducted a prospective nationwide, Web-based survey in which 2737 residents in their first postgraduate year (interns) completed 17,003 monthly reports that provided detailed information about work hours, work shifts of an extended duration, documented motor vehicle crashes, near-miss incidents, and incidents involving involuntary sleeping.

Results.—The odds ratios for reporting a motor vehicle crash and for reporting a near-miss incident after an extended work shift, as compared with a shift that was not of extended duration, were 2.3 (95 percent confidence interval, 1.6 to 3.3) and 5.9 (95 percent confidence interval, 5.4 to 6.3), respectively. In a prospective analysis, every extended work shift that was scheduled in a month increased the monthly risk of a motor vehicle crash by 9.1 percent (95 percent confidence interval, 3.4 to 14.7 percent) and increased the monthly risk of a crash during the commute from work by 16.2 percent (95 percent confidence interval, 7.8 to 24.7 percent). In months in which interns worked five or more extended shifts, the risk that they would fall asleep while driving or while stopped in traffic was significantly increased (odds ratios, 2.39 [95 percent confidence interval, 2.31 to 2.46] and 3.69 [95 percent confidence interval, 3.60 to 3.77], respectively).

Conclusions.—Extended-duration work shifts, which are currently sanctioned by the Accreditation Council for Graduate Medical Education, pose safety hazards for interns. These results have implications for medical residency programs, which routinely schedule physicians to work more than 24 consecutive hours.

▶ What were the activities of the interns on their nights off? The assumption is that nights off are used for rest, study, etc. If that is the case, interns have changed a great deal from my era when nights off emphasized "relaxation." We were on call every other night, so 50% of the workforce was in the hospital. In addition, you were only responsible for patients whose histories you knew. You could usually count on getting some sleep or predicting when you would not. As on call has gone to every fourth or fifth night, the workforce in the hospital has been reduced by 50% or greater, and the intern is guaranteed to be up all night. Consequently, if late nights occur on nights off, an increase in accidents would be expected. The answer is to increase the workforce at night with physician extenders who can screen calls for the on-duty physician.

In today's system in which an intern is expected to be up 24 to 36 hours straight even if it's every fourth night, I would not have chosen surgery as a career. I was lucky. I did my training in an institution with every other night call, excellent call rooms, free meals at night, buddies to share the experience with, and before level I trauma units and organ transplantation programs existed. I was seldom up 24 hours straight and could enjoy nights off and nights on call with equal enthusiasm—but that was a long time ago.

E. M. Copeland III, MD

Prospective, Blinded Evaluation of Accuracy of Operative Reports Dictated by Surgical Residents

Novitsky YW, Sing RF, Kercher KW, et al (Carolinas Med Ctr, Charlotte, NC)
Am Surg 71:627-632, 2005 1–3

Introduction.—Incomplete or inaccurate operative notes result in delayed, reduced, or denied reimbursement. Deficient reports may be more common when dictated by the surgical residents. We performed a blinded study to assess the accuracy of residents' dictations and their effect on the appropriate level of coding for reimbursement. A prospective, blinded study was performed comparing operative reports dictated by senior surgical residents (postgraduate years 3, 4, and 5) to reports dictated by attending surgeons. All residents had previously undergone group instruction on the importance and structure of operative notes. The trainees were blinded to the fact that the attending surgeons were dictating the operative reports on a separate dictation system. The dictations were analyzed by faculty reimbursement billing personnel for accuracy and completeness. Fifty operative reports of general surgical procedures dictated by both surgical residents and attending physicians were reviewed. A total of 97 CPT codes were used to report services rendered. Residents' dictations resulted in incorrect coding in 14 cases (28% error rate). The types of inaccuracies were a completely missed procedure (4) and insufficient documentation for an appropriate CPT code and/or modifier (10). All deficiencies occurred in complex, multicode, and/or laparoscopic cases. Sixty-seven per cent of late dictations were incomplete. The financial analysis revealed that deficiencies in resident dictations would have reduced the reimbursement by $18,200 (9.7%). For cases with deficient dictations, 29.5 per cent of charges would have been missed, delayed, or denied if the resident-dictated note was used to justify charges. Operative reports dictated by surgical residents are often incomplete or inaccurate, likely leading to reduced or delayed reimbursement. Dictations of complex, multicode, or laparoscopic surgeries, especially if delayed beyond 24 hours, are likely to contain significant deficiencies that affect billing. Attending surgeons may be better equipped to dictate complex cases. Formal housestaff education, mentorship by the attending faculty, and ongoing quality control may be paramount to minimize documentation errors to ensure appropriate coding for the services rendered.

► I have dictated my own operative records for some time because I get paid more for the procedure. It shocks me that all surgeons do not do the same. There was a time when we had sufficient money in the system that collecting all money allocated to a procedure was not a high priority. Having the resident dictate the operative report was thought to be a teaching tool, but it really isn't unless the report is reviewed by the attending surgeon and reviewed with the resident who dictated it. This seldom happened, so having the resident dictate the operative report was really just a convenience for the attending surgeon. I guess there are still a few of us around who remember those days and have not changed our ways to make more money and avoid liability.

E. M. Copeland III, MD

American Surgical Association Blue Ribbon Committee Report on Surgical Education: 2004

Debas HT, Bass BL, Brennan MF, et al (UCSF Global Health Sciences)

Ann Surg 241:1-8, 2005 1–4

Background.—American surgical education has produced some of the best-trained and most competent surgeons in the world. There has been little change in the structure of surgery residency since its formulation by Hallstead in the early 20th century. However, in recent years, several forces for change have begun to affect medical education, in general, and surgical training, in particular. Findings of the American Surgical Association Blue Ribbon Committee on Surgical Education, which was established in June 2002, are presented. The purpose of the committee was to examine the many forces affecting health care and to make recommendations regarding changes needed in surgical education to enhance the training of surgeons to serve the surgical needs of the United States and to maintain the high standard of training and research in surgery into the 21st century.

Overview.—At one time, it was predicted that there would be an excess of physicians by 2010; however, now it appears that a shortage of physicians will occur. Increasingly, students are selecting specialties with more controllable lifestyles than general surgery. In addition, the attrition rate among general surgery residencies is nearly 20%, again due primarily to lifestyle concerns of residents. More major changes will occur in surgical practice as much of clinical care continues to shift from the inpatient hospital setting to the outpatient setting; in addition, the length of stay for inpatients is decreasing. Surgical care is transitioning from discipline-based practice to disease-based practice; in this scenario, the surgeon will increasingly work as part of a team of experts. Surgical training needs to be adjusted to prepare surgeons to be leaders of these multidisciplinary teams.

Conclusions.—The development of a new surgical education system is recommended—a system that functions in the context of patient care. Implementation of this new system will require major redesign of surgery residency training and allocation of enough resources to achieve the desired outcomes.

▶ The members of the Blue Ribbon Committee are to be congratulated on their willingness to address the ever-mounting issues of surgical education. The change in surgical career development is a train hurtling down the track and can only be steered, not redirected. We have fought fragmentation for years and are now forced to accept it. There are or will be surgeons who leave after 5 to 7 years of training to do only breast, endocrine, or hernia surgery in their first jobs. In fact, fellowships after surgical training now exist in at least 2 of these areas. How long does it take to train someone in these limited skills? (Not long!) Do they require broad-based surgical training? (No!) The general surgeon of yesterday will be represented in the future by the trauma or emergency surgeon.

Should we focus our attention on training those surgeons who will require an in-depth knowledge of anatomy, physiology, and critical care? (Yes!) Making surgery more attractive to medical students through mentoring and education is a goal I embrace, but will it overcome the lifestyle issues of the current generation and recreate the broad-based general surgeon capable of practicing alone in a rural location? (Probably not!) Urbanization may eliminate the need for this individual but not during my lifetime. I predict that on-the-job training for the junior associate is going to be increasingly necessary by the senior partners unless there is room in the practice for someone who can devote full time to a limited area of general surgery.

The recommendations of the Blue Ribbon Committee will go a long way toward fixing the system or preventing its "fracture." Unfortunately, many recommendations require new money or redirecting currently budgeted money for educational purposes—wonderful ideas theoretically but ones with realistic limitations. I hope the people with the money are listening!

E. M. Copeland III, MD

Disciplinary Action by Medical Boards and Prior Behavior in Medical School

Papadakis MA, Teherani A, Banach MA, et al (Univ of California, San Francisco; Federation of State Med Boards, Dallas; Thomas Jefferson Univ, Philadelphia; et al)

N Engl J Med 353:2673-2682, 2005 1–5

Background.—Evidence supporting professionalism as a critical measure of competence in medical education is limited. In this case–control study, we investigated the association of disciplinary action against practicing physicians with prior unprofessional behavior in medical school. We also examined the specific types of behavior that are most predictive of disciplinary action against practicing physicians with unprofessional behavior in medical school.

Methods.—The study included 235 graduates of three medical schools who were disciplined by one of 40 state medical boards between 1990 and 2003 (case physicians). The 469 control physicians were matched with the case physicians according to medical school and graduation year. Predictor variables from medical school included the presence or absence of narratives describing unprofessional behavior, grades, standardized-test scores, and demographic characteristics. Narratives were assigned an overall rating for unprofessional behavior. Those that met the threshold for unprofessional behavior were further classified among eight types of behavior and assigned a severity rating (moderate to severe).

Results.—Disciplinary action by a medical board was strongly associated with prior unprofessional behavior in medical school (odds ratio, 3.0; 95 percent confidence interval, 1.9 to 4.8), for a population attributable risk of disciplinary action of 26 percent. The types of unprofessional behavior most strongly linked with disciplinary action were severe irresponsibility (odds ratio, 8.5; 95 percent confidence interval, 1.8 to 40.1) and severely diminished capacity for self-improvement (odds ratio, 3.1; 95 percent confidence interval, 1.2 to 8.2). Disciplinary action by a medical board was also associated with low scores on the Medical College Admission Test and poor grades in the first two years of medical school (1 percent and 7 percent population attributable risk, respectively), but the association with these variables was less strong than that with unprofessional behavior.

Conclusions.—In this case–control study, disciplinary action among practicing physicians by medical boards was strongly associated with unprofessional behavior in medical school. Students with the strongest association were those who were described as irresponsible or as having diminished ability to improve their behavior. Professionalism should have a central role in medical academics and throughout one's medical career.

► The current emphasis on professionalism in both medical school and residency is justified by the results of this study. The question, of course, is what to do when unprofessional behavior is identified. Irresponsibility and a restricted ability for self-improvement go together, and the latter means the former cannot be corrected. These are character flaws that have developed over a long period of time. It would be nice to identify these flaws before admission to medical school, and attention should be focused here. The responsibility of weeding out these people, however, rests with the medical profession at all levels. We have erred on the side of assuming that a medical degree is documentation of appropriate behavior. I would suggest that we take a directly opposite approach, that is, we should suspend physicians who have a documented character flaw and not reinstate them until the flaw has been corrected, and even then, not until after a long probationary period. Standardized testing may need to be utilized more in the future because direct contact with both medical students and residents has become somewhat limited by work hour restrictions. The lazy can hide among the enthusiastic and go unnoticed. Consequently, these flaws may not be picked up until residency, and then workforce issues help protect these people. The place that exposure is greatest is in the practice environment after residency. All hospitals should have a strict code of professionalism with severe restriction of practice and required reporting to the National Practitioner Data Bank. On the other end, before gaining hospital privileges, all credentialing committees should be required to check the applicant with the Data Bank.

E. M. Copeland III, MD

Has Implementation of the 80-Hour Work Week Made a Career in Surgery More Appealing to Medical Students?

Arnold MW, Patterson AF, Tang L (Ohio State Univ, Columbus)
Am J Surg 189:129-133, 2005 1–6

Background.—This study was conducted to determine if a surgical career became more appealing to medical students with the resident work week limited to 80 hours.

Methods.—At the start and conclusion of each surgery clerkship rotation, students completed a survey addressing perception of surgeons, and surgery as a career. They were divided into the control groups (rotations before July 2003; n = 109) and the experimental group (rotations after July 2003; n = 108).

Results.—Students in the experimental group had a significantly more favorable impression of a surgeon's lifestyle and work hours than those in the control group. This was especially true of female students post-rotation, who responded more positively to the statement that a surgical career would allow for a good balance between professional and personal life (1.87 vs 2.45, P <.01).

Conclusion.—The new Accreditation Council for Graduate Medical Education (ACGME) regulation has had a positive impact on students' perceptions of the surgeon's lifestyle, but does not necessarily increase their interest in a surgical career.

► Students at Ohio State University have a 6-week rotation in general surgery, which is a time much longer than many medical schools. Thus, the students surveyed did have an adequate time to evaluate the 2 time periods. When residents were working 100 hours per week, the students were more likely to believe that surgery is a rewarding career, that surgeons have big egos, and that surgeons are demanding of hospital personnel. My interpretation of these data is different from the authors. In the experimental group, the residents worked 30 fewer hours. I think this decrease lessened the intensity of longitudinal patient care and lessened the residents' feelings of responsibility for the patient. A more "laid back" resident is a less demanding one, appears to be less egotistical, and may be preoccupied with having more fun doing something other than surgery. I may be old-fashioned, but if I am right, the surgeon of the immediate future will look nothing like the surgeon of the immediate past. They will not have introjected into their professional personalities the need to know the status of their patients at all times and will experience little guilt if they miss the results of a test, have a beeper malfunction while on call, or decide to continue their leisure activity when paged to see a patient.

Until proven otherwise, I would prefer to have a sleepy resident who knows my history rather than an uninformed one whose responsibility for me is momentary.

E. M. Copeland III, MD

Impact of Work-Hour Restrictions on Residents' Operative Volume on a Subspecialty Surgical Service

Spencer AU, Teitelbaum DH (Univ of Michigan, Ann Arbor)

J Am Coll Surg 200:670-676, 2005 1–7

Background.—Whether the 80 hours per week limit on surgical residents' work hours has reduced the number or variety of cases performed by residents is unknown.

Study Design.—We quantified residents' operative experience, by case category, on a pediatric surgical service. The number of senior and junior residents' cases were compared between residents from the year before (n = 47) and after (n = 44) the 80-hour limit. Residents also completed a questionnaire about their operative and educational experience. As an additional dimension of the educational experience, resident participation in clinic was assessed. Student's *t*-test was used.

Results.—Total number of cases performed either by senior (before, 1.58 ± 0.42 versus after, 1.84 ± 0.82 cases/day) or junior (before, 0.70 ± 0.21 versus after, 0.71 ± 0.15) residents has not changed (p = NS). Senior residents' vascular access and endoscopy rate increased; other categories remained stable. Residents' perception of their experience was unchanged. But residents' participation in outpatient clinic was significantly decreased (before, 66.0% ± 14.7% versus after, 17.0% ± 19.9% of clinics covered, $p < 0.005$).

Conclusions.—The 80-hour limit has had minimal impact on residents' operative experience, in case number and variety, and residents' perceptions of their educational experience. Residents' reduction in duty hours may have been achieved at the expense of outpatient clinic experiences.

▶ The average number of cases done by a resident is determined in any program by the number of operations divided by the number of residents. Emphasis on continuity of care by the Surgical Residency Review Committee (RRC) before July 1, 2003 dictated that residents must participate in the preoperative and postoperative care of their patients. Because so much of this care had shifted to the outpatient setting, residents had required involvement in the "real time" workup of the patient preoperatively and were expected to manage both the short- and long-term complications of their procedures as outpatients. We may now be producing surgeons who are technically competent but not judgmentally sound—at least this was one of the fears of the RRC when continuity of care was mandated. We could be returning to the old preceptorial system in which residents show up in the operating room, check the schedule, and divide up the cases, knowing little or nothing about the patients. During my years as a member of the RRC, we worked hard to avoid such a system that we thought would produce only a surgical technician. Could we possibly have been wrong?

E. M. Copeland III, MD

Long-term Survival Is Superior After Resection for Cancer in High-Volume Centers

Fong Y, Gonen M, Rubin D, et al (Mem Sloan-Kettering Cancer Ctr, New York)

Ann Surg 242:540-547, 2005 1–8

Background.—A number of studies have demonstrated that surgical resection at high-volume centers is associated with improved short-term perioperative outcome. Whether long-term results after resection of visceral malignancies are superior at high-volume centers is largely unknown.

Methods.—All patients who were subjected to pancreatectomy or hepatectomy for cancer in the years 1995 and 1996 were identified in the National Medicare database. Data extracted and examined include demographics, comorbidities, and long-term survival. All survival was confirmed through 2001, providing actual 5-year survival. Long-term survival was examined as related to hospital volume.

Results.—In the study period, there were 2592 pancreatectomies and 3734 hepatectomies performed at 1101 and 1284 institutions, respectively. High-volume center was defined as >25 cases/y. By this definition, there were 10 high-volume centers for pancreatectomy and 12 centers for hepatectomy performing 11% (n = 291) of the pancreatectomies and 12% (n = 474) of the hepatectomies in this study period. Comparison by log-rank demonstrated superior survival for patients resected at high-volume centers (pancreatectomy: $P = 0.001$; hepatectomy: $P = 0.02$). This was confirmed by multivariate analysis. All analyses included an adjustment for within-center correlation.

Conclusion.—Superior long-term survival is associated with complex visceral resections for cancer at high-volume centers.

► This is another in the growing mass of literature reporting better results of major operations in high-volume hospitals. I believe the data, but most of it comes from authors in high-volume hospitals (although I am not sure whether that makes any difference when a Medicare database is used). I would like to see at least one of these studies put together by someone from a low-volume hospital.

E. M. Copeland III, MD

Effects of a Malpractice Crisis on Specialist Supply and Patient Access to Care

Mello MM, Studdert DM, DesRoches CM, et al (Harvard School of Public Health, Boston; Harvard Med School, Boston; Harris Interactive, Inc, New York; et al)

Ann Surg 242:621-628, 2005 1–9

Objective.—To investigate specialist physicians' practice decisions in response to liability concerns and their perceptions of the impact of the malpractice environment on patient access to care.

Summary Background Data.—A perennial concern during "malpractice crises" is that liability costs will drive physicians in high-risk specialties out of practice, creating specialist shortages and access-to-care problems.

Methods.—Mail survey of 824 Pennsylvania physicians in general surgery, neurosurgery, orthopedic surgery, obstetrics/gynecology, emergency medicine, and radiology eliciting information on practice decisions made in response to rising liability costs.

Results.—Strong majorities of specialists reported increases over the last 3 years in patients' driving distances (58%) and waiting times (83%) for specialist care or surgery, waiting times for emergency department care (82%), and the number of patients forced to switch physicians (89%). Professional liability costs and managed care were both considered important contributing factors. Small proportions of specialists reported that they would definitely retire (7%) or relocate their practice out of state (4%) within the next 2 years; another third (32% and 29%, respectively) said they would likely do so. Forty-two percent of specialists have reduced or eliminated high-risk aspects of their practice, and 50% are likely to do so over the next 2 years.

Conclusions.—Our data suggest that claims of a "physician exodus" from Pennsylvania due to rising liability costs are overstated, but the malpractice situation is having demonstrable effects on the supply of specialist physicians in affected areas and their scope of practice, which likely impinges upon patients' access to care.

▶ This study comes from a highly concentrated area of liability crisis but represents the eventual outcome for other areas of the country if the crisis is not reversed. The patterns of practice are already being altered as physicians begin to protect themselves from liability. HMOs created an access issue because patients could not select their preferred physician. Not until enough people had been affected by HMO methodology did the system get changed. The same will be true for malpractice reform. Not until the voting public is negatively affected by limitation of specialty care will the system change. If this prediction is true, then things are going to get worse before they get better. Hopefully, they will get worse in pockets around the country so that the reasons for limitation of specialty care can be evaluated by entities that have the power to change the system. Texas and California have been proactive, and personal communication has indicated that both the number of suits and the settlements have been reduced. In fact, some medical malpractice defense attorneys have had to widen their scope of practice to make a living. This is not a bad thing.

E. M. Copeland III, MD

Potential Targets to Encourage a Surgical Career

Brundage SI, Lucci A, Miller CC, et al (Stanford Univ, Calif; MD Anderson Cancer Ctr, Houston; Univ of Texas-Houston)

J Am Coll Surg 200:946-953, 2005 1–10

Background.—Our goal was to identify factors that can be targeted during medical education to encourage a career in surgery.

Study Design.—We conducted a cross-sectional survey of first and fourth year classes in a Liaison Committee on Medical Education-accredited medical school. Students scored 19 items about perceptions of surgery using a Likert-type scale. Students also indicated their gender and ranked their top three career choices.

Results.—There were 121 of 210 (58%) first year and 110 of 212 (52%) fourth year students who completed the survey. First year students expressed a positive correlation between surgery and career opportunities, intellectual challenge, performing technical procedures, and obtaining a residency position, although length of training, work hours, and lifestyle during and after training were negatively correlated with choosing surgery. Fourth year student responses correlated positively with career and academic opportunities, intellectual challenge, technical skills, role models, prestige, and financial rewards. Factors that correlated negatively were length of training, residency lifestyle, hours, call schedule, and female gender of the student respondent. Forty-four percent of first year male students expressed an interest in surgery versus 27% of fourth year male students ($p < 0.04$). Eighteen percent of first year female students expressed an interest in surgery versus 5% of fourth year female students ($p < 0.006$).

Conclusions.—Lifestyle issues remain at the forefront of student concerns. Intellectual challenge, career opportunities, and technical skills are consistently recognized as strengths of surgery. Additionally, fourth year students identify role models, prestige, and financial rewards as positive attributes. Emphasizing positive aspects may facilitate attracting quality students to future careers in surgery.

▶ This article comes from only 1 medical school and may not reflect the professional biases of medical students in general. Nevertheless, the fall off in interest in surgery as a career between the first and fourth years is an important observation and is indicative, at least in the institution studied, that the surgical faculty are not taking advantage of an innate surgical interest in their entering students. Also, these students' concern about debt was minimal, which is a frequently cited reason for not choosing a surgical career. Thus, a lack of external motivation toward a surgical career and lifestyle demands are the reasons for the decrease in interest between the first and fourth years. Surgery is essentially a hobby that allows one to make a living and provide a useful service to mankind. Most people spend hours on their hobby with no compensation and work on it well into the night. The "fun" part of surgery and an innate interest (and an aptitude for anatomy) attracted me to the profession. I suspect that limited work hours has attracted more students to surgery as a profession, but I predict that those students that genuinely enjoy the art and craft of the discipline will be frustrated by the limitations of work hours, much as I would have been.

E. M. Copeland III, MD

Predictors of Surgery Resident Satisfaction With Teaching by Attendings: A National Survey

Ko CY, Escarce JJ, Baker L, et al (RAND, Santa Monica, Calif)

Ann Surg 241:373-380, 2005 1–11

Objective.—To identify factors that predict fourth- and fifth-year surgical resident satisfaction of attending teaching quality.

Summary Background Data.—With the training of surgical residents undergoing major changes, a key issue facing surgical educators is whether high-quality surgeons can still be produced. Innovative techniques (eg, computer simulation surgery) are being developed to substitute partially for conventional teaching methods. However, an aspect of training that cannot be so easily replaced is the faculty-resident interaction. This study investigates resident perceptions of attending teaching quality and the factors associated with this faculty-resident interaction to identify predictors of resident educational satisfaction.

Methods.—A national survey of clinical fourth- and fifth-year surgery residents in 125 academically affiliated general surgery training programs was performed. The survey contained 67 questions and addressed demographics, hospital, and service characteristics, as well as surgery, education, and clinical care-related factors. Univariate analyses were performed to describe the characteristics of the sample; multivariate analyses were performed to evaluate the factors associated with resident educational satisfaction.

Results.—The response rate was 61.5% (n = 756). Average age was 32 years; most were male (79%), white (72%), and married (69%); 42% had children. Ninety-five percent of respondents graduated from U.S. medical schools, and the average debt was $80,307. Of 20 potentially mutable factors, 6 variables had positive associations with resident education satisfaction and 7 had negative associations. Positive factors included the resident being the operating surgeon in major surgeries, substantial citing of evidence-based literature by the attending, attending physicians giving spontaneous or unplanned presentations, increasing the continuity of care, clinical teaching aimed at the chief resident level, and having clinical decisions made together by both the attending and resident. There were 7 negative factors such as overly supervising in surgery, being interrupted so much that teaching was ineffective, and attending physicians being rushed and/or eager to finish rounds.

Conclusion.—This study identifies several factors that were associated with resident educational satisfaction. It offers the perspective of the learners (ie, residents) and, importantly, highlights mutable factors that surgery faculty (and departments) may consider changing to improve surgery resident education and satisfaction. Improving such satisfaction may help to produce a better product.

▶ This study was done before the implementation of the 80-hour workweek affected the fourth and fifth year residents who participated. When negative experiences were reported, only a small percentage of residents were exposed to them. Several of the positive experiences will be negatively affected by the 80-hour paradigm. Because time in the clinic has been curtailed in many programs, continuity of care may become a thing of the past, as will be some preoperative joint decision making because this exercise often occurs in the clinic. We must guard against having surgical residencies becoming primarily preceptorial, that is, where surgical technique but not surgical judgment is taught. Preoperative conferences may replace the interaction of the attending physician, patient, and resident in the clinic. Let's hope so.

E. M. Copeland III, MD

Preoperative Risk Factors and Surgical Complexity Are More Predictive of Costs Than Postoperative Complications: A Case Study Using the National Surgical Quality Improvement Program (NSQIP) Database

Davenport DL, Henderson WG, Khuri SF, et al (Univ of Kentucky, Lexington; Univ of Colorado, Denver; Natl Surgical Quality Improvement Program, West Roxbury, Mass)

Ann Surg 242:463-471, 2005 1–12

Objective.—This single-center study tested the hypothesis that preoperative risk factors and surgical complexity predict more variation in hospital costs than complications.

Background.—Complications after surgical operations have been shown to significantly increase hospital cost. The impact on complication-related costs of preoperative risk factors is less well known.

Methods.—The National Surgical Quality Improvement Program (NSQIP) preoperative risk factors, surgical complexity, and outcomes, along with hospital costs, were analyzed for a random sample of 5875 patients on 6 surgical services. Operation complexity was assessed by work RVUs (Centers for Medicare and Medicaid Services Resource Based Relative Value Scale). The difference in mean hospital costs associated with all variables was analyzed. Multiple linear regression was used to determine the cost variation associated with all variables separately and combined.

Results.—Fifty-one of 60 preoperative risk factors, work RVUs, and 22 of 29 postoperative complications were associated with higher variable direct costs ($P < 0.05$). Linear regressions showed that risk factors predicted 33% ($P < 0.001$) of cost variation, work RVUs predicted 23% ($P < 0.001$), and complications predicted 20% ($P < 0.001$). Risk factors and work RVUs together predicted 49% of cost variation ($P < 0.001$) or 16% more than risk factors alone. Adding complications to this combined model modestly increased prediction of costs by 4% for a total of 53% ($P < 0.001$).

Conclusion.—Preoperative risk factors and surgical complexity are more effective predictors of hospital costs than complications. Preoperative intervention to reduce risk could lead to significant cost savings. Payers and regulatory agencies should risk-adjust hospital cost assessments using clinical information that integrates costs, preoperative risk, complexity of operation, and outcomes.

▶ The obvious message here is to reduce preoperative risk factors so that complications from complex surgical procedures and, therefore, costs can be reduced. This is a laudable goal that, hopefully, all of us try to attain. Many preoperative risk factors cannot be further reduced. The example given by the authors is diabetes that is already controlled by medication but, nevertheless, remains a risk factor for costs. That payers and regulatory agencies should incorporate preoperative risk factors into hospital cost assessments is the new message and was unavailable until the NSQIP was moved into the private sector, which was an accomplishment aided by the American College of Surgeons. All surgeons should embrace NSQIP because, through this methodology, the correct data for costs, morbidity, and mortality will be obtained. Possibly pay for performance will be based on NSQIP data. For those of us who care for patients who need complicated operations but who have a disproportionate number of preoperative risk factors, these data are extremely valuable. NSQIP is a hospital-based program with some associated costs to the hospital. Consequently, not all hospital administrators are going to embrace the methodology (unless forced to do so for pay for performance). For now, it may require the surgeons on the staff to strongly recommend the program.

E. M. Copeland III, MD

Progressive Specialization Within General Surgery: Adding to the Complexity of Workforce Planning

Stitzenberg KB, Sheldon GF (Univ of North Carolina, Chapel Hill)

J Am Coll Surg 201:925-932, 2005 1–13

Background.—Although most general surgeons receive comparable training leading to Board certification, the services they provide in practice may be highly variable. Progressive specialization is the voluntary narrowing of scope of practice from the breadth of skills acquired during training; it occurs in response to patient demand, rapid growth of medical knowledge, and personal factors. Progressive specialization is increasingly linked to fellowship training, which generally abruptly narrows a surgeon's scope of practice. This study examines progressive specialization by evaluating trends in fellowship training among general surgeons.

Study Design.—Because no database exists that tracks trainees from medical school matriculation through entrance into the workforce, data from multiple sources were compiled to assess the impact of progressive specialization. Trends in overall number of trainees, match rates, and proportion of international medical graduates were analyzed.

Results.—The proportion of general surgeons pursuing fellowship training has increased from > 55% to > 70% since 1992. The introduction of fellowship opportunities in newer content areas, such as breast surgery and minimally invasive surgery, accounts for some of the increase. Meanwhile, interest in more traditional subspecialties (ie, thoracic and vascular surgery) is declining.

Conclusions.—Progressive specialization confounds workforce projections. Available databases provide only an estimate of the extent of progressive specialization. When surgeons complete fellowships, they narrow the spectrum of services provided. Consequently, as the phenomenon of progressive specialization evolves, a larger surgical workforce will be needed to provide the breadth of services encompassed by the primary components of general surgery.

► Narrowing the scope of practice has been a goal of surgeons for years. For example, many obstetricians give up deliveries when they can make a living with scheduled gynecologic surgery. Similarly, older general surgeons often have limited their practice to breast, hernias, and/or vascular access. This specialization was the result of many years of service to the community and recognized local expertise. Now fellowships in limited areas of general surgery brand the young surgeon as an expert, and a period of time in the community providing what I will call "general practice general surgery" no longer is required. In fact, many surgical groups in large cities have found that they need a female breast surgeon in their group to maintain their competitiveness among patients with breast diseases. The numbers of surgeons willing to provide "general practice general surgery" is rapidly shrinking, and no provisions have been made to replace these individuals (other than with specialists who may not be available). The hospital policy of requiring general surgeons younger than a certain age to take emergency calls was a good one and assured that those who chose to specialize during the day had to remain competent for the general surgical cases done during the night. I think that we will soon need a new surgical specialty called GENERAL SURGERY to fill the void left by the surgical specialist.

E. M. Copeland III, MD

Surgeon Contribution to Hospital Bottom Line: Not All Are Created Equal

Resnick AS, Corrigan D, Mullen JL, et al (Univ of Pennsylvania, Philadelphia)

Ann Surg 242:530-539, 2005 1–14

Objective.—We hypothesized that surgeon productivity is directly related to hospital operating margin, but significant variation in margin contribution exists between specialties.

Summary Background Data.—As the independent practitioner becomes an endangered species, it is critical to better understand the surgeon's importance to a hospital's bottom line. An appreciation of surgeon contribution to hospital profitability may prove useful in negotiations relating to full-time employment or other models.

Methods.—Surgeon total relative value units (RVUs), a measure of productivity, were collected from operating room (OR) logs. Annual hospital margin per specialty was provided by hospital finance. Hospital margin data were normalized by dividing by a constant such that the highest relative hospital margin (RHM) in fiscal year 2004 expressed as margin units (mu) was 1 million mu. For each specialty, data analyzed included RHM/OR HR, RHM/case, and RHM/RVU.

Results.—Thoracic (34.55 mu/RVU) and transplant (25.13 mu/RVU) were the biggest contributors to hospital margin. Plastics (–0.57 mu/RVU), maxillofacial (1.41 mu/RVU), and gynecology (1.66 mu/RVU) contributed least to hospital margin. Relative hospital margin per OR HR for transplant slightly exceeded thoracic (275.74 mu vs 233.94 mu) at the top and plastics and maxillofacial contributed the least (–3.83 mu/OR HR vs 9.36 mu/OR HR).

Conclusions.—Surgeons contribute significantly to hospital margin with certain specialties being more profitable than others. Payer mix, the penetration of managed care, and negotiated contracts as well as a number of other factors all have an impact on an individual hospital's margin. Surgeons should be fully cognizant of their significant influence in the marketplace.

► This excellent study differs from many others in its category because actual dollars collected are reported. The reader will immediately understand why some services with limited educational responsibility within a medical school framework get relatively more hospital resources (eg, neurosurgery) than those services with the bulk of medical school educational responsibility (eg, general surgery). In the days of plenty, to maintain a balanced educational experience, surgical chairs knew that some services would be chronic money losers, not because the faculty members weren't working but because reimbursement for their work was poor. Cross-subsidization occurred within the departmental structure, and no hospital money was needed to meet the annual departmental budget. No longer is this the case; consequently, the job of a department chair is very different than in the recent past. Many are now middle managers with little autonomy. Dependence on hospital revenue to meet the medical school mission can create tension between the hospital and the medical school and within divisions in a department in which cross-subsidization is no longer possible. Compounding this issue is the ever-increasing salaries of academic surgeons. The chair has 2 important means of managing a department: money and space. In the new paradigm, more loyalty could easily be given to the hospital than to the department; likewise, the dean is caught between the need for money from the hospital mission (often responding to an outside board of directors who are bottom-line–oriented—check out hospital administrators salaries and incentive programs) and the educational mission of the medical school. The educational health care systems that figure this new paradigm out and can cooperate will be the strong ones of the future. It is an excellent opportunity for second-tier systems to rise to the top. It will be interesting to see if any rise to the challenge or continue to function in the way that made them second tier.

E. M. Copeland III, MD

The Impact of Aviation-Based Teamwork Training on the Attitudes of Health-Care Professionals

Grogan EL, Stiles RA, France DJ, et al (Vanderbilt Univ, Nashville, Tenn; Crew Training Internatl, Memphis, Tenn)

J Am Coll Surg 199:843-848, 2004 1–15

Background.—Both the Institute of Medicine and the Agency for Healthcare Research and Quality suggest patient safety can be enhanced by implementing aviation Crew Resource Management (CRM) in health care. CRM emphasizes six key areas: managing fatigue, creating and managing teams, recognizing adverse situations (red flags), cross-checking and communication, decision making, and performance feedback. This study evaluates participant reactions and attitudes to CRM training.

Study Design.—From April 22, 2003, to December 11, 2003, clinical teams from the trauma unit, emergency department, operative services, cardiac catheterization laboratory, and administration underwent an 8-hour training course. Participants completed an 11-question End-of-Course Critique (ECC), designed to assess the perceived need for training and usefulness of CRM skill sets. The Human Factors Attitude Survey contains 23 items and is administered on the same day both pre- and posttraining. It measures attitudinal shifts toward the six training modules and CRM.

Results.—Of the 489 participants undergoing CRM training during the study period, 463 (95%) completed the ECC and 338 (69%) completed the Human Factors Attitude Survey. The demographics of the group included 288 (59%) nurses and technicians, 104 (21%) physicians, and 97 (20%) administrative personnel. Responses to the ECC were very positive for all questions, and 95% of respondents agreed or strongly agreed CRM training would reduce errors in their practice. Responses to the Human Factors Attitude Survey indicated that the training had a positive impact on 20 of the 23 items ($p < 0.01$).

Conclusions.—CRM training improves attitudes toward fatigue management, team building, communication, recognizing adverse events, team decision making, and performance feedback. Participants agreed that CRM training will reduce errors and improve patient safety.

► It is a little scary that this type of training is relatively new in the airline industry, and the public will be surprised that it is not part of the fabric of the operative experience. The concept that the surgeon is the "captain of the ship" and responsible for anything that goes wrong is no longer true. There was a time when I knew every facet of the patient's course in real-time and was the central repository for all information. In the new health care paradigm, I am forced to rely on other health care providers not always directly under my control to ensure that "all is well" in the perioperative period. Communication and a willingness to speak up are now of utmost importance for patient safety as the care of the patient becomes more diffused in the team atmosphere. I still practice the "old style" of medicine and insist as much as possible to have all the data at my fingertips. In the new paradigm when physician lifestyle and limited work hours take on more importance, the knowledge of the patient's situation may be fragmented among several health care providers. Hopefully, they will communicate! Especially if I am the patient!

E. M. Copeland III, MD

The Training Needs and Priorities of Male and Female Surgeons and Their Trainees

Saalwachter AR, Freischlag JA, Sawyer RG, et al (Univ of Virginia, Charlottesville; Johns Hopkins Hosp, Baltimore, Md)

J Am Coll Surg 201:199-205, 2005 1–16

Background.—Over the past decade, interest in general surgery careers has declined and the number of female medical school graduates has increased. This study was performed to identify the needs of both male and female surgical trainees and to guide design of training programs because attracting medical students to, and maintaining residents in, general surgery training programs can be difficult without a clear understanding of the training needs and priorities of both men and women. We hypothesized that men and women would express similar training priorities, yet have subjectively different experiences.

Study Design.—Medical students, surgical residents, fellows, and fully trained surgeons affiliated with at least one of four major surgical societies were asked to complete a level-specific survey located on the American College of Surgeons Web site.

Results.—There were 4,308 respondents (76% men). Men and women selected similar reasons for choosing a surgical career and residency program and criteria critical to a successful residency program, with women placing greater emphasis on clerkship experience and faculty diversity. There were no statistically significant differences between the men and women's perceptions of their own training. Although, when asked to evaluate whether certain aspects of training were comparable for male and female residents, women were statistically less likely to agree that their experiences were comparable with those of their male colleagues.

Conclusions.—Male and female surgical residents, fellows, and trained surgeons identified almost identical training needs and priorities yet women perceived disparate treatment.

▶ It is comforting to know that male and female surgeons selected the same reasons for becoming surgeons. Most of us "aging" academic surgeons have been recruiting favorite students into surgery for some time, and it would be disquieting to find that we had to drastically change our strategy. I have always thought that male and female students enter surgery for the same reasons, and the results of this survey demonstrate me to be accurate.

I would like to have those programs that discriminate against women residents identified. This complaint has been around for a long time without specific institutional examples for those of us who either are too naive to notice the discrimination or do not have it in our institutions. Is it possible that women are more sensitive to the same treatment given to men, and the problem is then one of perception? If that were the case, then women would be asking for preferential treatment compared with men.

The most disturbing results from this survey are that only 75% of male and female surgeons would choose surgery again, and, similarly, only 75% would recommend the profession of surgery to medical students. A 25% dissatisfaction rate seems high to me and may be at the heart of the problem of recruiting and retention of surgical residents. With this dissatisfaction rate, the chance of encountering a disgruntled surgeon is almost 100%, and such a person is not going to be very supportive during times when a trainee is having a "bad day." Culling these dissatisfied surgeons from contact with students and residents in the formative years might be the best solution to recruiting and retention.

E. M. Copeland III, MD

2 Trauma

Introduction

Despite the continuing evolution of trauma care systems, 46.7 million Americans still have no access to a trauma center within an hour after injury. Conversely, 42.8 million Americans have access to 20 or more level I or II trauma centers within 1 hour from their home. Selecting the location of trauma centers based on geographic need and sharing trauma care resources across states will be important in the future. Funding of trauma care remains an important consideration to both hospitals and physicians. The recent nationally publicized threats of closures of urban trauma centers due to high costs, combined with an awakening among trauma and critical care societies and surgeons that their specialty is in danger of extinction, speaks for the need to evaluate the dichotomy of hospital and surgeon reimbursement for trauma care. Creating an emergency general surgery service is one opportunity to increase the operative productivity of trauma surgeons. Transferring the emergency surgery population to a service attuned to the care of patients in emergency situations such as trauma seems ideally suited. Also, the ability to increase the elective general surgery volumes for colleagues practicing non-emergency specialties can be obtained. The perceived increased malpractice risks attributed to trauma patient care discourages participation in trauma call duties and may influence career choices for surgeons and subspecialists. This perception may or may not be the case, as careful review of the malpractice cases at one institution revealed no difference in incidence between trauma and elective cases.

Abdominal compartment syndrome continues to occur in critically ill patients after intra-abdominal trauma or massive resuscitation. Marked bowel edema is usually present, and gut dysfunction in this setting has been described. Despite these problems, it is possible to provide enteral nutrition safely in most patients in the setting of an open abdomen. Long-term parenteral nutrition may not be required, as is practiced by some. Those patients who survive damage control surgery or decompressive laparotomy for abdominal compartment syndrome requiring temporary abdominal closure may be left with massive abdominal wall hernias. The combined efforts of trauma surgeons and plastic surgeons in a multidisciplinary approach may improve the patient's outcome from an abdominal wall reconstruction. The use of a components separation approach with or without mesh insertion is often of value.

Trauma surgeons generally support the concept of implementation of programs to screen injured patients for the presence of alcohol abuse and dependence. Both the CDC and the National Traffic Safety Administration have recommended routine trauma center screening. The uniform accident and sickness policy provision law is a legal statute that allows insurance carriers to exclude coverage for alcohol and drug-related injuries. Nearly 1 in 4 trauma surgeons reported denials of insurance claims due to this policy. Both legislators and trauma surgeons endorse revision of these policies. Many screening tools exist for identification of patients with alcohol-related problems. Even a single simple question can be asked to identify these patients with a relatively high degree of certainty.

The availability of recombinant factor VIIa as an adjunctive therapy for bleeding in trauma patients has been described, but the appropriateness of the use of this agent needs to be carefully evaluated. Overuse of this product comes at a significant financial cost, and those patients who would benefit most from this therapy would best be prospectively identified. Predictors of futility of this treatment include profound metabolic acidosis and elevated prothrombin time, as well as multicavitary injuries and advanced age. Patients who sustain major trauma while receiving warfarin may bleed more seriously from their injuries, particularly when head trauma occurs. Reluctance to continue anticoagulation treatment after the traumatic injuries have been resolved is common. In patients where long-term warfarin treatment was discontinued after major trauma, there was no increased risk of stroke or myocardial infarction, but the patients did have an increased risk of venous thromboembolism.

Recent changes in military capabilities and doctrine have resulted in a change in the pattern of casualties returning to the continental United States during military conflicts. Critical care air transport teams have made the air evacuation of critically ill patients a routine process. Critically ill and ventilator-dependent casualties may be returned to the United States as early as 3 days after injury and receive a more definitive approach to resolution of their traumatic injuries.

Contrast-enhanced sonography is a novel imaging technique that may be useful in the assessment of abdominal emergencies. This technique makes the detection of bleeding with extravasation possible to identify using relatively standard ultrasound equipment. This technique may, with further development, be applicable to the care of trauma patients. Selective clinical management of patients with anterior abdominal stab wounds remains controversial. In the absence of shock, peritonitis, or evisceration, an alternative strategy for management of stable patients may include serial clinical assessments for evidence of bleeding or hollow viscus injury. A report included in this year's selections describes this approach, which should continue to be evaluated in larger series.

All-terrain vehicles continue to impart a substantial risk in all age groups, particularly for teenagers below the driving age who receive little training and adult supervision. Safety equipment is rarely used, and this population is more likely to engage in risky behavior while riding an all-terrain vehicle. Unlike their 3-wheeled counterparts, relatively little has been done to decrease the injury rates from these vehicles through product regulation or legislation.

There is a bimodal distribution of traumatic brain injury with respect to age. The deleterious effect of age is particularly pronounced in patients older than 70 years. These older patients have a poorer functional status at discharge and improve less at 1 year compared with younger patients. Deterioration and recovery potential begins to appear in patients between 45 and 59 years of age.

David W. Mozingo, MD

Access to Trauma Centers in the United States

Branas CC, MacKenzie EJ, Williams JC, et al (Univ of Pennsylvania, Philadelphia; Johns Hopkins Bloomberg School of Public Health, Baltimore, Md; Johns Hopkins Whiting School of Engineering, Baltimore, Md; et al)
JAMA 293:2626-2633, 2005 2–1

Context.—Previous studies have reported that the number and distribution of trauma centers are uneven across states, suggesting large differences in access to trauma center care.

Objective.—To estimate the proportion of US residents having access to trauma centers within 45 and 60 minutes.

Design and Setting.—Cross-sectional study using data from 2 national databases as part of the Trauma Resource Allocation Model for Ambulances and Hospitals (TRAMAH) project. Trauma centers, base helipads, and block group population were counted for all 50 states and the District of Columbia as of January 2005.

Main Outcome Measures.—Percentages of national, regional, and state populations having access to all 703 level I, II, and III trauma centers in the United States by either ground ambulance or helicopter within 45 and 60 minutes.

Results.—An estimated 69.2% and 84.1% of all US residents had access to a level I or II trauma center within 45 and 60 minutes, respectively. The 46.7 million Americans who had no access within an hour lived mostly in rural areas, whereas the 42.8 million Americans who had access to 20 or more level I or II trauma centers within an hour lived mostly in urban areas. Within 45 and 60 minutes, respectively, 26.7% and 27.7% of US residents had access to level I or II trauma centers by helicopter only and 1.9% and 3.1% of US residents had access to level I or II centers only from trauma centers or base helipads outside their home states.

Conclusion.—Selecting trauma centers based on geographic need, appropriately locating medical helicopter bases, and establishing formal agreements for sharing trauma care resources across states should be considered to improve access to trauma care in the United States.

► In many areas of the United States, residents do not have timely access to trauma centers that could save their lives. In other areas there may be too many trauma centers, possibly leading to inefficiencies and lower patient volumes per center. Critical to the development of effective trauma systems is the designation or verification of trauma center hospitals equipped to treat the most seriously injured patients. The number of trauma centers has increased over the past decade; however, the geographic distribution of these centers is variable. This important study identified that 46.7 million Americans have no access to a trauma center within an hour following injury. Most of these live in rural areas. Conversely, 42.8 million Americans have access to 20 or more level I or II trauma centers within an hour, mostly living in urban areas. Another important finding in this study is that distance and land area metrics can lead to potentially misleading impressions of access. Depending on the maturity of the trauma system, using the western United States as an example, even the greater distances between centers can be overcome with mature transport capabilities. Selecting trauma centers based on geographic need and establishing formal agreements for sharing trauma care resources across states will be important for the future of trauma care.

D. W. Mozingo, MD

Trauma System Structure and Viability in the Current Healthcare Environment: A State-by-State Assessment

Mann NC, MacKenzie E, Teitelbaum SD, et al (Univ of Utah, Salt Lake City; Johns Hopkins Univ, Baltimore, Md; Health Resources and Services Administration)

J Trauma 58:136-147, 2005 2–2

Objective.—Anecdotal reports suggest that some state trauma systems are struggling to remain solvent while others appear stable in the current health care environment. The purpose of this research is to characterize the current structure and viability of state trauma systems in the U.S.

Methods.—Expert panels were convened in all 50 states to characterize the current structure of trauma care and to identify strengths, weakness, opportunities and threats facing trauma care delivery in each state.

Results.—States continue to value the formalization of trauma systems. System operations, evaluation/research methods and trauma leadership are highly valued by states with mature systems. However, all states consider their trauma system severely threatened by inadequate funding and difficulty recruiting and retaining physicians and nurses.

Conclusion.—Trauma care systems are valued and demonstrate potential for future expansion. However, economic shortfalls and retention of medical personnel threaten the viability of current systems across the U.S.

▶ Although trauma systems have proven to be effective in delivering the needed healthcare, neither public opinion nor economic issues favor further enhancement of the trauma system concept. In fact, trauma systems face growing public apathy and economic shortfalls that have resulted in the closure of several established trauma centers and many others strain to remain solvent. Information for this report was gained by convening expert panels in all 50 states to characterize the current structure of trauma care. When considering state responses together or dividing into groups, financial issues were considered both a prevalent weakness and the leading threat to trauma systems. This economic instability was associated with a pervasive concern regarding a recruitment and retention of trauma care providers, especially physicians and nurses.

D. W. Mozingo, MD

Trauma/Critical Care Surgeon: A Specialist Gasping for Air

Rodriguez JL, Christmas AB, Franklin GA, et al (Univ of Louisville, Ky)

J Trauma 59:1-7, 2005 2–3

Background.—In the last 10 years, trauma/critical care has become less attractive because of the decreasing surgical caseload, the nocturnal work hours, and the economics of the practice. Nevertheless, during the same period, the number of verified trauma centers has significantly increased. This study assesses the economic drive behind this dichotomy.

Methods.—Over a 1-year period, we collected financial data on 1,907 trauma patients for both Level I trauma centers and trauma/critical care surgeons. Financial data, including payor source, cost, reimbursement, margin, and reimbursement-to-charge and reimbursement-to-direct cost ratios, were calculated.

Results.—For commercial- and government-insured patients, the reimbursement-to-direct cost ratio was 2-and 35-fold greater, respectively, for the trauma centers than for the trauma/critical care surgeons. For uninsured patients, the addition of local government funds allowed the trauma center to cover direct cost with no margin. In contrast, even with the addition of supplemental salary dollars from the institution, for every dollar in direct cost generated by the trauma/critical care surgeons in caring for uninsured patients, they recovered 55 cents, or a loss of 45 cents per direct cost dollar spent.

Conclusion.—The economic dichotomy that exists between trauma centers and trauma/critical surgeons is significant. It drives institutional growth and, at the same time, discourages surgeons from entering the subspecialty. As physician reimbursement decreases and the number of uninsured patients increases, this economic dichotomy will amplify. Over the next decade, without a significant adjustment, the subspecialty is in danger of extinction.

► A significant economic dichotomy exists between trauma centers and trauma/critical care surgeons. Trauma/critical care has become less attractive because of a decreasing surgical case load, night time work hours, and the poor economics of this type of practice. Conversely, the number of verified trauma centers has significantly increased. Recently, there have been several nationally publicized threats of closures of urban trauma centers attributable to either the malpractice insurance crisis or high operating losses as a result of the significant increase in underfunded patients. There has also been an awakening among trauma and critical care societies and surgeons that the specialty is in danger of extinction because of the relative inability to attract young dedicated individuals. Analysis for the hospital's reimbursement for trauma care included in this report demonstrates that, despite the prevalence of underinsured patients, the hospital is able to more than cover the cost of the trauma population. It is inevitable that within a short period, in the absence of financial restructuring and commitment of governmental agencies, that trauma centers and trauma surgeons will not be able to exist in their current roles.

D. W. Mozingo, MD

Creating an Emergency General Surgery Service Enhances the Productivity of Trauma Surgeons, General Surgeons and the Hospital

Austin MT, Diaz JJ Jr, Feurer RD, et al (Vanderbilt Univ, Nashville, Tenn)

J Trauma 58:906-910, 2005 2–4

Background.—Several models that integrate trauma and emergency general surgery (EGS) have been proposed to provide a diverse and challenging operative practice for trauma surgeons and improve recruitment. In July 2002, our institution established a 24/7 EGS consult service, staffed primarily by critical care/trauma surgeons (CCTS). The objective of this report was to evaluate the impact of this new service on CCTS, general surgeons (GS) and the hospital.

Methods.—All admissions to CCTS and GS from July 1, 2000 to June 30, 2003 were reviewed by querying hospital and physician databases for demographics, diagnoses, operative intervention(s), and resource utilization. Data were analyzed using nonparametric methods.

Results.— 9,405 admissions were identified, with GS and EGS admissions increasing over time. In July 2002, EGS became a separate service and captured 26% of GS admissions. Hospital-wide trauma admissions remained stable despite a slight decrease in trauma admissions to CCTS. A decrease in trauma operations by CCTS was offset by an increased EGS operative volume. EGS included "bread and butter" GS procedures including appendectomies and cholecystectomies and complex surgical procedures. EGS patients were often sicker with more than 50% requiring ICU admission compared with GS admissions of which only 10% required ICU care. (Table 1 is included in full-text article.)

Conclusions.—Departmental restructuring to include an EGS service: 1) increased CCTS volume despite decreased CCTS trauma admissions and operations; 2) increased elective GS volume; 3) generated increased use of ICU and operating room resources; and 4) demonstrated that CCTS with broad operative GS backgrounds and critical care knowledge can effectively staff an EGS service.

► Trauma care has changed dramatically over the past decade. Since the epidemic of gun-related violence in the early 1990s, the rate of penetrating trauma has been declining. In addition, safer vehicles and strict enforcement of helmet laws for motorcyclists and seat belt laws for automobiles have improved highway safety. The trend toward nonoperative management of blunt solid organ trauma has also contributed to the decline in surgical cases. This selection reviews the establishment of a trauma and EGS service in the setting of a level I trauma center. This program allowed CCTSs to increase operative volume during a time when trauma admissions and trauma-related operations were declining. Also realized was the ability to increase the elective general surgery volumes of their colleagues no longer involved in EGS. In addition, it was noted that a greater proportion of the EGS patients require ICU admissions than the typical elective general surgery patient, a situation ideally suited to the surgeon with added qualifications in surgical critical care.

D. W. Mozingo, MD

Trauma Surgery Malpractice Risk: Perception Versus Reality
Stewart RM, Johnston J, Geoghegan K, et al (Univ of Texas at San Antonio)
Ann Surg 241:969-977, 2005 2–5

Objective.—We set out to compare the malpractice lawsuit risk and incidence in trauma surgery, emergency surgery, and elective surgery at a single academic medical center.

Summary and Background Data.—The perceived increased malpractice risk attributed to trauma patients discourages participation in trauma call panels and may influence career choice of surgeons. When questioned, surgeons cite malpractice risk as a rationale for not providing trauma care. Little data substantiate or refute the perceived high trauma malpractice risk. We hypothesized that the malpractice risk was equivalent between an elective surgical practice and a trauma/emergency practice.

Methods.—Three prospectively maintained institutional databases were used to calculate and characterize malpractice incidence and risk: a surgical operation database, a trauma registry, and a risk management/malpractice database. Risk groups were divided into elective general surgery (ELECTIVE), urgent/emergent, nontrauma general surgery (URGENT), and trauma surgery (TRAUMA). Malpractice claims incidence was calculated by dividing the total number of filed lawsuits by the total number of operative procedures over a 12-year period.

Results.—Over the study period, 62,350 operations were performed. A total of 21 lawsuits were served. Seven were dismissed. Three were granted summary judgments to the defendants. Ten were settled with payments to the plaintiffs. One went to trial and resulted in a jury verdict in favor of the defendants. Total paid liability was $4.7 million ($391,667/year). Total legal defense costs were $1.3 million ($108,333/year). The ratio of lawsuits filed/operations performed and incidence in the 3 groups is as follows: ELECTIVE 14/39,080 (3.0 lawsuits/100,000 procedures/year), URGENT 5/17,958, (2.3 lawsuits/100,000 procedures/year), and TRAUMA 2/5312 (3.1/100,000 procedures/year). During the study period, there were an estimated 49,435 trauma patients evaluated. The incidence of malpractice lawsuits using this denominator is 0.34 lawsuits/100,000 patients/year.

Conclusions.—These data demonstrate no increased risk of lawsuit when caring for trauma patients, and the actual risk of a malpractice lawsuit was low.

► Trauma care is perceived by many as a high malpractice risk specialty. This perceived increased malpractice risk attributed to trauma patients discourages participation in trauma call duties and may influence the career choice of surgeons and subspecialists. Though this is a common perception, little data are available to support this notion. In this selection, a single level I trauma center evaluated the malpractice risk between an elective general surgery-based practice and a trauma/emergency surgery practice. The authors found no increased risk of lawsuit when caring for trauma patients and that the actual risk of a malpractice lawsuit was low at 0.34 lawsuits per 100,000 patients per year. This study represents a single institution's experience and must be considered in that light. A broader exploration of this issue is needed.

D. W. Mozingo, MD

Postinjury Abdominal Compartment Syndrome Does Not Preclude Early Enteral Feeding After Definitive Closure

Cothren CC, Moore EE, Ciesla DJ, et al (Univ of Colorado, Denver)

Am J Surg 188:653-658, 2004 2–6

Background.—Critically injured patients are susceptible to the abdominal compartment syndrome (ACS), which requires decompressive laparotomy with delayed abdominal closure. Previous work by the University of Texas Houston group showed impaired gut function after resuscitation-associated gut edema. The purpose of this study was to determine if enteral nutrition was precluded by the intra-abdominal hypertension and bowel edema of the ACS.

Methods.—Patients developing postinjury ACS from January 1996 to August 2003 at our level-I trauma center were reviewed. Patient demographics, time to definitive abdominal closure, and institution and tolerance of enteral nutrition were evaluated.

Results.—Thirty-seven patients developed postinjury ACS during the study period; 26 men and 11 women with a mean age of 36 ± 4 and injury severity score of 33 ± 4. Mean intra-abdominal pressure before decompression was 32 ± 3 mm Hg, and concurrent mean peak airway pressure was 50 ± 4 cm oxygen. Enteral feeding was never started in 12 patients; 4 died within 48 hours of admission, 7 required vasoactive agents until their death, and 1 developed an enterocutaneous fistula requiring parenteral nutrition. Enteral feeding was initiated in the remaining 25 patients: 13 had feeds started within 24 hours of abdominal closure; 5 were fed with open abdomens; and 7 had a delay because of vasopressors (n = 2), multiple trips to the operating room (n = 2), paralytics (n = 2), and increased intra-abdominal pressures (n = 1). Once advanced, enteral feeding was tolerated in 23 (92%) of the 25 patients with attainment of goal feeds in a mean of 3.1 ± 1 days.

Conclusions.—Despite the bowel edema and intra-abdominal hypertension related to the ACS, early enteral feeding is feasible after definitive abdominal closure.

► ACS occurs in critically injured patients after intraabdominal trauma or massive resuscitation, relief of which is most often accomplished by laparotomy and temporary closure of the abdomen. Marked bowel edema is usually present and gut dysfunction in this setting has been described. A single institution's experience was reviewed in 37 patients who had postinjury ACS develop that required decompressive laparotomy. The delivery of enteral nutrition was accomplished in 25 of these patients who survived the immediate postinjury period. Feedings were tolerated once the abdomen was closed in most patients; however, some were fed in the face of a persistent open abdomen without complications. Enteral access in these patients was obtained by needle catheter jejunostomy placement at the time of abdominal closure or bowel coverage. Management of patients with the ACS and open abdomen is complex. Conclusions from this study suggest that long-term total parenteral nutrition is not required in this subset of patients and that effective alimentation can be provided via the enteral route.

D. W. Mozingo, MD

Multidisciplinary Approach to Abdominal Wall Reconstruction After Decompressive Laparotomy for Abdominal Compartment Syndrome

Hultman CS, Pratt B, Cairns BA, et al (Univ of North Carolina, Chapel Hill)

Ann Plast Surg 54:269-275, 2005 2–7

Introduction.—Decompressive laparotomy for abdominal compartment syndrome has been shown to reduce mortality in critically ill patients, but little is known about the outcome of abdominal wall reconstruction. This study investigates the role of plastic surgeons in the management and reconstruction of these abdominal wall defects.

Methods.—We performed a retrospective review of 82 consecutive critically ill patients who underwent decompressive laparotomy for abdominal compartment syndrome, at a university level 1 trauma center, from April 2000 to May 2004. Patients reconstructed by trauma surgeons alone (n = 15) were compared with patients reconstructed jointly with plastic surgeons (n = 12), using Student t test and χ^2 analysis.

Results.—Eighty-two patients underwent decompressive laparotomy for abdominal compartment syndrome, yielding 50 survivors (61%). Of the 27 patients who underwent abdominal wall reconstruction, 6 had early primary fascial repair, and 21 had staged reconstruction with primary fascial closure (n = 4), components separation alone (n = 3), components separation with mesh (n = 10), or permanent mesh only (n = 4). Compared with patients whose reconstruction was performed by trauma surgeons, patients who underwent a combined approach with plastic surgeons were older (50.5 versus 31.7 years, $P < 0.05$), had more comorbidities ($P < 0.001$), were less likely to have a traumatic etiology ($P < 0.001$), had a longer delay to reconstruction (407 versus 119 days, $P < 0.05$), and were more likely to undergo components separation ($P < 0.05$). Mean follow-up of 11.5 months revealed 2 recurrent hernias in the combined reconstruction group, both of which were successfully repaired.

Conclusions.—A multidisciplinary approach is essential to the successful management of abdominal wall defects after decompressive laparotomy for abdominal compartment syndrome. Although carefully selected patients can undergo early primary fascial repair, most of reconstructed patients had staged closure of the abdominal wall via components separation, with a low rate of recurrent hernia. High-risk patients with large defects and comorbidities appear to benefit from the involvement of a plastic surgeon.

▶ Those patients who survive damage control surgery or decompressive laparotomy for abdominal compartment syndrome require temporary closure of the abdominal wound, followed by later definitive reconstruction of the abdominal wall. The most challenging cases involve patients whose abdomen cannot be closed in the ensuing days after decompression but are left with skin grafts over a mound of granulating bowel and omentum. In addition to problems with activities of daily living, these patients with large abdominal wall hernias are at risk for obstruction, bowel infarction, cellulitis, and fistula formation. This report presents an experience with abdominal wall reconstruction after decompressive laparotomy for abdominal compartment syndrome. The combined efforts of trauma surgeons and plastic surgeons resulted in successful management of these complex cases. Central to the theme was the use of a components separation approach with or without mesh insertion. Older patients with larger hernia defects and more frequent comorbidities appear to benefit greatly from this multidisciplinary approach.

D. W. Mozingo, MD

Effect of the Uniform Accident and Sickness Policy Provision Law on Alcohol Screening and Intervention in Trauma Centers

Gentilello LM, Donato A, Nolan S, et al (Univ of Texas, Dallas; Harvard Med School, Boston; Univ of California at San Diego; et al)

J Trauma 59:624-631, 2005 2–8

Background.—Alcohol screening and intervention in trauma centers are widely recommended. The Uniform Accident and Sickness Policy Provision Law (UPPL) exists in most states, and allows insurers to refuse payment for treatment of injuries in patients with a positive alcohol or drug test. This article analyzed the UPPL's impact on screening and reimbursement, measured the knowledge of legislators about substance use problems in trauma centers, and determined their opinions about substance use-related exclusions in insurance contracts for trauma care.

Methods.—A nationwide survey of members of the American Association for the Surgery of Trauma was conducted. A separate survey of legislators who are members of the Senate, House, or Assembly and serve in some leadership role on committees responsible for insurance in their state was also performed.

Results.—Ninety-eight trauma surgeon and 56 legislator questionnaires were analyzed. Surgeons' familiarity with the UPPL was limited; only 13% believed they practiced in a UPPL state, but 70% actually did. Despite lack of knowledge of the statute, 24% reported an alcohol- or drug-related insurance denial in the past 6 months. This appeared to affect screening practices; the majority of surgeons (51.5%) do not routinely measure blood alcohol concentration, even though over 91% believe blood alcohol concentration testing is important. Most (82%) indicated that if there were no insurance barriers, they would be willing to establish a brief alcohol intervention program in their center. Legislators were aware of the impact of substance use on trauma centers. They overwhelmingly agreed (89%) that alcohol problems are treatable, and 80% believed it is a good idea to offer counseling in trauma centers. As with surgeons, the majority (53%) were not sure whether the UPPL existed in their state, but they favored prohibiting alcohol-related exclusions by a 2:1 ratio, with strong bipartisan support.

Conclusions.—The study documents strong support for screening and intervention programs by both trauma surgeons and legislators. Surgeons experience alcohol-related insurance denials but are not familiar with the state law that sanctions this practice. A majority of legislators are also not familiar with the UPPL but support elimination of insurance statutes that allow exclusion of coverage for trauma care on the basis of intoxication.

► A program to screen injured patients for the presence of an alcohol problem and providing a brief intervention to those with a positive result has been shown to reduce subsequent alcohol use, hospital readmissions and related consequences. Trauma surgeons generally support the implementation of such programs in their trauma centers. A number of federal agencies have also recommended routine trauma center screening and intervention including the Centers for Disease Control and Prevention and the National Traffic Safety Administration. The majority of trauma centers currently do not provide this service, however. The UPPL is a legal statute that allows insurance carriers to exclude coverage for alcohol- and drug-related injuries. The UPPL was developed as a model law by the National Association of Insurance Carriers in 1947. Overall, 39 states have adopted the UPPL model and 4 adopted it with minor modifications. In this survey, recent alcohol-related denials of insurance claims were reported by nearly 1 of 4 surgeons. The legislators surveyed support elimination of the insurance statutes that allow such exclusions in coverage. Reports by the Institute of Medicine, court decisions and actions by both federal and state governments have changed the view of alcohol and drug problems from a moral one requiring punishment to one that considers the role of medical, genetic, environmental and social factors. The trauma surgeons and legislators responding to this survey also endorsed this viewpoint and agreed that the archaic law based on moral claims should be changed.

D. W. Mozingo, MD

Use of a Single Question to Screen Trauma Patients for Alcohol Dependence

Reed DN Jr, Saxe A, Montanez M, et al (Michigan State Univ, East Lansing; McLaren Regional Med Ctr, Flint, Mich)

J Trauma 59:619-623, 2005 2–9

Background.—Alcohol-dependent trauma patients are known to be at future risk for both recidivism and mortality. Psychological tools exist to screen for alcohol-dependent disorders, and among patients with alcohol-dependent disorders, a brief intervention has been shown to modify behavior. However, the training involved and time required to administer these tools may decrease their utility. We explored the possibility that yet simpler screening tools could be used.

Methods.—A prospective consecutive study was designed whereby all adult patients admitted to the trauma service were asked to participate in the study. If consent was obtained, one trained member of the research team would apply a standard alcohol-misuse screening tool (i.e., the Alcohol Use Disorders Identification Test [AUDIT]). One hundred forty-nine patients met criteria and agreed to participate. Fully completed questionnaires were then subjected to statistical analysis.

Results.—Among the 149 participating patients, 36% were women and 64% were men, and 146 had blood alcohol levels (BALs) drawn. Those 146 patients form the basis of this report. Fifty-seven of the 146 (39%) patients had positive BALs and, among them, 74% of men and 54% of women recorded screening results consistent with harmful or dependent drinking. Among those with negative blood alcohol levels, 8% of women and 13% of men had scores consistent with harmful or dependent drinking by the AUDIT score. In both groups of patients, a cutoff of three or more drinks per day as a response to question 2 on the AUDIT (i.e., "On a typical day when you are drinking, how many drinks do you have?") correlated strongly with scores on the entire screening tool (AUDIT) in identifying those at risk for alcohol misuse.

Conclusion.—It may be reasonable to substitute a single question for the entire AUDIT screening instrument to screen for those at risk for alcohol misuse. If so, this single question could easily be incorporated into the history taken among patients admitted to a trauma service. Confirmation with a larger study is recommended.

► In the past decade, brief intervention has been shown to reduce hazardous drinking in a variety of settings. A main concern about brief intervention has been the difficulty in identifying patients most likely to benefit given the time and effort required for screening. An ideal screening tool would be simple to use and capture the at-risk patients. The lack of screening skills by the surgeons and the time commitment involved in administering lengthy questionnaires has been a major impediment to success of these screening programs. This selection identifies a single question from a 10-item screening tool to identify those at risk for alcohol misuse. Such a simple question would be appropriate to introduce in the social history for each admission to a trauma service.

D. W. Mozingo, MD

Recombinant Factor VIIa as Adjunctive Therapy for Bleeding Control in Severely Injured Trauma Patients: Two Parallel Randomized, Placebo-Controlled, Double-Blind Clinical Trials

Boffard KD, for the NovoSeven Trauma Study Group (Johannesburg Hosp, South Africa; et al)

J Trauma 59:8-18, 2005 2–10

Background.—Uncontrolled bleeding is a leading cause of death in trauma. Two randomized, placebo-controlled, double-blind trials (one in blunt trauma and one in penetrating trauma) were conducted simultaneously to evaluate the efficacy and safety of recombinant factor VIIa (rFVIIa) as adjunctive therapy for control of bleeding in patients with severe blunt or penetrating trauma.

Methods.—Severely bleeding trauma patients were randomized to rFVIIa (200, 100, and 100 μg/kg) or placebo in addition to standard treatment. The first dose followed transfusion of the eighth red blood cell (RBC) unit, with additional doses 1 and 3 hours later. The primary endpoint for bleeding control in patients alive at 48 hours was units of RBCs transfused within 48 hours of the first dose.

Results.—Among 301 patients randomized, 143 blunt trauma patients and 134 penetrating trauma patients were eligible for analysis. In blunt trauma, RBC transfusion was significantly reduced with rFVIIa relative to placebo (estimated reduction of 2.6 RBC units, $p = 0.02$), and the need for massive transfusion (>20 units of RBCs) was reduced (14% vs. 33% of patients; $p = 0.03$). In penetrating trauma, similar analyses showed trends toward rFVIIa reducing RBC transfusion (estimated reduction of 1.0 RBC units, $p = 0.10$) and massive transfusion (7% vs. 19%; $p = 0.08$). Trends toward a reduction in mortality and critical complications were observed. Adverse events including thromboembolic events were evenly distributed between treatment groups.

Conclusion.—Recombinant FVIIa resulted in a significant reduction in RBC transfusion in severe blunt trauma. Similar trends were observed in penetrating trauma. The safety of rFVIIa was established in these trauma populations within the investigated dose range.

► Recombinant activated coagulation factor VII is currently approved in North America and most other regions of the world for the treatment of bleeding in hemophilia patients. Although investigational use of rFVIIa in trauma patients has shown promising results, the data supporting the use within this population have been limited to case series and anecdotal reports. This selection describes 2 large randomized placebo-controlled double-blind trials to evaluate the efficacy and safety of this treatment as an adjunct for control of bleeding in patients with severe blunt or penetrating trauma. In patients with blunt trauma, blood transfusion was significantly reduced with treatment relative to placebo and the need for massive transfusion was also reduced. There were less differences noted in patients with penetrating trauma. Improvements in clinical outcomes did not reach statistical significance. Patient selection is a critical factor in determining the efficacy of this therapy. Overuse of this product comes at a significant financial cost.

D. W. Mozingo, MD

Determinants of Futility of Administration of Recombinant Factor VIIa in Trauma

Stein DM, Dutton RP, O'Connor J, et al (Univ of Maryland, Baltimore)
J Trauma 59:609-615, 2005 2–11

Background.—"Off-label" use of human coagulation factor VIIa (FVIIa) is presently restricted to patients in extremis at our institution. Although bleeding will diminish in most patients, some will still die early as a result of irreversible shock and/or rebleeding. Futile administration of FVIIa significantly increases the economic burden of this expensive therapy and therefore limits its availability. On the basis of both human and in vitro studies, profound acidosis may be expected to predict lack of response. In addition, the depth of hemorrhagic shock, as defined by the degree of hypoperfusion over a given period of time, may be predictive of failure of FVIIa administration. We hypothesized that retrospective review of FVIIa use would identify variables associated with clinical futility.

Methods.—Characteristics of patients receiving FVIIa for acute traumatic hemorrhage were identified. Patients were retrospectively stratified into two groups; those who died as a result of acute hemorrhagic shock (nonresponders) and those in whom hemostasis was achieved and sustained (responders). Demographics, laboratory values, transfusion requirements, and outcomes were recorded for all patients. Data were analyzed using the Student's t test to identify the clinical characteristics of nonresponders and stepwise logistic regression was then used to identify independently predictive factors. A classification and regression tree analysis was conducted to develop a decision tree on the basis of our results.

Results.—Eighty-one patients received FVIIa therapy over a 3-year period. Among the 46 patients treated for acute hemorrhage, there were 26 with blunt and 20 with penetrating mechanisms of trauma. Average age was 35 ± 15 years, 72% were male, and the average Injury Severity Score was 36 ± 15. Revised Trauma Score (RTS), lactate, and preadministration prothrombin time (PT) each predicted lack of response ($p < 0.05$ for each). RTS and PT were independently predictive of failure of response. An RTS of less than 4.09 and a PT of greater than or equal to 17.6 seconds were significantly associated with futile administration of FVIIa. Age was a significant factor in patients with a PT greater than or equal to 17.6 seconds, whereas ISS was significant in patients with an RTS greater than or equal to 4.09.

Conclusion.—Profound acidosis and coagulopathy may predict failure of FVIIa therapy. Depth of hemorrhagic shock, as described by the RTS, was also associated with futile administration. These variables should be considered as potential contraindications to the use of FVIIa. Earlier administration of FVIIa, before the development of massive blood loss and severe shock, may increase the rate of clinical response.

► This study seeks to identify that subset of patients not responding to therapy with recombinant factor VIIa after trauma. By comparing those patients who died as a result of acute hemorrhagic shock and those in whom hemostasis was achieved, certain clinical variables were found to be more common in the group that died. Patients with profound hemorrhagic shock as evidenced by a low revised trauma score, elevated prothrombin time, or profound metabolic acidosis were unlikely to respond. Multicavitary injuries and advancing age also predicted futility. Although the number of patients studied in this retrospective review is small, it sets a starting point for examination of patient selection criteria for this form of therapy.

D. W. Mozingo, MD

Prognostic Implications of Warfarin Cessation After Major Trauma: A Population-based Cohort Analysis

Hackam DG, Kopp A, Redelmeier DA (Univ of Toronto; Sunnybrook & Women's College, Toronto)

Circulation 111:2250-2256, 2005 2–12

Background.—Warfarin therapy is often withheld from elderly patients who fall or otherwise experience injury because of concerns regarding the long-term risk of hemorrhage in these individuals. We studied whether stopping warfarin after trauma is associated with a higher risk of subsequent adverse cardiovascular events.

Method and Results.—We conducted a retrospective, population-based, cohort study using linked administrative databases in the province of Ontario, Canada for the years 1992 to 2001. A total of 8450 elderly patients (age >65 years) who survived an incident of major trauma and were receiving warfarin before injury were followed up for a mean of 3.3 years. During the 6-month interval after trauma, 1827 (22%) patients discontinued warfarin, whereas 6623 (78%) patients continued warfarin. Warfarin cessation was not associated with an increased risk of subsequent stroke (hazard ratio [HR] 0.99, 95% CI 0.82 to 1.21) or myocardial infarction (HR 0.94, 95% CI 0.74 to 1.20) but was associated with a lower risk of major hemorrhage (HR 0.69, 95% CI 0.54 to 0.88) and a higher risk of venous thromboembolism (HR 1.59, 95% CI 1.07 to 2.36). Adjustment for baseline demographics, stroke risk factors, other comorbidities, and characteristics of the trauma did not materially change these findings. On-treatment analyses yielded similar results.

Conclusions.—Cessation of warfarin in elderly patients after major trauma was not associated with an increased risk of arterial thrombotic events but was associated with a significantly increased risk of venous thromboembolism.

► Patients who sustain major trauma while receiving warfarin may bleed more seriously from their injuries, particularly when head trauma occurs. The potential protection from stroke and other thrombotic events supports reinstitution of long-term anticoagulation; however, the occurrence of trauma may be a marker of poor functional status or unreliable patient behavior that could compromise the benefits of long-term anticoagulation. In this study, the discontinuation of long-term warfarin use after major trauma was not associated with an increased risk of stroke or myocardial infarction. Patients did, however, have a significant increase in the risk of venous thromboembolism. It is important therefore to carefully weigh the risks of hemorrhage and venous thromboembolism in deciding whether to continue anticoagulation in elderly patients after trauma.

D. W. Mozingo, MD

The Evaluation of Casualties From Operation Iraqi Freedom on Return to the Continental United States From March to June 2003

Montgomery SP, Swiecki CW, Shriver CD (Womack Army Med Ctr, Fort Bragg, NC; Walter Reed Army Med Ctr, Washington, DC)

J Am Coll Surg 201:7-13, 2005 2–13

Background.—Most seriously wounded US Army casualties from the Iraqi theater of operations come through Walter Reed Army Medical Center on their return to the United States. General surgery and orthopaedic surgery services have developed a multidisciplinary team approach to triage and treatment of incoming casualties.

Study Design.—Prospective database of returning casualties to Walter Reed Army Medical Center from Operation Iraqi Freedom (OIF) from March 1 to July 1, 2003.

Results.—Of 294 casualties seen, 119 were triaged to inpatient status and treated within 1 hour of arrival; mean age 26.6 ± 6.2 years (range 23 to 37). Time from original battlefield injury was a mean of 8 days (range 3 to 28 days). Forty-six (39%) sustained gunshot wounds, 37 (31%) sustained blast and shrapnel injuries, and 41 (34%) had blunt/motor vehicle collision mechanisms. There were a total of 184 wounded locations in these 119 casualties; of these, there were 29 head and neck, 25 chest, 20 abdomen, 74 lower extremity, and 36 upper extremity. Twenty-eight casualties (23%) required emergent surgical procedures on the night of arrival. Another 30

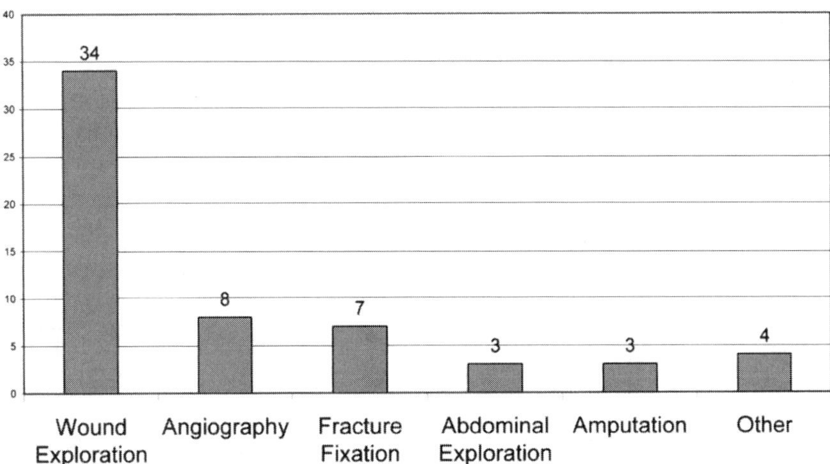

FIGURE 3.—Types of operations performed within 48 hours of arrival. There were two more knee amputations and one through the knee amputation. Other represents thoracoscopy (video-assisted thoracic surgery) with decortication (2), tracheostomy (1), and pseudoaneurysm repair (1). (By permission of the Journal of the American College of Surgeons, from Montgomery SP, Swiecki CW, Shriver CD: The evaluation of casualties from Operation Iraqi Freedom on return to the continental United States from March to June 2003. *J Am Coll Surg* 201:7-13, 2005.)

(25%) required an urgent surgical procedure within 48 hours of arrival (Fig 3).

Conclusions.—Followup surgical procedures were urgently or emergently required in 43% of admitted battlefield casualties from OIF on transfer to Level V care in the continental United States. The injury pattern of wounds from this engagement is described. The Walter Reed Army Medical Center system of incoming battlefield casualty evaluation using multidisciplinary teams is successful in expediting care and ensuring evaluation of the full range of potential injuries.

► Recent changes in military capabilities and doctrine have resulted in a change in the pattern of casualties returning to the continental United States during military conflicts. Patients are returning to the United States more quickly, and patients have a much higher acuity than those from earlier conflicts. The development of critical care air transport teams has markedly changed patient transportation practices. These teams comprise nurses, physicians, and support staff trained in intensive care medicine. There is rapid patient movement through the evacuation chain as soon as patients are stable for transport and often before definitive care has been accomplished. Critically ill and ventilator-dependent casualties move through the evacuation chain to the United States as early as 3 days after injury. Many still have injuries in evolution and require close evaluation and frequent operative management.

D. W. Mozingo, MD

Real-Time, Contrast-Enhanced Sonography: A New Tool for Detecting Active Bleeding

Catalano O, Sandomenico F, Raso MM, et al (S Maria delle Grazie Hosp, Pozzuoli, Italy)
J Trauma 59:933-939, 2005 2–14

Background.—Active contrast medium extravasation is a known angiographic and computed tomographic sign of ongoing, potentially life-threatening hemorrhage. Sonography (US) is frequently the first imaging option for screening patients with abdominal emergencies. Because of the current possibilities of low-mechanical-index, real-time, contrast-specific systems, it is possible to detect contrast leakage by using US. The purpose of this article is report our pilot experience in the evaluation of active traumatic and nontraumatic bleeding with contrast-enhanced US.

Methods.—In a 2-year period, we performed 153 consecutive emergent contrast-enhanced US studies. Traumatic emergencies accounted for 83 examinations and nontraumatic emergencies accounted for 70. We used the contrast-specific mode Contrast Tuned Imaging and the contrast medium SonoVue. A 2.4- to 4.8-mL contrast medium bolus was injected with continuous US acquisition, starting immediately after contrast injection and lasting 1 to 6 minutes.

Results.—Contrast extravasation was found in 20 cases (13%). These included spleen injury (n = 8), liver injury (n = 3), kidney injury (n = 1), abdominal aortic aneurysm rupture (n = 5), splenic angiosarcoma rupture (n = 1), postsurgical bleeding after abdominal aortic aneurysm repair (n = 1), and postsplenectomy bleeding (n = 1). Active extravasation appeared as a round, hyperechoic pool or as a fountain-like, hyperechoic jet.

Conclusion.—Our retrospective clinical study shows for the first time how US can detect contrast medium extravasation, a significant indicator of active hemorrhage and of need for prompt surgical or interventional treatment.

▶ This clinical study shows how contrast-enhanced sonography, a novel imaging technique, can be useful in the assessment of abdominal emergencies. When solid organ injury was suspected by conventional US examination, a sulfur hexafluoride microbubble contrast agent was injected rapidly via a peripheral vein in a volume of 2.4 to 4.8 mL. Continuous scanning started immediately after injection and lasts 1 to 6 minutes. Contrast extravasation was found in 20 cases of 153 examinations. They were able to identify extravasation associated with splenic injury, liver injury, and kidney injury. In addition, nontraumatic emergency conditions such as abdominal aortic aneurysm rupture and postoperative bleeding were demonstrated. A technique such as this may more quickly identify those patients needing prompt surgical or invasive radiologic procedures.

D. W. Mozingo, MD

Selective Clinical Management of Anterior Abdominal Stab Wounds

Tsikitis V, Biffl WL, Majercik S, et al (Brown Med School, Providence, RI)

Am J Surg 188:807-812, 2004 2–15

Background.—The optimal management of clinically stable patients with anterior abdominal stab wounds (AASWs) is debated. We implemented a protocol of serial clinical assessments to determine the need for laparotomy. The purpose of this study was to determine whether the approach is safe and effective.

Methods.—Records of patients sustaining AASWs from 1999 to 2003 were reviewed.

Results.—Seventy-seven patients sustained AASWs. Twenty-five were taken directly to the operating room because of hypotension (5), evisceration (7), or peritonitis (15). Seventeen patients had diagnostic peritoneal lavage (DPL) for associated thoracoabdominal wounds and 5 had local wound exploration (LWE) off protocol. The remaining 30 patients were managed with serial clinical assessments and were discharged uneventfully.

Conclusion.—Patients sustaining AASWs who present without hypotension, evisceration, or peritonitis may be managed safely under a protocol of serial clinical evaluations. This approach should be compared with LWE/DPL in a prospective, randomized multicenter trial.

► Multiple approaches to manage patients with AASWs have been promoted ranging from mandatory laparotomy to local wound exploration and DPL. In the absence of shock, peritonitis, or evisceration, this selection describes an alternative strategy for management of stable patients with AASWs, namely, that of serial clinical assessments looking for evidence of ongoing bleeding or hollow viscus injury. In this series, 30 patients not requiring immediate treatment were all safely observed through hospital discharge. Two thirds of the patients were seen in follow-up clinic. The ultimate outcome of the remaining third being unknown. The authors proposed that a larger series is needed in a prospective randomized trial to compare the safety and cost effectiveness of this approach with one that uses local wound exploration and DPL.

D. W. Mozingo, MD

Unsafe at Any Age: A Retrospective Review of All-Terrain Vehicle Injuries in Two Level I Trauma Centers From 1995 to 2003

Smith LM, Pittman MA, Marr AB, et al (Louisiana State Univ, Shreveport and New Orleans; Henry Ford Hosp, Detroit; Univ of South Carolina, Mobile, Ala; et al)

J Trauma 58:783-788, 2005 2–16

Background.—All-terrain vehicles (ATVs) are popular recreational and utility vehicles. In 1984, Cogbill published an article regarding three-wheelers. These are no longer manufactured, but the injury and death rate with four-wheeled ATVs is high and disproportionately affects young riders.

Methods.—We conducted a retrospective review at two Level I trauma centers from January 1994 to April 2003. Statistical analysis was performed using the SAS V8.2 program. Values of $p < 0.05$ were significant.

Results.—Two hundred eight patients were identified. There were no differences identified in demographics, mechanism, types of injury, Injury Severity Score (ISS), or Glasgow Coma Scale (GCS) score. Seventy-five percent were male and 84% were white. The mean age was 23 ± 13 years. The average ISS was 12.3 ± 9 and the mean GCS score was 13.1 ± 3.7. Injury mechanisms were loss of stability (33%), separation of rider from ATV (32%), and ATV versus stationary object (27%). ISS for ages 12 to 15 years was significantly higher than for other ages (14.5 vs. 11.5, $p = 0.04$, Wilcoxon rank sum test) and included more major head injuries (40.4% vs. 21.8%, $p = 0.09$, Wilcoxon rank sum test). They experienced fewer spinal fractures (3.9% vs. 15.4%, $p = 0.03$) and pelvic injuries (0% vs. 9%, $p = 0.02$, Wilcoxon rank sum test). The GCS score in this group was lower (12.3 vs. 13.4, $p = 0.03$, Wilcoxon rank sum test).

Conclusion.—Adolescent ATV riders have more severe injuries and more head injuries than other age groups. Prevention efforts should target this group.

► The increasing use of ATVs for both recreation and occupational purposes has outpaced public safety awareness and government and industry regulation. This translates into a significant risk of death and injury for riders. Appearing on the market in 1971, ATVs have been associated with literally thousands of deaths and hundreds of thousands of injuries. Only 21 states have helmet and safety equipment regulations. The cost of ATV injuries is estimated to currently exceed 6.5 billion dollars annually. In this selection, the experiences of 2 level I trauma centers were examined over a 9-year period. They identified 318 patients with injury or death attributable to an ATV-related crash. Two hundred eight of these patients were identified as having sufficient data in the medical records to include for statistical analysis. Adolescent ATV riders had higher injury severity scores and a higher number of head injuries than any other age group. ATVs continue to be a substantial risk in all age groups but particularly for teenagers below the driving age who receive little training and adult supervision. They rarely use safety equipment and are more likely to engage in risky behavior while riding an ATV.

D. W. Mozingo, MD

Recovery at One Year Following Isolated Traumatic Brain Injury: A Western Trauma Association Prospective Multicenter Trial

Livingston DH, Lavery RF, Mosenthal AC, et al (UMDNJ–New Jersey Med School, Newark; Univ of California, San Francisco; Univ of Washington, Seattle; et al)

J Trauma 59:1298-1304, 2005 2–17

Background.—Age has been shown to be a primary determinant of survival following isolated traumatic brain injury (TBI). We have previously reported that patients ≥65 years who survived mild TBI have decreased functional outcome at 6 months compared with younger patients. The purpose of this study was to further investigate the effect of age on outcome at 1 year in all patients surviving isolated TBI.

Methods.—The Western Trauma Association multicenter prospective study included all patients sustaining isolated TBI defined as Abbreviated Injury Scale score for Head ≥ 3 with an Abbreviated Injury Scale score in any other body area ≤ 1. Outcome data included discharge disposition, Glasgow Outcome Scale (GOS) score (1 = dead to 5 = full recovery) and modified Functional Independence Measure (FIM) score measuring feeding, expression, and locomotion (1 = total dependence to 4 = total independence) for each component at discharge and 1 year.

Results.—In all, 295 patients were enrolled with a follow-up of 82%, resulting in 241 study patients. An additional five patients died from non-TBI causes and were excluded. The mean and median times for the last follow-up in the 236 remaining patients were 307 and 357 days, respectively. Patients were divided into four age ranges: 18 to 29 years (n = 66), 30 to 44 years (n = 54), 45 to 59 years (n = 50), and ≥60 years (n = 65). More severe TBIs, as measured by admitting Glasgow Coma Scale (GCS), were observed in the youngest group compared with all others but there were no differences in mean GCS between the remaining three groups. There were no differences in neurosurgical intervention between the groups. Age was a major determinant in the outcome at discharge and last follow-up. Patients over 60 years discharged with a GOS ≤4 were less likely to improve at 1 year than all other groups (37% versus 63 to 85%; $p \leq 0.05$). Patients between 18 and 29 years of age had the lowest mean Glasgow Outcome Scale and discharge FIM scores, which correlated with the low admission GCS. Despite the increased severity of TBI, this group had the best FIM score at 1 year. In contrast, patients older than 60 years had the least improvement and had a significantly lower final FIM score at 1 year compared with all other groups.

Conclusion.—Older patients following isolated TBI have poorer functional status at discharge and make less improvement at 1 year compared with all other patients. These worse outcomes occur despite what appears to be less severe TBI as measured by a higher GCS upon admission. Differences in outcome begin to appear even in patients between 45 and 59 years. Further investigations with more detailed outcome instruments are required to better understand the qualitative limitations of a patient's recovery and to devise strategies to maximize functional improvement following TBI. Age is an exceedingly important parameter affecting recovery from isolated TBI.

► There is a bimodal distribution of TBI with respect to age. In males the incidence peaks between the ages of 15 and 24 years and then again after age 75 years. A similar bimodal pattern is seen in women. The deleterious effect of age is particularly pronounced in patients older than 70 years and in those presenting with GCS score below 8. Though the functional outcome at the time of trauma center discharge has been well characterized, less is known about the long-term functional recovery of TBI delineated by patient age. This study demonstrates that older patients have poorer functional status at discharge and make less improvement at 1 year compared with all other patients. These worse outcomes occur despite a less severe TBI as measured by a higher GCS on admission. The deterioration in recovery potential begins to appear in patients between 45 and 59 years. Further investigations that use more detailed analysis are required to better understand the qualitative limitations of patients' recovery and to investigate strategies to maximize functional outcome in these patients.

D. W. Mozingo, MD

3 Burns

Introduction

After the events of September 11, 2001, the disaster response to a burn mass casualty situation has received heightened awareness in the burn community. Burn centers are limited in supply in contrast to trauma centers, and they continue to close due to economic pressures. These centers are a unique national resource with highly specialized burn care systems to address the complex nature of these injuries. As such, the American Burn Association proposed a disaster management plan describing the important role of the American Burn Association in interacting with federal agencies regarding mass casualty burn disaster preparedness. Four other selections report on individual centers' experiences in caring for burn mass casualty victims, ranging from direct reports of the care of patients after September 11 in both New York and Washington, DC, to a thoughtful discussion of the care of patients after the Rhode Island nightclub fire, a pharmaceutical plant explosion, and a boiler room explosion aboard a cruise ship. Burn centers and State Departments of Health around the nation have received grant funding for development of burn mass casualty response programs, and these selections highlight the enormous use of resources related to these types of disasters.

In addition to major trauma, the abdominal compartment syndrome has been recognized in the resuscitated burn patient as a serious complication. Intra-abdominal pressures rise during resuscitation in proportion to the fluid volume administered when crystalloid resuscitation is employed. Colloid containing resuscitations reduce fluid requirements and edema and have lower intra-abdominal pressures during their resuscitation compared with the crystalloid counterpart. The effect seems to be directly related to total volume administered. The combined injury of burn and mechanical trauma occurs infrequently in patients admitted to burn centers. Analysis of data from the National Trauma Data Bank showed a dramatic increase in the risk of death for patients with combined burn and mechanical trauma compared with the trauma-only and burn-only groups. Future studies are needed to prospectively evaluate these patients to determine the impact of mechanical injuries on burn survival as well as such analysis of smoke inhalation injury on the survival in patients with concomitant mechanical trauma. Much is known about the importance of nutritional support in burn care. In elderly patients there is a well-known increase in morbidity and mortality related to age as well as the presence of comorbid factors. The incidence of protein energy malnutrition in the geriatric burn population was more than 60% in a series. Half were characterized as moderately to severely malnourished. With the anticipated increase in the population of elderly patients in the near future, more attention should be paid to the impact of such findings in these patients. Throughout the trauma literature, an association has been demonstrated between females and an increased mortality from mechanical trauma. A study confirmed these findings in a large series of burn patients. Women had increased odds of mortality after burn injury but demonstrated a differential effect of age on associated mortality as well. In contradistinction, an animal model demonstrates that while male sex hormones potentiate lung and gut injury in a combined model of burn and hemorrhage, female sex hormones reduce this and organ injury.

The psychological burden in addition to the physical burden of injury plays a major role in the recovery of patients after burns. Complementing wound closure and early care efforts with early interventions designed to reduce the initial psychological distress has been demonstrated to accelerate both physical and psychosocial recovery in patients sustaining major burns.

Long-term studies regarding the actuarial survival in patients who survive a major burn are lacking. It is unknown whether the prolonged period of critical illness sustained by patients with extreme injuries plays a role in ultimate lifespan. A series was reported which demonstrated that the rate of accidental or violent death was an order of magnitude higher than that predicted in the typical population. The higher risk for accidental death after survival from burn was mainly encountered in the younger population.

A number of interesting reports relate to care of the burn wound or the physiology of wounds and scars. Hypertrophic scarring remains an important problem in the postburn recovery period, and little progress in this area has been made in part due to the lack of a reliable animal model for study. The red duroc pig had previously been described to make hypertrophic scar similar to the human counterpart in histologic appearance. This tissue also has now been shown to have changes in growth factor expression and nitric oxide production in a very similar manner to human hypertrophic scars, potentially enabling this model to be useful in future studies. Hypertrophic scarring of the face can be a catastrophic event after burn injury. Biologic or synthetic dressings are known to decrease some scarring in relationship to shortening the healing time in second-degree burns as well as providing barriers to bacteria. The use of human cadaver allograft in patients with facial burns resulted in no infection and complete re-epithelialization by 10 days post-burn, and no hypertrophic scarring was observed at 3 and 6 months after burn injury. This approach, although encumbering the risk and cost of allograft use, seems useful to prevent excessive scar. The Versajet™, a new hydrosurgery system that was initially applied to the debridement of chronic wounds and traumatically devitalized tissue, has now been reported in use with burn wound excision. The stream of pressurized saline functions somewhat like a knife and may be used in smaller concave areas or on complex 3-dimensional structures such as the ears and webspaces, areas in which traditional knives are difficult to use for excision.

Finally, though not related to burn injury per se, this chapter contains an interesting report of an open-label study to evaluate the safety and efficacy of tissue plasminogen activator (TPA) in the treatment of severe frostbite. Although compared with historic controls, the objective findings and rate of digit salvage were markedly improved in the patients treated with TPA. The relatively small numbers of these patients make a large-scale study difficult to perform, but this suggests that this may be an effective treatment in this setting.

David W. Mozingo, MD

Disaster Management and the ABA Plan

ABA Board of Trustees and the Committee on Organization and Delivery of Burn Care (Chicago)

J Burn Care Rehabil 26:102-106, 2005 3–1

Background.—In response to the terrorist attacks of September 11, 2001, the American Burn Association (ABA) developed the ABA Plan for the management of mass burn casualties resulting from mass disasters and terrorist attacks. Information included in the ABA Plan includes the extent of burn injuries in mass disasters and terrorist acts; the importance of appropriate triage and surge capacity policy; the rationale for treating burn patients in burn centers rather than trauma centers; the critical role of burn centers in the local, regional, and federal response to mass burn casualty situations; and the important role of the ABA in interacting with federal agencies and other entities in preparing for mass burn casualty disasters.

Overview.—In most traumatic events, approximately 25% to 30% of victims will require burn care treatment. About one third of persons hospitalized in New York City after the September 11 attack had severe burn injuries. The attack on that date at the Pentagon resulted in 11 burn patients, a high proportion of those injured. The most efficient and cost-effective care for these patients is available at burn centers. Burn injuries often require a prolonged course of treatment—50 days is the average ICU stay for a patient with a 50% body surface area burn. Burn centers are not the same as trauma centers; there are only 312 burn care centers in the United States, representing just 1897 burn beds. Burn centers have been specifically recognized in federal bioterrorism legislation because of the availability of highly specialized burn care systems established to handle the complex treatment of burn injuries. Most burn surgeons have the expertise to treat both burn and trauma victims, but the reverse is not necessarily the case; thus, unique benchmarks are needed to ensure that the needs of burn-injured patients are addressed in the event of a terrorism incident. The ABA has the capability to respond within hours with burn resource information for federal and state agencies, as was demonstrated after the September 11, 2001 terrorist attacks and in preparations for the war in Iraq.

► In the aftermath of September 11, the ABA and its members were made acutely aware of the lack of a well-designed national plan for responding to burn-related disasters. The limited number of patients treated from the terrorist attacks on the World Trade Center and Pentagon, though taxing individual institutions, did not stress the burn care system on a national level. Burn centers are in limited supply, and in contrast to trauma centers, burn centers continue to close because of economic pressures. They are a unique national resource with highly specialized burn care systems to address the complex nature of these injuries. This selection outlines the unique, critical role that burn centers play in local, regional, and federal responses to mass burn casuality situations and defines the important role of the ABA in interacting with federal agencies regarding mass burn casualty disaster preparedness.

D. W. Mozingo, MD

A Regional Burn Center's Response to a Disaster: September 11, 2001, and the Days Beyond

Yurt RW, Bessey PQ, Bauer GJ, et al (Weill Cornell Med Ctr, New York)
J Burn Care Rehabil 26:117-124, 2005 3–2

Background.—Almost immediately after the first plane struck the World Trade Center on September 11, 2001, hospitals throughout New York City's metropolitan area began to prepare for large numbers of casualties in accordance with established disaster planning. However, it soon became apparent that the event overwhelmed usual emergency medical services, as patients began arriving throughout the city by whatever means available. The William Randolph Hearst Burn center, like other facilities in the area, made substantial adjustments to its usual operations—adjustments that remained in place for nearly 2 months. There have been several reports of the distribution and care of burn-injured victims, but there has been no published review specific to the care of patients with burn injury. The logistic and organizational ways in which the burn centers and other institutions responded to the challenges that presented themselves on September 11, 2001 and in the ensuing months were summarized.

Methods.—A literature review and retrospective study of prospectively collected data at a regional burn center were conducted. Medical records were also reviewed. Data also were collected for assessment of the impact of the disaster on patient care and the response of the burn team. In addition, data were collected to assess the response in light of alternative methods for caring for large numbers of burn-injured patients.

Results.—The facilities in the New York City metropolitan area had 120 burn care beds. These facilities were prepared for massive numbers of casualties, but it soon became apparent that the extent of the effects on medical centers would be much less than anticipated. Only two thirds of the burn-injured patients who required hospital admission were admitted to designated burn centers, and only 28% of burn-injured patients initially were triaged to the 5 burn centers that were within a 20-mile radius of Ground Zero. The care provided at the study center was made possible by the fact that it was a "disaster-ready" facility and by supplementation of personnel from resources provided by The National Disaster Medical System. Outcomes at this burn center exceeded the predictions of logistic regression analysis.

Conclusions.—It is recommended that the American Burn Association continue not only to maintain a national database on bed availability but also to aid in identifying ways to triage large numbers of patients within and outside a region during and immediately after a disaster when emergency medical services transportation is limited and under control of law enforcement and the military.

▶ This selection details the patient influx and workload ramifications for the William Randolph Hearst Burn Center, New York Presbyterian, Weill Cornell Medical Center in New York City after the terrorist attack on the World Trade Center towers. This report summarizes the organizational and logistic ways in which this center and other institutions responded to the challenges of providing care for multiply injured and burn patients. A detailed description of the national response is also presented. The authors recommended that the American Burn Association continue in its efforts to maintain a national database on burn bed availability and to assist in identifying ways of triaging large numbers of patients within and outside a region during and after a disaster when transportation capabilities are limited.

D. W. Mozingo, MD

The Pentagon Attack of September 11, 2001: A Burn Center's Experience

Jordan MH, Hollowed KA, Turner DG, et al (Washington Med Ctr, Washington, DC)

J Burn Care Rehabil 26:109-116, 2005 3–3

Introduction.—On September 11, 2001, an airplane flown by terrorists crashed into the Pentagon, causing a mass casualty incident with 189 deaths and 106 persons treated for injuries in local hospitals. Nine burn victims and one victim with an inhalation injury only were transported to the burn center hospital. The Burn Center at Washington Hospital Center admitted and treated the acute burn patients while continuing its mission as the regional burn center for the Washington DC region. Eight of the nine burn patients survived. Lessons learned include 1) A large-volume burn center hospital can absorb nine acute burns and maintain burn center and hospital operations, but the decision to keep or transfer burn patients must be tempered with the reality that several large burns can double or triple the work load for 2 to 3 months. 2) Transfer decisions should have high priority and be timely to ensure optimum care for the patients without need for movement of medical personnel from one burn center to another. 3) The reserve capacity of burn beds in the United States is limited, and the burn centers and the American Burn Association must continue to seek recognition and support from Congress and the federal agencies for optimal preparedness.

► A similar scene is encountered at the Washington Hospital Burn Center after the crash of American Airlines Flight 77 into the Pentagon. The hospital's response is detailed in this selection, and costs associated with provision of this care enumerated. As in the case of the burn care delivered in New York, assistance of the Federal Emergency Management Agency (FEMA) in the form of burn nurses from other states, were required. The experience in this setting combined with the patient care delivered in New York City raised the questions as to when should patients be considered for transfer from one burn facility to another to provide more reasonable workloads for the hospital staff. Though a typical burn center may treat several hundred patients per year, these patients usually arrive one at a time. As detailed in this selection, workload dramatically increases when patients present in multiple numbers to the same burn center.

D. W. Mozingo, MD

Lessons Learned From a Nightclub Fire: Institutional Disaster Preparedness

Mahoney EJ, Harrington DT, Biffl WL, et al (Brown Med School, Providence, RI)

J Trauma 58:487-491, 2005 3–4

Background.—On February 20, 2003, a nightclub fire caused a multiple casualty disaster, with 215 victims requiring treatment at area hospitals. In this report, we describe the events, the surgical response at our trauma center, and the lessons learned in institutional disaster preparedness.

Methods.—Information regarding the fire was obtained from public access media and state governmental and hospital reports. Patient information was obtained through review of our trauma registry, patient records, and questionnaires sent to regional hospitals.

Results.—Four hundred thirty-nine patrons were in the building at the time of the fire, of whom 96 died at the scene. One hundred people ultimately died. Two hundred fifteen patients were evaluated at area hospitals: 64 at our trauma center and 151 at 15 other area facilities. Seventy-nine patients were admitted: 47 to our center and 32 to other hospitals. Eight patients were transferred from Rhode Island Hospital (RIH) to other Level I trauma centers. Twenty-eight (60%) of the patients admitted to RIH were intubated for inhalation injury. For patients admitted to RIH, the extent of the total body surface burn was less than 20% in 33 patients (70%), 21% to 40% in 12 patients (26%), and greater than 40% in 2 patients (4%). The average age was 31 years (range, 18-43 years). Previous disaster planning drills facilitated a quick institutional response directed by a surgeon. The trauma floor of the hospital, which normally consists of a 10-bed trauma intensive care unit (ICU), an 11-bed step-down unit, and a 22-bed medical-surgical floor, was cleared of patients and converted into a 21-bed burn ICU and a 34-bed acute burn ward. Surgical residents were mobilized into teams assigned to the emergency department, ICUs, and surgical floors. In addition to the in-house trauma attending already present, four additional surgical staff members were called in to help man the emergency department and burn wards. Two operating rooms became dedicated burn rooms where 23 cases were performed the first week. In total, 43 operative procedures and 9 bedside tracheostomies were performed over 8 weeks. Over the first 4 weeks, 132 bronchoscopies were performed for diagnostic purposes and pulmonary toilet. There were no deaths.

Conclusion.—Disaster planning as well as personnel and institutional commitment resulted in an optimal response to a multiple casualty incident. Still, lessons were learned that will further improve readiness for future disasters.

► This selection outlines the course of care for 215 victims requiring treatment at area hospitals. In addition to the excellent patient care described herein, this reference serves as a testament to the individual and institutional commitment to disaster planning that resulted in an optimal response in this incident. Critical components of the disaster plan for this institution are outlined, including the assignment of an experienced trauma surgeon to directly oversee patient triage, and the formulation of trauma teams to treat the most critically injured patients. The team, composed of a senior surgical resident, a trauma nurse, and a respiratory therapist, ensured an accurate assessment and prompt resuscitation of the patient from the time of arrival in the emergency department through ICU admission. Surgical attendings were assigned to key areas of the hospital. Experienced attendings were immediately present and available to oversee the care of the severely injured patients 24 hours per day. The treatment was prompt and accurate. The successful management of this large number of patients is a testament to prior planning and to the institutional and personal commitment of the hospital staff.

D. W. Mozingo, MD

Managing a Combined Burn Trauma Disaster in the Post-9/11 World: Lessons Learned From the 2003 West Pharmaceutical Plant Explosion

Cairns BA, Stiffler A, Price F, et al (Univ of North Carolina, Chapel Hill)

J Burn Care Rehabil 26:144-150, 2005 3–5

Introduction.—At 1:37 pm on January 29, 2003, an explosion occurred at the West Pharmaceutical chemical plant in Kinston, North Carolina. The explosion killed three people at the scene and resulted in more than 30 admissions to area hospitals. The disaster resulted in 10 critically ill burn patients, who were all intubated with inhalation injuries, many with combined burn and trauma injuries. All 10 critically injured patients were admitted to a tertiary care facility 100 miles away with both a Level I trauma center and a verified burn center. Ultimately, 7 of 10 patients survived (a mortality rate of 30%), and none were transferred to another trauma or burn center. This article analyzes the unique challenges that combined burn and trauma patients present during a disaster, critically examines the response to this disaster, describes lessons learned, and presents recommendations that may improve the response to such disasters in the future.

► An important aspect of disaster management that has not received significant attention is the issue of optimal triage, evacuation, and care of patients with both burn and traumatic injuries. In the United States, combined burn and traumatic injury is relatively rare, making up less than 5% of admissions to burn centers and less than 1% of all trauma center admissions. The authors thoughtfully analyzed problems with scene triage, patient transport, and communication difficulties arising for some 8 hours after the disaster. They also examined whether a single center should have treated all critically injured patients and elaborated on plans of the American Burn Association and other trauma organizations in defining intercenter cooperation and defining appropriate surge capacity.

D. W. Mozingo, MD

A Burn Mass Casualty Event Due to Boiler Room Explosion on a Cruise Ship: Preparedness and Outcomes

Tekin A, Namias N, O'Keeffe T, et al (Univ of Miami, Fla)

Am Surg 71:210-215, 2005 3–6

Introduction.—The purpose of this study was to review our experience with a mass casualty incident resulting from a boiler room steam explosion aboard a cruise ship. Experience with major, moderate, and minor burns, steam inhalation, mass casualty response systems, and psychological sequelae will be discussed. Fifteen cruise ship employees were brought to the burn center after a boiler room explosion on a cruise ship. Eleven were triaged to the trauma resuscitation area and four to the surgical emergency room. Seven patients were intubated for respiratory distress or airway protection. Six patients had >80 per cent burns with steam inhalation, and all of these died. One of the 6 patients had 99 per cent burns with steam inhalation and died after withdrawal of support within the first several hours. All patients with major burns required escharotomy on arrival to trauma resuscitation. One patient died in the operating room, despite decompression by laparotomy for abdominal compartment syndrome and pericardiotomy via thoracotomy for cardiac tamponade. Four patients required crystalloid, 20,000 mls/m^2-27,000 mls/m^2 body surface area (BSA) in the first 48 hours to maintain blood pressure and urine output. Three of these four patients subsequently developed abdominal compartment syndrome and died in the first few days. The fourth patient of this group died after 26 days due to sepsis. Five patients had 13-20 per cent bums and four patients had less than 10 per cent burns. Two of the patients with 20 per cent burns developed edema of the vocal cords with mild hoarseness. They improved and recovered without

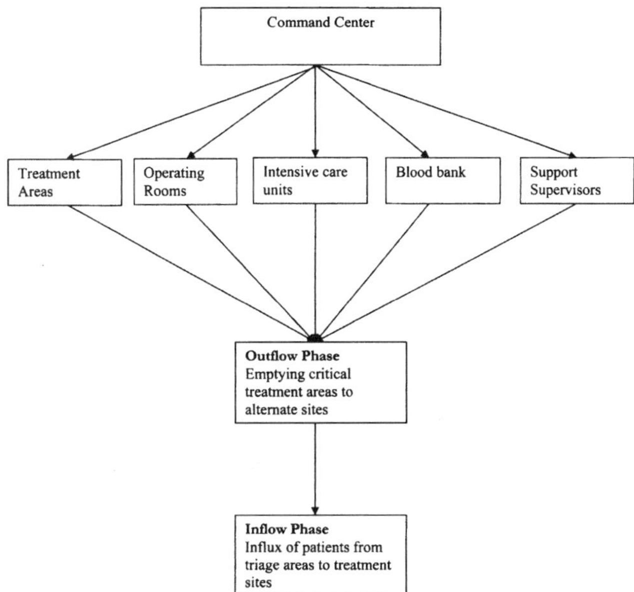

FIGURE 2.—UM/JMH disaster organization and objectives. (Courtesy of Tekin A, Namias N, O'Keeffe T, et al: A burn mass casualty event due to boiler room explosion on a cruise ship: Preparedness and outcomes. *Am Surg* 71:210-215, 2005.)

intubation. The facility was prepared for the mass casualty event, having just completed a mass casualty drill several days earlier (Fig 2). Twenty-six beds were made available in 50 minutes for anticipated casualties. Fifteen physicians reported immediately to the trauma resuscitation area to assist in initial stabilization. The event occurred at shift change; thus, adequate support personnel were instantaneously to hand. Our mass casualty preparation proved useful in managing this event. Most of the patients who survived showed signs of post-traumatic stress syndrome, which was diagnosed and treated by the burn center psychology team. Despite our efforts at treating large burns (>80%) with steam inhalation, mortality was 100 per cent. Fluid requirements far exceeded those predicted by the Parkland (Baxter) formula. Abdominal compartment syndrome proved to be a significant complication of this fluid resuscitation. A coordinated effort by the facility and preparation for mass casualty events are needed to respond to such events.

▶ The final selection involving burn disaster management describes the care of 15 cruise ship employees treated in a regional burn center after a boiler room explosion aboard ship. Six of the patients cared for had greater than 80% burn with steam inhalation injury. Steam inhalation differs from smoke inhalation in that the amount of heat carried by the steam has 4000 times the heat carrying capacity of air. In this regard, inhalation injury is very severe and survival less common. A description of the center's initiation of their mass casualty plan and details of patient care are presented. A number of patients from this accident developed the abdominal compartment syndrome and had a high mortality rate. In the past, before recognition of this problem, these patients with extensive burns would have likely died during resuscitation and considered to have succumbed to resuscitation failure. Our current knowledge of the pathophysiology of this problem permits the use of decompressive laparotomy to reduce the intraabdominal hypertension; however, patients with extensive burns rarely survive this treatment.

D. W. Mozingo, MD

A Prospective, Randomized Evaluation of Intra-abdominal Pressures With Crystalloid and Colloid Resuscitation in Burn Patients

O'Mara MS, Slater H, Goldfarb IW, et al (Univ of California, Sacramento; Temple Univ, Pittsburgh, Pa)

J Trauma 58:1011-1018, 2005 3–7

Background.—The volume of resuscitation in burn patients has been shown to correlate with intra-abdominal pressure (IAP). Limiting volume may reduce consequences of IAP and abdominal compartment syndrome. Colloid resuscitation has been previously shown to limit the volume required initially after burn.

Methods.—Thirty-one patients were prospectively followed. Inclusion criteria were a burn of 25% total body surface area with inhalation injury or 40% total body surface area without. Patients received crystalloid (Parkland formula) or plasma resuscitation. IAP was measured by means of urinary bladder transduction.

Results.—Mean age, area of burn, and baseline IAP were not different. Urine output was maintained. There was a greater increase in IAP with crystalloid (26.5 vs. 10.6 mm Hg, $p < 0.0001$). Two patients in the plasma group developed IAP greater than 25 mm Hg; only one patient in the crystalloid group maintained IAP less than 25 mmHg. More fluid volume was required with crystalloid resuscitation, 0.26 L/kg, versus 0.21 L/kg ($p < 0.005$). Correlation was seen in both groups between volume of fluid and IAP (crystalloid, $r^2 = 0.351$; plasma, $r^2 = 0.657$; all patients, $r^2 = 0.621$).

Conclusion.—Plasma-resuscitated patients maintained an IAP below the threshold of complications of intra-abdominal hypertension. This appears to be a direct result of the decrease in volume required. Lower fluid volume regimens should be given consideration as the incidence and consequences of intra-abdominal hypertension in burn patients continue to be defined.

▶ Development of the abdominal compartment syndrome has been recognized in the resuscitated burn patient as a serious complication. In studies of crystalloid resuscitation, IAP rises in proportion to fluid volume. In general, colloid resuscitation has been shown to reduce fluid requirements and edema; however, without a clear influence on improving outcome or decreased mortality. In this study, 31 patients were prospectively monitored during their resuscitation with a crystalloid formula or plasma resuscitation. Patients receiving the plasma resuscitation had lower IAPs; however, when both groups were combined, the pressure was directly related to the total volume infused regardless of resuscitation strategy. This translated to a 0.475 L/kg of fluid resuscitation being required to raise the IAP to 25 mm Hg. In this small group of patients, differences in survival could not be ascertained. The power of such a study would require large numbers of patients for evaluation.

D. W. Mozingo, MD

The Impact of Combined Trauma and Burns on Patient Mortality

Hawkins A, MacLennan PA, McGwin G Jr, et al (Univ of Alabama at Birmingham)

J Trauma 58:284-288, 2005 3–8

Background.—Combined trauma and burn injuries are uncommon and seldom studied. There is a presumption that these patients fare worse than their trauma- and burn-only counterparts, but the mortality risk has not been quantified.

Methods.—This was a retrospective cohort study using the 1994 to 2002 National Trauma Data Bank. Trauma- and burn-only patients were categorized according to Injury Severity Score (ISS) and burn severity (percentage body surface area burned [BSAB]), respectively, and combined trauma-burn patients were similarly categorized. Risk ratios (RRs) and 95% confidence intervals (CIs) were calculated comparing combined trauma-burn mortality to trauma-only and burn-only patients by corresponding trauma or burn severity. RRs were adjusted for age, gender, and ISS or burn severity.

Results.—Compared with minor trauma-only patients (ISS of 1-15), patients with minor trauma, when combined with burn injury, had significantly increased mortality (RR, 4.04; 95% CI, 3.51-4.66). Similarly, relative to minor burn-only patients (BSAB of 1-25%), combined trauma-burn patients with minor burns (RR, 5.00; 95% CI, 3.54-7.06) had significantly increased mortality. For combined trauma-burn patients with more severe burns or trauma, small but significant increased mortality risks were seen relative to major trauma-only patients (ISS of 26+; RR, 1.26; 95% CI, 1.05-1.51) and major burn-only patients (BSAB of 76+; RR, 1.45; 95% CI, 1.15-1.82).

Conclusion.—The large increased risk of death for those with combined minor injuries is of clinical interest because the majority of combined patients fall into this category. Future research should characterize specific causes and types of injury of increased mortality in the patient with combined injuries.

▶ The combined burn and trauma patient presents major challenges in clinical management and resource use. For this reason, such patients are referred to major trauma centers where greater resources are available. Despite the multidisciplinary management approach, morbidity is increased compared with trauma-only and burn-only patients. This study relied on data from the National Trauma Data Bank and identified 5462 patients with combined burn/trauma injury. The authors identified a dramatic increase in the risk of death for combined burn and trauma when compared with those of trauma-only and burn-only groups. Although this study evaluates the largest number of patients with combined burn and trauma to date, the authors did not attempt to characterize specific causes and types of injuries or the cause of increased mortality in the combined trauma and burn patient. Importantly, the potential impact of smoke inhalation injury was not assessed as it is not explicitly defined in the National Trauma Data Bank. The alarmingly poor outcomes identified through this research suggests that future studies be directed toward filling the information gaps in the National Trauma Data Bank to permit a more thorough assessment of outcomes with combined injury.

D. W. Mozingo, MD

The Incidence and Impact of Pre-Existing Protein Energy Malnutrition on Outcome in the Elderly Burn Patient Population

Demling RH (Harvard Med School, Boston)

J Burn Care Rehabil 26:94-100, 2005 3–9

Introduction.—Protein energy malnutrition (PEM) and involuntary weight loss is a common problem in the elderly population. Our purpose was to determine the incidence and the effect on outcome of PEM in the elderly burn patient population. A chart review and review of the burn data registry was undertaken to determine the incidence and effect of PEM in patients older than 65 years of age with major burns from 1% to 30% TBSA. PEM was diagnosed using standard physiological and biochemical markers. Data were compared with those from a well-nourished elderly burn group to assess the impact. Of the 123 patients studied, we found that PEM was present in 61%. There was a significant increase in infection rate, decrease in the rate of healing of a standard skin graft donor site, and an increase in length of stay in the PEM group compared with the nourished elderly burn group. Mortality with PEM was 17% compared with 9% without PEM, a significant increase. We conclude that PEM is a common comorbid factor in the elderly burn population that increases morbidity and mortality.

▶ Increased morbidity and mortality in elderly burn patients is related as much to the presence of comorbid factors as to the burn injury. Because the elderly population is rapidly increasing, more attention to the factors that alter the outcome of burn injury is warranted. Involuntary weight loss and malnutrition are recognized as significant risk factors for hospital inpatients. The subsequent morbidity may include increased infections, impaired healing, weakness, and disability. The authors of this study found that the incidence of protein energy malnutrition in the geriatric burn population was more than 60%. Of these, half were characterized as moderately to severely malnourished. They also demonstrated a significant increase in infections, mainly pulmonary, in the moderate to severely malnourished population.

D. W. Mozingo, MD

The Association Between Sex and Mortality Among Burn Patients as Modified by Age

George RL, McGwin G Jr, Schwacha MG, et al (Univ of Alabama at Birmingham)

J Burn Care Rehabil 26:416-421, 2005 3–10

Introduction.—Although an increased risk of death among female patients suffering thermal injury has been noted, the differential influence of age has received little attention. Because experimental evidence suggests that sex hormones influence the immune response to thermal injury, an age-related sex influence on patient mortality is biologically plausible as the hormone milieu changes with the onset of menopause. The goal of this study was to estimate the association between sex and mortality after thermal injury in a large, population-based sample. The National Trauma Data Bank yielded data for more than 6200 burn patients 20 years of age or older. Logistic regression was used to calculate mortality odds ratios (OR) with 95% confidence intervals (CIs) for men relative to women, both overall and by age. Adjustments for age, race, burn etiology, percent body surface area burned, comorbid conditions, and inhalation injury were performed. For the overall study population, the adjusted risk of death was approximately 30% lower for males (OR 0.67, 95% CI 0.52-0.87). Within age strata, the adjusted association was statistically significant only in those aged 20 to 34 years (OR 0.45; 95% CI 0.24-0.87); 35 to 49 years (OR 0.71; 95% CI 0.39-1.30); 50 to 64 years (OR 0.55; 95% CI 0.31-1.00); and 65 years or older (OR 0.85; 95% CI 0.57-1.27). The results of the present study not only indicate that women have an increased odds of mortality after thermal injury but also demonstrate a differential effect of age on the association between sex and mortality. On the basis of the findings of the present study as well as the results of experimental studies, further clinical research is needed to investigate the impact of sex hormones on mortality among burn patients.

▶ By using the National Trauma Data Bank, the authors conducted a retrospective study of more than 6200 thermally injured patients to investigate the association between sex and mortality and the function of age. Age-specific associations between sex and mortality have been observed previously in thermal and nonthermal injury. In addition, experimental models of trauma and hemorrhage have demonstrated a change in the relative proportion of immune cell subpopulations as well as the responsiveness of these cells, based on sex. Female sex has been associated with increased mortality from burn injury, although the strength of this association varies between studies. Early studies did not incorporate sex in models of burn mortality; however, more recently sex has been identified as an important burn mortality risk factor. This study confirms these findings in a large subset of patients, identifying that women have an increased odds of mortality after thermal injury but also demonstrate a differential effect of age on associated mortality.

D. W. Mozingo, MD

Sex Hormones Modulate Distant Organ Injury in Both a Trauma/ Hemorrhagic Shock Model and a Burn Model

Ananthakrishnan P, Cohen DB, Xu DZ, et al (Univ of Medicine and Dentistry of New Jersey, Newark)

Surgery 137:56-65, 2005 3–11

Background.—Emerging data suggest a gender dimorphism in resistance and susceptibility to distant organ injury after mechanical and thermal trauma. The aim of this study was to determine the role that testosterone and estradiol play in modulating resistance or susceptibility to distant organ injury, and whether their effects were associated with differences in the production of nitric oxide.

Methods.—Adult male, female, castrated male, and ovariectomized female Sprague-Dawley rats were given intraperitoneal pentobarbital sodium anesthesia and subjected to trauma/sham shock or trauma/hemorrhagic shock (T/HS). A second set of animals were subjected to a 40% total body surface area, third-degree burn or sham burn. At 3 hours after resuscitation, plasma levels of nitrite/nitrate were measured, and the extent of lung injury (permeability to Evans Blue dye and neutrophil sequestration by myeloperoxidase) and intestinal injury (morphology) were determined.

Results.—Proestrus females showed resistance to lung and gut injury after both T/HS and burns, and had low levels of nitrite/nitrate production. This resistance to injury was abrogated by ovariectomy with an associated increase in nitric oxide production. Males showed increased lung and gut injury after both T/HS and burns associated with increased production of nitrite/nitrate. Castration decreased susceptibility to both lung and gut injury, and decreased production of nitrite/nitrate. A correlation was noted between intestinal and lung injury, and both intestinal and lung injury correlated with plasma nitrite/nitrate levels.

Conclusions.—Male sex hormones potentiate, while female hormones reduce T/HS and burn-induced lung and gut injury. Production of nitric oxide is associated with increased lung and gut injury after T/HS and burns.

► The authors of this selection explore the sex differences in resistance and susceptibility to distant organ injury after mechanical and thermal trauma. In particular, they evaluated the role of testosterone and estradiol in modulating resistance or susceptibility to distant organ injury notably in the lung and the gut. Their results show that the male sex hormones potentiate, whereas female hormones reduce lung and gut injury in the experimental animal subjected to trauma and hemorrhage or burn injury. They have also linked increased nitric oxide production to the increased susceptibility to organ injury in this model. Additional studies will be required to determine whether similar changes occur in patients.

D. W. Mozingo, MD

Burden of Burn: A Norm-Based Inquiry Into the Influence of Burn Size and Distress on Recovery of Physical and Psychosocial Function

Fauerbach JA, Lezotte D, Hills RA, et al (Johns Hopkins Univ, Baltimore, Md; Univ of Colorado, Denver; Univ of Texas, Dallas; et al)

J Burn Care Rehabil 26:21-32, 2005 3–12

Introduction.—This prospective, longitudinal study examined the influence of baseline physical and psychological burden on serial assessments of health-related quality of life among adults with major burns from three regional burn centers (n = 162). Physical burden groups were defined by % TBSA burned: <10%, 10% to 30%, or >30%. Psychological burden groups were defined by in-hospital distress using the Brief Symptom Inventory Global Severity Index T-score with scores of < 63 or ≥ 63. Analyses compared groups across level of burden and with published normative data. Assessments reflected health and function (Short Form 36) during the month before burn, at discharge, and at 6 and 12 months after burn. Physical functioning was significantly more impaired and the rate of physical recovery slower among those with either large physical burden or large psychological burden. Notably, psychosocial functioning also was more impaired and the rate of psychosocial recovery slower among those with greater psychological burden. These results suggest that, in addition to aggressive wound closure, interventions that reduce in-hospital distress may accelerate both physical and psychosocial recovery.

▶ This study was designed to examine the degree of impairment and rate of recovery among individuals who experience a major burn with differing levels of physical and psychologic burdens. Injury factors such as extent of burn, pain, and length of stay in the ICU are associated with quality of life. A significant measure of the degree of recovery from severe burn injury is health-related quality of life that is defined as the subjective perception of function and well-being. This study examined the influence of baseline physical and psychologic burden on serial assessments of quality of life in adult burn patients. In this large-scale multicenter study, important findings included that complementing wound closure and resuscitation efforts with early interventions designed to reduce initial psychologic distress may accelerate both physical and psychosocial recovery of individuals sustaining major burn injury. Also, substantial suffering from acute psychologic stress as well as its prolonged association with poor recovery may warrant a more aggressive approach to early mental health assessment and intervention after burn injury.

D. W. Mozingo, MD

High Risk for Accidental Death in Previously Burn-Injured Adults

Onarheim H, Vindenes HA (Haukeland Univ, Bergen, Norway)
Burns 31:297-301, 2005 3–13

Introduction.—This study investigated the long-term mortality in 1182 burn patients admitted at a single burn centre in 1984-2003. One thousand and forty-nine patients were discharged alive, of which 999 (95.2% of all discharged) were available for follow-up (mean observation time: 9.6 ± 5.5 (S.D.) years). One hundred and twenty-two patients had died after discharge but before follow-up. For 111 patients, the official information recorded from their death certificates revealed that 83 patients (mainly in the higher age groups) had died due to a variety of natural causes. Twenty-three patients (M:F = 18:5) (age: 37.7 ± 11.3 years), previously hospitalised for burns, had later suffered accidental or violent deaths, including suicide (5), assault (2), and deaths related to substance and/or alcohol abuse (12). Additionally, five other deaths were recorded as sudden death, with no additional specific information as to the cause of death. This study shows that the rates of accidental or violent death in previously burned adult patients (around 40 deaths per 1000 years at risk) may be an order of magnitude higher than that in the average Norwegian population.

► Outcome studies related to burn injury typically address data such as in-hospital mortality or length of stay relative to the extent of burn. Other problems such as scarring, cosmetic results, or eventual needs for reconstructive procedures are also commonly addressed. Recently, a focus on various aspects related to quality of life has been addressed, particularly after severe injury. Burn patients may differ from other populations with regard to risky activities or preexisting psychiatric or mental illness. Also, the frequency of unemployment and alcohol or drug use may be higher in this population. This study evaluated the cause of death of 111 patients of 999 discharges where death occurred in the follow-up period. This study shows that the rate of accidental or violent death was an order or magnitude higher than predicted in the typical population. The higher risk for accidental death was mainly encountered in the younger patient population. Only 2 of the accidental deaths were recognized in patients older than 50 years. There was no relation between the extent of burn and subsequent risk for accidental death.

D. W. Mozingo, MD

Changes in VEGF and Nitric Oxide After Deep Dermal Injury in the Female, Red Duroc Pig—Further Similarities Between Female, Duroc Scar and Human Hypertrophic Scar

Zhu KQ, Engrav LH, Armendariz R, et al (Univ of Washington, Seattle)
Burns 31:5-10, 2005 3–14

Introduction.—Despite decades of research, our understanding of human hypertrophic scar is limited. A reliable animal model could significantly increase our understanding. We previously confirmed similarities between scarring in the female, red, Duroc pig and human hypertrophic scarring. The purpose of this study was to: (1) measure vascular endothelial growth factor (VEGF) and nitric oxide (NO) levels in wounds on the female Duroc; and (2) to compare the NO levels to those reported for human hypertrophic scar. Shallow and deep wounds were created on four female Durocs. VEGF levels were measured using ELISA and NO levels with the Griess reagent. VEGF and NO levels were increased in deep wounds at 10 days when compared to shallow wounds ($p < 0.05$). At 15 weeks, VEGF and NO levels had returned to the level of shallow wounds. At 21 weeks, VEGF and NO levels had declined below baseline levels in deep wounds and the NO levels were significantly lower ($p < 0.01$). We found that VEGF and NO exhibit two distinctly different temporal patterns in shallow and deep wounds on the female Durocs. Furthermore, NO is decreased in female, Duroc scar as it is in human, hypertrophic scar further validating the usefulness of the model.

► In this selection, the authors further explore the validity of the female red Duroc pig model of hypertrophic scarring as related to hypertrophic scarring in the human counterpart. They had previously reported similarities in clinical appearance, histology time to healing, and immunohistochemistry of growth factor expression. Little progress has been made in dealing with the clinical problems of hypertrophic scars because of the lack of a viable animal model for this problem. The results presented in this experiment demonstrate that changes in growth factors and NO confirm the similarity to human hypertrophic scarring. They found that VEGF and NO levels vary according to the depth of the wound and described a distinct temporal progression. These findings, including the elevated NO levels, further confirm the validity of the Duroc model of hypertrophic scarring.

D. W. Mozingo, MD

Treatment of Second Degree Facial Burns With Allografts—Preliminary Results

Horch RE, Jeschke MG, Spilker G, et al (Friedrich-Alexander-Univ, Freiburg, Germany; City of Cologne Hosp, Cologne-Merheim, Germany; Univ of Texas, Galveston)

Burns 31:597-602, 2005 3–15

Introduction.—Facial burns are very common and have significant clinical impact. However, the treatment regimen for superficial to deep facial burns is not well defined. The purpose of this study was to investigate the effects of cadaver skin grafting in deep partial thickness facial burns in comparison to standard care.

In a prospective open study design severely injured patients with superficial and deep partial thickness burns were randomized into the group receiving open treatment with silversulfadiazine (standard $n = 5$) or into the group receiving early superficial debridement followed by coverage with glycerolized cadaver skin ($n = 5$). The outcome measures were time and quality of wound healing, and incidence of hypertrophic scarring at 3 and 6 months post burn.

There were no significant differences in demographics between groups. In the group treated with the allogenic material time to reepithelialization was 10.5 days, while it was 12.4 days in the silversulfadiazine group ($p < 0.05$). Scar quality was found to be significantly improved in the allogenic treatment group. Three and 6 months postburn there were no patients with significant hypertrophic scarring in the allogenic group while there were two patients who developed hypertrophic scars in the silversulfadiazine group ($p < 0.05$). In this study, we demonstrated that glycerolized cadaver allograft skin represents a superior biological dressing for shallow and deep partial thickness facial burns. This is in concordance with other reports on scalds. It would be worthwhile to perform more clinical studies with a larger number of patients to further evaluate the effect and function of allogenic skin for facial burns.

▶ Disfiguring and hypertrophic scarring of the face after superficial or deep partial thickness burns has serious clinical, psychologic, and functional impact in burn patients. Facial burns are common occurring in 30% to 50% of minor to moderate burns and in more than 50% of large burns. The majority of facial burns are partial thickness in nature, and because of the difficulty and complexity of wound care, most patients with partial thickness wounds to the face, require hospital care. Healing time is of major importance in these wounds. Wounds that typically remain open after 10 days postburn have an increased risk of infection and scar formation. This selection describes a single center's experience in managing partial thickness burns of the face with superficial debridement, followed by application of human cadaver allograft compared with conventional topical antimicrobial therapy. The use of biologic and synthetic dressings is well known in burn care. Their ability to diminish pain, prevent desiccation of vital structures, decrease bacterial load, and decrease evaporative water loss have been described previously. In this study, the investigators demonstrated that wound coverage with the use of allografts resulted in no infection, good re-epithelialization by 10 days postburn, and no hypertrophic scar formation at 3 and 6 months after burn injury. Although the number of patients included in the study is small, the results speak for continued evaluation of this aggressive approach toward healing of facial burns.

D. W. Mozingo, MD

The Versajet™ Water Dissector: A New Tool for Tangential Excision

Klein MB, Hunter S, Heimbach DM, et al (Univ of Washington, Seattle)

J Burn Care Rehabil 26:483-487, 2005 3–16

Introduction.—Goulian and Watson knives work well for tangential burn excision on large flat areas. They do not work well in small areas and in areas with a three-dimensional structure. The Versajet Hydrosurgery System

(Smith and Nephew, Key Largo, FL) is a new waterjet-powered surgical tool designed for wound excision. The small size of the cutting nozzle and the ability to easily maneuver the water dissector into small spaces makes it a potentially useful tool for excision of burns of the eyelids, digits and web spaces. The Versajet Hydrosurgery System contains a power console that propels saline through a handheld cutting device. This stream of pressurized saline functions as a knife. We have used the Versajet for burn excision in 44 patients. Although there is a learning curve for both surgeons using and operating room staff setting up the device, the Versajet provides a relatively facile method for excision of challenging aesthetic and functional areas.

▶ The authors describe the application of the Versajet hydrosurgery system to burn wound excision. This is a relatively new tool that provides a high-pressure water jet capable of cutting tissue. Water dissection works by the Venturi effect. A jet of saline solution propelled by a power console travels across the operating window of a handheld piece and then into a suction collector. The stream of pressurized saline solution functions like a knife. The debrided tissue is then aspired into the suction receptacle. The power of the dissecting device can be adjusted to permit less cutting power on more delicate areas and shallower burns. The small size of the cutting nozzle is actually an advantage when excising areas with a concavity or 3-dimensional structure such as the ears, eyelids, and webspaces of the hand. The handheld Goulian and Watson knives have long been the preferred tools for burn excision. These knives allow for rapid excision of large surface areas of eschar; however, they are not well suited to some anatomic areas. The Versajet Water Dissector may provide a faster and more precise method of excising critical and difficult-to-access areas.

D. W. Mozingo, MD

An Open-Label Study to Evaluate the Safety and Efficacy of Tissue Plasminogen Activator in Treatment of Severe Frostbite

Twomey JA, Peltier GL, Zera RT (Hennepin County Med Ctr, Minneapolis)

J Trauma 59:1350-1355, 2005 3–17

Background.—Severe frostbite can have devastating consequences with loss of limbs and digits. One of the mechanisms of cold injury to human tissue is vascular thrombosis. The effect of tissue plasminogen activator (tPA) and heparin in limb and digit preservation in severe frostbite patients has not been previously studied.

Methods.—Intra-arterial (6 patients) or intravenous (i.v., 13 patients) tPA and IV heparin were used in patients with severe frostbite. All patients between January 1, 1989 and February 1, 2003 with severe frostbite not improved by rapid rewarming, with absent Doppler pulses in distal limb or digits, without perfusion by Technetium (Tc) 99m three-phase bone scan, and no contraindication to tPA use were eligible. Efficacy was assessed on the basis of predicted digit amputation before therapy, given the clinical and Tc-99m scan results, versus partial or complete digits removed.

Results.—There were no complications with i.v. tPA. Two patients with intra-arterial tPA had bleeding complications. We know from historical Tc-99m scan data which digits were at risk for amputation. In this study, there were 174 digits at risk in 18 patients and only 33 were amputated.

Conclusion.—Intravenous tPA and heparin after rapid rewarming is safe and reduced predicted digit amputations considerably. Patients with no response to thrombolytic therapy were those with more than 24 hours of cold exposure, warm ischemia times greater than 6 hours, or evidence of multiple freeze-thaw cycles. Our algorithm for treatment of severe frostbite now includes use of i.v. tPA for patients without contraindications.

► Vascular injury and resulting thrombosis appear to be one of the important mechanisms in determining the overall tissue impact of cold exposure. The use of rapid rewarming addresses mainly the ice crystal phase of cellular damage and does not improve already damaged and thrombosed vessels. Late thrombosis may also occur up to 16 hours after rewarming. This study evaluates the effect of tPA and heparin in limb and digit preservation after severe frostbite. Early studies used intra-arterial infusion, whereas later experience indicated that IV infusion was equally effective. The results of patients treated were compared with historical controls. Both the Tc-99m blood-flow scans and clinical parameters were improved in patients receiving tPA and heparin. This would be an extremely difficult population of patients to study in a prospective manner because of their relative infrequency of presentation. This clinical experience suggests that this treatment is safe and may improve outcomes from frostbite.

D. W. Mozingo, MD

4 Critical Care

Introduction

In recent years, an enormous emphasis has been placed on patient safety and the prevention of avoidable medical errors and complications. Critical care units provide life-saving care for the sickest of patients who are also at risk for these events and errors. These events can be characterized as system-related problems or individual performance failures. Most serious medical errors involve the ordering or execution of treatments, particularly medications. Protocol-based treatments applied in the ICU setting may also decrease errors, morbidity, and mortality by assuring best practices and eliminating lapses in treatment. Such protocols as the ARDS network protocol have been associated with a reduced hospital mortality. Methods to report event incidence in the ICU related to system factors and failure help identify potential areas of improvement. Incidence-reporting systems based on contributing factors, limiting factors, and preventive factors, though tedious and manpower-intensive to track, often result in improvement of outcome. Six Sigma is a data-driven quality improvement methodology that seeks to improve outcomes by eliminating the variation within a process. Six Sigma refers to a statistical defect rate of 6 standard deviations or 3.4 defects per million events. Application of this strategy to reduce the incidence of catheter-related bloodstream infections resulted in a marked drop in catheter-related infections.

The diagnosis and treatment of ventilator-associated pneumonia continues to be a problem in ICUs. More than one half of patients with closed head injury requiring mechanical ventilation will develop this complication. The accurate diagnosis of ventilator-associated pneumonia is often difficult. Culturing bronchoalveolar lavage fluid or deep endotracheal aspirates are options in this setting; however, bronchoalveolar lavage is often more specific and seems to lessen the spectrum of antibiotics needed for coverage of the organisms. There seems to be no difference in mortality rates related to the type of diagnostic procedure performed; however, invasive approaches to ventilator-associated pneumonia affect antibiotic use and prescribing.

Insulin resistance is a central feature of stress metabolism in critically ill patients. This process has been described in the past as a pathophysiologic adaptation to ensure adequate substrate supply to non–insulin-dependent vital tissue such as the brain. New information suggests that hyperglycemia in the basal state is mainly accounted for by an increase in endogenous glucose production, suggesting the presence of hepatic insulin resistance. Normoglycemia, achieved by the administration of insulin during feeding, suppresses endogenous glucose production, and peripheral glucose uptake is not increased despite the presence of pharmacologic concentrations of insulin in the circulation.

Endocrine abnormalities have been described in critically ill patients, and adrenal insufficiency is increasingly recognized in this population even though the classic signs are typically not present. Patients with this problem may also have hyperthyroidism in 12% of cases. There is much controversy regarding the levels of cortisol that are considered adequate in septic shock. Adrenocortical stimulation tests are often used, but there is no standardized definition of a normal response in the critically ill. Low-dose tests can identify a subgroup of patients in septic shock with inadequate adrenal reserve and worse outcome. This group may be missed by higher dose stimulation tests.

Recombinant human erythropoietin has been shown to decrease the need for blood transfusion in critically ill patients; however, the reductions were modest at best. To avoid one transfusion-related adverse event, more than 5000 patients would need to be treated with this product. More than 28,000 would require treatment to avoid a serious transfusion-related event. Postoperative hemorrhage after major trauma surgery carries a high mortality rate. The use of recombinant factor VIIa may significantly decrease the total blood product transfusion requirement. This off-label use of this medication might be considered in trauma patients when coagulopathy and nonsurgical bleeding occur.

Intra-abdominal hypertension has been associated with increased morbidity and mortality in surgical and trauma patients. The occurrence of intraabdominal hypertension during the ICU stay is an independent predictor of mortality. Documentation of intra-abdominal pressure should be considered in the setting of renal or hepatic failure in patients with multiple organ failure syndromes.

Patients at risk for developing rhabdomyolysis include those with multisystem trauma, especially with extremity fractures and vascular injuries. Patients with electrical burns and deep circumferential thermal burns are also at risk. An algorithm has been developed to identify patients at risk for developing renal failure related to this problem, which also enables prompt treatment.

Candidal isolates account for a rising proportion of nosocomial bloodstream infections and are a common cause of catheter-related infection in surgical ICUs. Mortality is increased in surgical ICU patients with candidemia, although attributing the increase in mortality to this infection remains controversial. The use of fluconazole prophylaxis in critically ill surgical patients does result in a decrease in the rate of candidal infections, but an effect on mortality could not be demonstrated. The use of pulmonary artery catheters in the management of critically ill patients has been questioned repeatedly and remains a matter of controversy. Patients with indwelling intravascular catheters including the pulmonary catheter have a higher rate of embolic events, although the mechanism for this complication is unclear. Insertion of a pulmonary artery catheter caused a change in coagulation parameters as detected by thrombelastography. The time to initial fibrin formation was decreased, suggesting that the presence of this catheter in the circulation may induce a relative hypercoagulable state.

David W. Mozingo, MD

The Critical Care Safety Study: The Incidence and Nature of Adverse Events and Serious Medical Errors in Intensive Care

Rothschild JM, Landrigan CP, Cronin JW, et al (Harvard Med School, Boston)
Crit Care Med 33:1694-1700, 2005 4–1

Objective.—Critically ill patients require high-intensity care and may be at especially high risk of iatrogenic injury because they are severely ill. We sought to study the incidence and nature of adverse events and serious errors in the critical care setting.

Design.—We conducted a prospective 1-year observational study. Incidents were collected with use of a multifaceted approach including direct continuous observation. Two physicians independently assessed incident type, severity, and preventability as well as systems-related and individual performance failures.

Setting.—Academic, tertiary-care urban hospital.

Patients.—Medical intensive care unit and coronary care unit patients.

Interventions.—None.

Measurements and Main Results.—The primary outcomes of interest were the incidence and rates of adverse events and serious errors per 1000 patient-days. A total of 391 patients with 420 unit admissions were studied during 1490 patient-days. We found 120 adverse events in 79 patients (20.2%), including 66 (55%) nonpreventable and 54 (45%) preventable adverse events as well as 223 serious errors. The rates per 1000 patient-days for all adverse events, preventable adverse events, and serious errors were 80.5, 36.2, and 149.7, respectively. Among adverse events, 13% (16/120) were life-threatening or fatal; and among serious errors, 11% (24/223) were potentially life-threatening. Most serious medical errors occurred during the ordering or execution of treatments, especially medications (61%; 170/277). Performance level failures were most commonly slips and lapses (53%; 148/277), rather than rule-based or knowledge-based mistakes.

Conclusions.—Adverse events and serious errors involving critically ill patients were common and often potentially life-threatening. Although many types of errors were identified, failure to carry out intended treatment correctly was the leading category.

► Critical care units provide lifesaving care for the sickest patients, who are also at significant risk for adverse events and serious medical errors. The delivery of critical care presents significant safety challenges. This type of care is complex and requires urgent high-risk decision making. Also, critically ill patients may be particularly vulnerable to iatrogenic injury because of the severity and instability of their condition and the frequent need for high-risk interventions and medications. The authors describe a prospective 1-year observational study during which incidents were collected and analyzed by incident type, severity, and preventability. Such incidents were also characterized as system-related problems or individual performance failures. Most serious medical errors occurred during the ordering or execution of treatments, particularly medications. Although many types of errors were identified, failure to provide the intended treatment correctly was the leading cause.

D. W. Mozingo, MD

Clinical Implementation of the ARDS Network Protocol Is Associated With Reduced Hospital Mortality Compared With Historical Controls

Kallet RH, Jasmer RM, Pittet J-F, et al (Univ of California, San Francisco)

Crit Care Med 33:925-929, 2005 4–2

Objective.—To assess the impact of implementing a low tidal volume ventilation strategy on hospital mortality for patients with acute lung injury or acute respiratory distress syndrome.

Design.—Retrospective, uncontrolled study.

Setting.—Adult medical-surgical and trauma intensive care units at a major inner city, university-affiliated hospital.

Patients.—A total of 292 patients with acute lung injury or acute respiratory distress syndrome.

Interventions.—Between the years 2000 and 2003, 200 prospectively identified patients with acute lung injury/acute respiratory distress syndrome were managed by the ARDS Network low tidal volume protocol. A historical control group of 92 acute respiratory distress syndrome patients managed by routine practice from 1998 to 1999 was used for comparison.

Measurements and Main Results.—Patients managed with the ARDS Network protocol had a lower hospital mortality compared with historical controls (32% vs. 51%, respectively; $p = .004$). Multivariate logistic regression estimated an odds ratio of 0.32 (95% CI, 0.17-0.59; $p = .0003$) for mortality risk with use of the ARDS Network protocol. Protocol-managed patients had a lower tidal volume (6.2 ± 1.1 vs. 9.8 ± 1.5 mL/kg; $p < .0001$) and plateau pressure (27.5 ± 6.4 vs. 33.8 ± 8.9 cm H_2O; $p < .0001$) than historical controls.

Conclusion.—Adoption of the ARDS Network protocol for routine ventilator management of acute lung injury/acute respiratory distress syndrome patients was associated with a lower mortality compared with recent historical controls.

► The authors initiated the ARDS Network protocol using mechanical ventilation with a tidal volume of 6 mL/kg predicted body weight in their institution. During a 3-year period, 200 patients with a diagnosis of acute lung injury or ARDS were managed clinically with the low tidal volume protocol. This group was compared with a group of 112 patients with ARDS cared for in the 2 previous years. A significant survival advantage was seen in patients managed with the low tidal volume protocol. This study also enrolled patients who would not have been eligible for enrollment into the ARDS Network trial because of disease-related criteria. An improvement in survival was seen in this group as well.

D. W. Mozingo, MD

A System Factors Analysis of "Line, Tube, and Drain" Incidents in the Intensive Care Unit

Needham DM, Sinopoli DJ, Thompson DA, et al (Johns Hopkins Univ, Baltimore, Md)

Crit Care Med 33:1701-1707, 2005 4–3

Objective.—To analyze the system factors related to "line, tube, and drain" (LTD) incidents in the intensive care unit (ICU).

Design.—Voluntary, anonymous Web-based patient safety reporting system.

Setting.—Eighteen ICUs in the United States.

Patients.—Incidents reported by ICU staff members during a 12-month period ending June 2003.

Interventions.—None.

Measurements.—Characteristics of the incidents (defined as events that could/did cause harm), patients, and patient harm were described. Separate multivariable logistic regression analyses of contributing, limiting, and preventive system factors for LTD vs. non-LTD incidents were reported.

Main Results.—Of the 114 reported LTD incidents, >60% were considered preventable. One patient death was attributed to an LTD incident. Of patients experiencing LTD incidents, 56% sustained physical injury, and 23% had an anticipated increased hospital stay. Factors contributing to LTD incidents included occurrence in the operating room (odds ratio [OR], 3.50; 95% confidence interval [CI], 1.25-9.83), occurrence on a holiday (OR, 3.65; 95% CI, 1.12-11.9), patient medical complexity (OR, 3.68; 95% CI, 2.28-5.92), and age of 1-9 yrs (OR, 7.95; 95% CI, 3.29-19.2). Factors related to team communication were less likely to limit LTD incidents (OR, 0.28; 95% CI, 0.11-0.68), while clinician knowledge and skills helped prevent LTD incidents (OR, 1.80; 95% CI, 1.09-2.97).

Conclusions.—Patients are harmed by preventable LTD incidents. Relative to non-LTD events, these incidents occur more frequently during holidays and in medically complex patients and children. Focusing on these contributing factors and clinician knowledge and skills is important for reducing and preventing these hazardous events.

▶ ICU incidents involving invasive LTDs related to their placement, maintenance, or removal may result in catastrophic events. This study used a system factor approach to study patient safety, focusing on the conditions in which ICU staff worked to prevent and minimize medical errors. The incident reporting system was based on contributing factors, limiting factors, and preventive factors. Of the 114 reported incidents in this study, over 60% were considered preventable. Hospital holidays, patient complexity, and younger age were important contributing factors to these incidents. Provider knowledge and skill were also related to these incidents. Managers and clinicians should focus on these high-risk patients and incident characteristics and ensure that providers' skills are developed and maintained.

D. W. Mozingo, MD

Use of Corporate Six Sigma Performance-Improvement Strategies to Reduce Incidence of Catheter-related Bloodstream Infections in a Surgical ICU

Frankel HL, Crede WB, Topal JE, et al (Yale Univ, New Haven, Conn)
J Am Coll Surg 201:349-358, 2005 4–4

Background.—Corporate performance-improvement methodologies can outperform traditional ones in addressing ICU-based adverse events. My colleagues and I used Six Sigma methodology to address our catheter-related bloodstream infection (CR-BSI) rate, which considerably exceeded the nationally established median over a 9-year period. We hypothesized that use of Six Sigma methodology would result in a substantial and sustainable decrease in our CR-BSI rate.

Study Design.—All patients were directly cared for by a geographically localized surgical ICU team in an academic tertiary referral center. CR-BSIs were identified by infection control staff using CDC definitions. Personnel trained in Six Sigma techniques facilitated performance-improvement efforts. Interventions included barrier precaution kits, new policies for catheter changes over guide wires, adoption of a new site-preparation antiseptic, direct attending supervision of catheter insertions, video training for housestaff, and increased frequency of dressing changes. After additional data analysis, chlorhexidine-silver catheters were used selectively in high-risk patients. The impact of interventions was assessed by monitoring the number of catheters placed between CR-BSIs.

Results.—Before the intervention period, 27 catheters were placed, on average, between individual CR-BSIs, a CR-BSI rate of 11 per 1,000 catheter days. After all operations were implemented, 175 catheters were placed between line infections, an average CR-BSI rate of 1.7/1,000 catheter days, a 650% improvement ($p < 0.0001$) (Fig 5). Compared with historic controls, adoption of chlorhexidine-silver catheters in high-risk patients had a considerable impact (50% reduction; $p < 0.05$).

Conclusions.—This represents the first successful application of Six Sigma corporate performance-improvement method impacting purely clinical outcomes. CR-BSI reduction was highly substantial and sustained after other traditional strategies had failed.

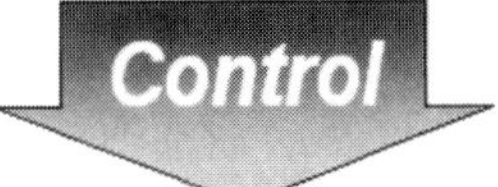

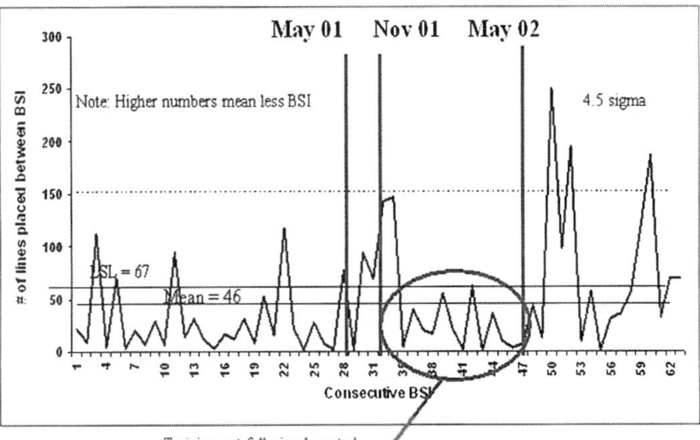

FIGURE 5.—Control chart of catheter-related bloodstream infections (*BSI*) at Yale New Haven Hospital surgical ICU, November 2001 and April 2002. (Reprinted from Frankel HL, Crede WB, Topal JE, et al: Use of corporate Six Sigma performance-improvement strategies to reduce incidence of catheter-related bloodstream infections in a surgical ICU. *J Am Coll Surg* 201:349-358, 2005. Copyright 2005, with permission from the American College of Surgeons.)

► Six Sigma, a corporate performance strategy developed by the Motorola Corporation, has been piloted in the health care arena focusing on areas of business operations, throughput, and case management. Six Sigma is a data-driven quality improvement methodology that seeks to improve outcomes by eliminating the variation within a process. Six Sigma refers to a statistical defect rate of 6 standard deviations or 3.4 defects per million events. The higher the Sigma number, the fewer the defects. Most medical processes operate in the realm of 3 to 4 Sigma or about 67,000 to 6000 errors per million events, respectively. In the study presented here, factors that contribute to the development of CR-BSIs are identified and displayed in a cause-and-effect diagram. The operations and procedures used to improve the metric were a combination of epidemiologic analyses and identification of those factors important to the process, including the need to change the standard process. Implementation of this Six Sigma program resulted in a drop in CR-BSIs of 11 per 1000 catheter days to 1.7 per 1000 catheter days. Although this strategy is rigorous and requires a significant personnel commitment, additional use of this methodology to improve outcomes in patient safety should be considered.

D. W. Mozingo, MD

The Effect of Ventilator-associated Pneumonia on the Prognosis of Head Trauma Patients

Kallel H, Chelly H, Bahloul M, et al (Service de Réanimation Médicale, Sfax, Tunisia)

J Trauma 59:705-710, 2005 4–5

Background.—To investigate the effect of ventilator-associated pneumonia (VAP) on the prognosis of head trauma patients.

Methods.—We performed a retrospective case-control study in which 57 head trauma patients with VAP were matched to 57 head trauma patients without VAP. Matching criteria were age (±5 years), Glasgow Coma Scale score (±2), Injury Severity Score (±5), Simplified Acute Physiology Score II (±5), and duration of exposure to mechanical ventilation.

Results.—The most causative organisms of VAP were *Pseudomonas aeruginosa*, and *Acinetobactor baumannii* (36.8% and 33.8% of isolated organisms, respectively). The duration of mechanical ventilation, intensive care unit stay, and hospital stay were significantly increased in case patients (13 ± 8.4, 24.5 ± 18, and 30.8 ± 18.6 days, respectively) compared with control patients (8.3 ± 4.3, 12.3 ± 8, and 20.3 ± 18.7 days, respectively). Mortality rate was also higher in case (29.8%) than in control (12.3%) patients ($p = 0.02$).

Conclusion.—We conclude that the occurrence of VAP caused by high-risk organisms in cranial trauma patients may increase the risk of death, the mechanical ventilation duration, the intensive care unit stay, and the hospital stay.

► Over one half of patients with closed head injury requiring mechanical ventilation will develop VAP. This high incidence may be explained by immunosuppression, and the need for emergency tracheal intubation and invasive therapeutics secondary to the brain injury. The investigators identified high-risk organisms, namely, *P aeruginosa*, *A baumannii*, and methicillin-resistant *Staphylococcus aureus*, which were associated with a higher mortality rate than infections caused by other organisms. The duration of mechanical ventilation, the ICU stay, the hospital stay, and the mortality rate were all increased in these patients.

D. W. Mozingo, MD

Prospective Comparison of Bronchoalveolar Lavage and Quantitative Deep Tracheal Aspirate in the Diagnosis of Ventilator Associated Pneumonia

Mondi MM, Chang MC, Bowton DL, et al (Wake Forest Univ, Winston-Salem, NC)

J Trauma 59:891-896, 2005 4–6

Background.—Ventilator associated pneumonia (VAP) is common in trauma patients, and accurate diagnosis of VAP may improve survival. With the risk of development of bacterial resistance, we also strive to minimize the use of unnecessary antibiotics. Recent studies suggest that quantitative deep endotracheal aspirate (QDEA) is adequate in VAP diagnosis. We currently use bronchoalveolar lavage (BAL) diagnosis. The purpose of this study was to examine the accuracy of QDEA as compared with BAL in diagnosing VAP in trauma patients.

Methods.—We prospectively compared the results of BAL and QDEA in intubated patients suspected of having VAP during an 8-month period. Indication for BAL was pulmonary infiltrate, systemic inflammatory response syndrome, and C-reactive protein >17 mg/dL at ≥48 hours after admission. Study patients underwent QDEA immediately before BAL, and quantitative cultures were compared for both specimens. The techniques differ in that QDEA involves the direct culture of sputum suctioned from the distal trachea, whereas BAL involves lavage of the bronchoalveolar tree with sterile saline, which is then cultured. VAP was diagnosed on BAL if $\geq 10^5$ cfu/mL was present on culture. The ability of QDEA to diagnose pneumonia was examined at cutoffs of $\geq 10^5$ cfu/mL and $\geq 10^4$ cfu/mL, as compared with BAL at $\geq 10^5$.

Results.—Sixty-one patients underwent BAL during this period, and 39 of these underwent both BAL and QDEA for the study. Of the 39 studied patients between March 16, 2002, and November 4, 2002, 20 (51%) were found to have VAP by BAL ($\geq 10^5$ cfu/mL). Using this cutoff for QDEA, 18 of 20 (90%) would have been correctly diagnosed. Using $\geq 10^4$ cfu/mL for QDEA, the rate of correct diagnosis would increase to 19 of 20 (95%). However, of the 19 who did not have pneumonia according to BAL, 6 (31%) would have been incorrectly diagnosed with VAP using the QDEA cutoff of $\geq 10^5$ cfu/mL. A QDEA cutoff of $\geq 10^4$ cfu/mL would result in the even higher false-positive rate of 8 of 19 patients (42%).

Conclusion.—Whereas most patients with pneumonia by BAL would have been diagnosed by QDEA, use of QDEA in treatment decisions would have led to needless antibiotic administration in 31% of VAP-negative patients at a cutoff of $\geq 10^5$ cfu/mL and 42% at $\geq 10^4$ cfu/mL. The use of QDEA in VAP diagnosis is limited because of the rate of over-diagnosis. With the increasing problems associated with excess antibiotic use, we believe these results support the use of BAL over QDEA in the diagnosis of VAP in the ventilated trauma patient.

► VAP remains a significant problem in the critically ill, resulting in increased morbidity, mortality, and cost. To date, issues regarding the diagnosis and therapy for VAP remain controversial. This study was undertaken to compare this group's standard methodology for diagnosis of VAP, BAL, with that of QDEA. Recent studies have suggested that QDEA is adequate in the diagnosis of VAP. QDEA has been proposed as a less invasive and less expensive means of obtaining a specimen for culture in a ventilated patient. The investigators found that most patients with pneumonia by BAL would have been diagnosed by QDEA; however, those patients with a positive QDEA and a negative BAL would have received needless antibiotic administration 31% of the time. In this setting, a diagnosis made by BAL seems most appropriate to avoid the unnecessary use of broad-spectrum agents.

D. W. Mozingo, MD

Invasive Approaches to the Diagnosis of Ventilator-Associated Pneumonia: A Meta-analysis

Shorr AF, Sherner JH, Jackson WL, et al (Walter Reed Army Med Ctr, Washington, DC; Washington Univ, St Louis)

Crit Care Med 33:46-53, 2005 4–7

Objective.—Ventilator-associated pneumonia remains a major challenge in the intensive care unit. The role for invasive diagnostic methods (e.g., bronchoscopy) remains unclear. We hypothesized that invasive testing would alter antibiotic management in patients with ventilator-associated pneumonia but would not necessarily alter mortality.

Design.—Meta-analysis of randomized, controlled trials of invasive diagnostic strategies in suspected ventilator-associated pneumonia and a separate pooled analysis of prospective, observational studies of the effect of invasive cultures on antibiotic utilization in ventilator-associated pneumonia.

Setting.—NA.

Patients.—Subjects enrolled in the various clinical trials identified.

Interventions.—None.

Measurements and Main Results.—We identified four randomized, controlled trials that included 628 patients. The overall quality of these studies was moderate (median Jadad score of 5) and there was both clinical and statistical heterogeneity among these trials. Ventilator-associated pneumonia was confirmed bronchoscopically in 44-69% of participants, with *Pseudomonas aeruginosa* and *Staphylococcus aureus* being the most frequently isolated pathogens. Most subjects (90.3%) received adequate antibiotics; however, in one trial there was a significant difference between the invasive and noninvasive arms with respect to this factor. Overall, an invasive approach did not alter mortality (odds ratio 0.89, 95% confidence interval 0.56-1.41). Invasive testing, though, affected antibiotic utilization (odds ratio for change in antibiotic management after invasive sampling, 2.85, 95% confidence interval 1.45-5.59). Five prospective observational studies examined invasive testing and included 635 subjects. These reports confirm that invasive sampling leads to modifications in the antibiotic regimen in more than half of patients (pooled estimate for rate of alteration in antibiotic prescription, 50.3%, 95% confidence interval 35.9-64.6%).

Conclusions.—Few trials have systematically examined the impact of diagnostic techniques on outcomes for patients suspected of suffering from ventilator-associated pneumonia. Invasive strategies do not alter mortality. Invasive approaches to ventilator-associated pneumonia affect antibiotic use and prescribing.

▶ This article was chosen because it reviews multiple trials regarding the diagnostic methodology for ventilator-associated pneumonia. Despite being a common and expensive nosocomial infection in the ICU, controversy exists about both the attributable mortality of this disease and appropriate management strategies. Four randomized controlled trials that included 628 patients are identified as well as 5 prospective observational studies examining invasive testing of 635 subjects. Analysis of these reports demonstrates that there is no mortality difference related to the diagnostic techniques; however, invasive approaches to ventilator-associated pneumonia affect antibiotic use and prescribing. It is important that physicians adopt procedures and protocols that help to ensure that patients with ventilator-associated pneumonia receive initially appropriate antibiotic therapy. The use of bronchoscopy does not represent a tool for increasing the rate of initially appropriate antibiotic selection; however, its use represents one option for attempting to balance the competing pressures to initiate therapy with broad-spectrum agents against the imperative to diminish antibiotic overuse.

D. W. Mozingo, MD

Intensive Insulin Treatment in Critically Ill Trauma Patients Normalizes Glucose by Reducing Endogenous Glucose Production

Thorell A, Rooyackers O, Myrenfors P, et al (Karolinska Institutet, Stockholm; Huddinge Univ, Stockholm)

J Clin Endocrinol Metab 89:5382-5386, 2004 4–8

Introduction.—Critical illness is associated with insulin resistance and hyperglycemia. Intensive insulin treatment to normalize blood glucose during feeding has been shown to improve morbidity and mortality in patients in intensive care. The mechanisms behind the glucose-controlling effects of insulin in stress are not well understood.

Six previously healthy, severely traumatized patients (injury severity score > 15) were studied early (24-48 h) after trauma. Endogenous glucose production (EGP) and whole-body glucose disposal (WGD) were measured (6,6-$^2H_2$-glucose) at basal, during total parenteral nutrition (TPN), and during TPN plus insulin to normalize blood glucose (TPN+I). Six matched volunteers served as controls.

At basal and TPN, concentrations of glucose and insulin were higher in patients ($P < 0.05$). During TPN+I, insulin concentrations were 30-fold higher in patients. At basal, WGD and EGP were 30% higher in patients ($P < 0.05$). During TPN, EGP decreased in both groups but less in patients, resulting in 110% higher EGP than controls ($P < 0.05$). Normoglycemia coincided with reduced EGP, resulting in similar rates in both groups. WGD did not change during TPN or TPN+I and was not different between the groups.

In conclusion, in healthy subjects, euglycemia is maintained during TPN at physiological insulin concentrations by a reduction of EGP, whereas WGD is maintained at basal levels. In traumatized patients, hyperglycemia is due to increased EGP. In contrast to controls, normalization of glucose concentration during TPN needs high insulin infusion rates and is accounted for by a reduction in EGP, whereas WGD is not increased.

▶ Insulin resistance is a central feature of stress metabolism in critically ill patients. With insulin resistance, glucose uptake is reduced in peripheral insulin-sensitive tissues, whereas EGP is increased, resulting in hyperglycemia. It has been suggested that this response is a pathophysiologic adaptation to ensure substrate supply to non–insulin-dependent vital tissues such as the brain. An increasing body of evidence strongly suggests that hyperglycemia is harmful by itself, and by controlling this hyperglycemia, major impacts on clinical outcome have been achieved. This study measured EGP and WGD in severely traumatized patients compared with matched volunteers. The investigators showed that hyperglycemia in the basal state is mainly accounted for by an increase in EGP, suggesting the presence of hepatic insulin resistance. In response to the administration of insulin during feeding, normoglycemia is achieved and maintained by suppression of EGP, whereas peripheral glucose uptake is not stimulated despite pharmacologic concentrations of insulin in the plasma. However, the observation that suppression of EGP by insulin is responsible for blood glucose lowering raises the possibility that reduced gluconeogenesis might be a mechanism by which insulin treatment renders positive clinical effects in states of stress.

D. W. Mozingo, MD

Relative Adrenal Insufficiency in Patients With Septic Shock: Comparison of Low-Dose and Conventional Corticotropin Tests

Siraux V, De Backer D, Yalavatti G, et al (Erasme Univ, Brussels, Belgium)

Crit Care Med 33:2479-2486, 2005 4–9

Objective.—To compare a low-dose (1 µg) corticotropin stimulation test with the more standard (250 µg) test for the diagnosis of relative adrenal insufficiency.

Design.—Diagnostic study.

Setting.—Thirty-one-bed mixed medico-surgical department of intensive care.

Patients.—Forty-six consecutive patients with septic shock.

Interventions.—Corticotropin stimulation tests (low-dose test, 1 µg, and standard 250-µg test), performed consecutively at an interval >4 hrs.

Measurements and Main Results.—In each test, serum cortisol levels were measured before (T0) and 30 (T30), 60 (T60), and 90 (T90) mins after corticotropin injection. The maximal increase in cortisol (Δmax) was calculated as the difference between T0 and the highest cortisol value at T30, T60, or T90 and considered as adequate if >9 µg/dL (250 nmol/L). Nonresponders to the low-dose test had a lower survival rate than responders to both tests (27 vs. 47%, $p = .06$; Kaplan Meier curves). Interestingly, nonresponders to high-dose test received hydrocortisone treatment and had a similar survival to responders. Multivariable logistic regression disclosed that the response to the combined low-dose test and high-dose test was an independent predictor of survival (odds ratio 28.91, 95% confidence interval 1.81-462.70, $p = .017$), whereas basal or maximal cortisol levels in both tests were not.

Conclusions.—The low-dose test identified a subgroup of patients in septic shock with inadequate adrenal reserve who had a worse outcome and would have been missed by the high-dose test. These patients may also benefit from glucocorticoid replacement therapy.

▶ Endogenous plasma cortisol concentrations are usually normal or increased in patients with sepsis as a protective response to stress. There is much controversy regarding the levels of cortisol that are considered adequate in septic shock. Very low levels have been associated with a higher mortality rate. The use of adrenocorticoid stimulation tests in patients with septic shock also remains controversial in the absence of a standarized definition of a normal adrenal response in the critically ill. In this study, the investigators compared the low-dose and conventional-dose corticotropin tests. They concluded that the low-dose test identified a subgroup of patients in septic shock with inadequate adrenal reserve and worse outcome. This group would have been missed by the high-dose test alone. Nonresponders to the low-dose test had a lower survival rate than responders to both tests. Further studies will need to be performed to determine whether the patients identified as nonresponders by the low-dose test also benefit from corticosteroid replacement.

D. W. Mozingo, MD

Number Needed to Treat and Cost of Recombinant Human Erythropoietin to Avoid One Transfusion-Related Adverse Event in Critically Ill Patients

Shermock KM, Horn E, Lipsett PA, et al (Johns Hopkins Univ, Baltimore, Md)
Crit Care Med 33:497-503, 2005 4–10

Objective.—To calculate the absolute risk reduction of transfusion-related adverse events, the number of patients needed to treat, and cost to avoid one transfusion-related adverse event by using erythropoietin in critically ill patients.

Design.—Number needed to treat with sensitivity analysis.

Setting.—Teaching hospital.

Patients.—Hypothetical cohort of critically ill patients who were candidates to receive erythropoietin.

Interventions.—Using vs. not using erythropoietin to reduce the need for packed red blood cell transfusions.

Measurements and Main Results.—We used published estimates of known transfusion risks: transfusion-related acute lung injury, transfusion-related errors, hepatitis B and C, human immunodeficiency virus, human T-cell lymphotropic virus, and bacterial contamination, stratified by severity. Based on the estimated risk and frequency of transfusions with and without erythropoietin, we calculated the absolute risk reduction of transfusion-related adverse events, the number needed to treat, and cost to avoid one transfusion-related adverse event by using erythropoietin. The estimated incidence of transfusion-related adverse event was 318 per million units transfused for all transfusion-related adverse events, 58 per million for serious transfusion-related adverse events, and 21 per million for likely fatal transfusion-related adverse events. The routine use of erythropoietin resulted in an absolute risk reduction of 191 per million for all transfusion-related adverse events, 35 per million for serious transfusion-related adverse events, and 12 per million for likely fatal transfusion-related adverse events. The number needed to treat was 5,246 to avoid one transfusion-related adverse event, 28,785 to avoid a serious transfusion-related adverse event, and 81,000 for a likely fatal transfusion-related adverse event. The total cost was $4,700,000 to avoid one transfusion-related adverse event, $25,600,000 to avoid one serious transfusion-related adverse event, and $71,800,000 to avoid a likely fatal transfusion-related adverse event. The magnitude of these results withstood extensive sensitivity analysis.

Conclusions.—From the perspective of avoidance of adverse events, erythropoietin does not appear to be an efficient use of limited resources for routine use in critically ill patients.

▶ The use of recombinant human erythropoietin has been shown to decrease the need for a blood transfusion in critically ill patients; however, the reductions were modest at best, with 3 transfusions in the placebo group compared with 2.4 in the group receiving recombinant human erythropoietin. Adverse events related to blood transfusions are rare, and with the advent of better screening techniques, the incidence of transfusion-related infections has been greatly reduced in the past decade. The investigators in this study sought to determine the number of patients and cost of recombinant human erythropoietin with respect to avoiding transfusion-related adverse events. They used published estimates of known transfusion risks including transfusion-related acute lung injury, transfusion-related clerical errors, viral infections, and bacterial contamination. The risk estimate was applied to a hypothetical ICU population. Based on the previously published response to erythropoietin, they calculated the number needed to treat was 5,246 to avoid 1 transfusion-related adverse event, and over 28,000 to avoid a serious transfusion-related adverse event. From the perspective of this approach, erythropoietin does not appear to be an efficient use of limited resources for routine use in the critically ill. Other confounding factors, namely that of blood transfusion–related immunosuppression and increased risk of infection, were not considered in this study.

D. W. Mozingo, MD

Recombinant Factor VIIa for the Treatment of Severe Postoperative and Traumatic Hemorrhage

Khan AZ, Parry JM, Crowley WF, et al (Michigan State Univ, Grand Rapids; Spectrum Health, Grand Rapids, Mich)

Am J Surg 189:331-334, 2005 4–11

Background.—The aim of this study was to determine the dose of recombinant factor VIIa (rFVIIa) that has been used in our institution to successfully control hemorrhage in trauma and postoperative patients.

Methods.—This was an 8-month retrospective cohort study of 13 patients with acute hemorrhage and no known history of coagulopathic disorders.

Results.—Administration of factor VIIa resulted in the cessation of life-threatening hemorrhage at dosages approximately one half those recommended for the management of hemophilia. After administration, there was a significant decrease in the total blood-product transfusion requirement ($P < 0.05$).

Conclusions.—The use of factor VIIa in patients with life-threatening hemorrhage is a safe and effective therapeutic modality when used as an adjunct to standard interventions for control of severe hemorrhage. Lower-dose regimens were as successful as higher-dose regimens previously reported. The results of this respective study of 13 patients suggests that recombinant factor VIIa therapy for control of life-threatening hemorrhage as an adjunct to standard interventions can be successful at doses <90 mg/kg.

▶ Trauma patients with uncontrolled bleeding and coagulopathy have high mortality rates, with most early deaths attributable to uncontrolled hemorrhage. The authors of this selection reviewed an 8-month retrospective cohort of 13 patients with acute hemorrhage who received rFVIIa. They determined that the dose required to curtail the life-threatening hemorrhage was approximately one half of that recommended for the management of hemophilia. After administration they noted a significant decrease in the total blood product transfusion requirement. The off-label use of this medication should be considered in the control of nonsurgical bleeding. Evaluation of the optimal dosage and patient selection will await randomized clinical trials.

D. W. Mozingo, MD

Incidence and Prognosis of Intraabdominal Hypertension in a Mixed Population of Critically Ill Patients: A Multiple-Center Epidemiological Study

Malbrain MLNG, Chiumello D, Pelosi P, et al (Ziekenhuis Netwerk Antwerpen, Belgium; Univ of Milan, Italy; Univ of Insubria, Varese, Italy; et al)

Crit Care Med 33:315-322, 2005 4–12

Objective.—Intraabdominal hypertension is associated with significant morbidity and mortality in surgical and trauma patients. The aim of this study was to assess, in a mixed population of critically ill patients, whether intraabdominal pressure at admission was an independent predictor for mortality and to evaluate the effects of intraabdominal hypertension on organ functions.

Design.—Multiple-center, prospective epidemiologic study.

Setting.—Fourteen intensive care units in six countries.

Patients.—A total of 265 consecutive patients admitted for >24 hrs during the 4-wk study period.

Interventions.—None.

Measurements and Main Results.—Intraabdominal pressure was measured twice daily via the bladder. Data recorded on admission were the patient demographics with Simplified Acute Physiology Score II, Acute Physiology and Chronic Health Evaluation II score, and type of admission; during intensive care stay, Sepsis-Related Organ Failure Assessment score and intraabdominal pressure were measured daily together with fluid balance. Nonsurvivors had a significantly higher mean intraabdominal pressure on admission than survivors: 11.4 ± 4.8 vs. 9.5 ± 4.8 mm Hg. Independent predictors for mortality were age (odds ratio, 1.04; 95% confidence interval, 1.01-1.06; $p = .003$), Acute Physiology and Chronic Health Evaluation II score (odds ratio, 1.1; 95% confidence interval, 1.05-1.15; $p < .0001$), type of intensive care unit admission (odds ratio, 2.5 medical vs. surgical; 95% confidence interval, 1.24-5.16; $p = .01$), and the presence of liver dysfunction (odds ratio, 2.5; 95% confidence interval, 1.06-5.8; $p = .04$). The occurrence of intraabdominal hypertension during the intensive care unit stay was also an independent predictor of mortality (relative risk, 1.85; 95% confidence interval, 1.12-3.06; $p = .01$). Patients with intraabdominal hypertension at admission had significantly higher Sepsis-Related Organ Failure Assessment scores during the intensive care unit stay than patients without intraabdominal hypertension.

Conclusions.—Intraabdominal hypertension on admission was associated with severe organ dysfunction during the intensive care unit stay. The mean intraabdominal pressure on admission was not an independent risk factor for mortality; however, the occurrence of intraabdominal hypertension during the intensive care unit stay was an independent outcome predictor.

▶ Intra-abdominal hypertension has been associated with increased morbidity and mortality in surgical and trauma patients. Increased intra-abdominal pressure can induce moderate to severe organ failure, mainly through a direct mechanical effect, and if untreated, mortality is increased. Sustained increases in pressure above 20 mm Hg negatively affect respiratory, cardiovascular, splanchnic, neurologic, and renal function. This study followed up 265 consecutive patients admitted for greater than 24 hours during the 4-week study. Fourteen ICUs contributed to data collection. The investigators found that intra-abdominal hypertension on admission was associated with severe organ dysfunction during the remainder of the ICU stay. The occurrence of intra-abdominal hypertension during the ICU stay was also an independent predictor of mortality. A major difference in this study compared with previous reports is that the investigators considered a threshold of 12 mm Hg as a definition of intra-abdominal hypertension. Although this study does not prove whether an increase of intra-abdominal pressure is directly or indirectly related to mortality, the presence of intra-abdominal hypertension should be considered in the setting of renal or hepatic failure in patients with multiple organ failure.

D. W. Mozingo, MD

Rhabdomyolysis and Secondary Renal Failure in Critically Ill Surgical Patients

Sharp LS, Rozycki GS, Feliciano DV (Emory Univ, Atlanta, Ga)

Am J Surg 188:801-806, 2004 4–13

Background.—Rhabdomyolysis accounts for up to 28% of the causes of posttraumatic acute renal failure requiring dialysis. Clinically significant rhabdomyolysis is poorly characterized biochemically and difficult to diagnose.

Methods.—A retrospective review of all surgical, trauma, burn, and pediatric surgical patients admitted to Grady Memorial Hospital in Atlanta, GA, from January 1995, through April 2002 was performed. Patients were screened for serum creatinine, base deficit, serum creatine kinase (CK) ≥1,000, presence of myoglobinuria, or if they had a clinical diagnosis of rhabdomyolysis by an attending surgeon.

Results.—The sequential addition of admission laboratory values for serum creatinine ≥1.5 mg/dL (positive predictive value [PPV] = 33%), base deficit ≤−4 (PPV = 52%), serum CK level ≥5,000 U/L (PPV = 80%), and myoglobinuria increases the ability to predict which patients will develop dialysis-requiring acute renal failure after an episode of rhabdomyolysis. Patients with maximum CK ≥5,000 are also at increased risk for persistent renal insufficiency (Cr ≥2.0 mg/dL).

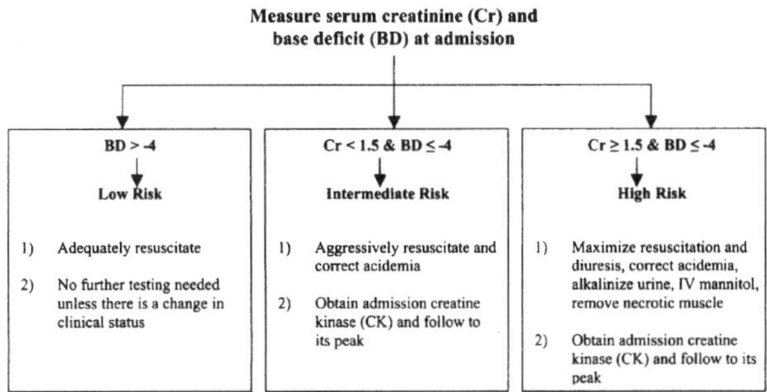

FIGURE 1.—Algorithm for managing surgical/trauma patients at risk of developing acute renal failure (ARF) after rhabdomyolysis. (Courtesy of Sharp LS, Rozycki GS, Feliciano DV: Rhabdomyolysis and secondary renal failure in critically ill surgical patients. *Am J Surg* 188:801-806, 2004. Copyright 2004, with permission from Excerpta Medica Inc.)

Conclusions.—An algorithm for testing at-risk surgical patients was developed and may aid in the early diagnosis of clinically significant rhabdomyolysis (Fig 1).

► Patients at risk of developing rhabdomyolysis include those with multisystem trauma, especially with extremity fractures and vascular injuries, with acute vascular occlusion, and with crush injuries. Patients with significant electrical burns and with deep, circumferential thermal burns are also at risk. The authors of this selection reviewed their experience at a trauma and burn center where patients were screened for serum Cr, base deficit, serum CK, and for the presence of myoglobinuria. A useful clinical algorithm was developed including testing on admission and again at 18 to 24 hours after admission. The initial laboratory results can guide the physician as to the need to measure serum CK. Patients with a serum Cr of 1.5 mg/dL or greater and a base deficit of −4 or less would be considered in the high-risk group. Evaluation of the authors' treatment algorithm in a prospective manner would help validate their recommendations.

D. W. Mozingo, MD

Fluconazole Prophylaxis in Critically Ill Surgical Patients: A Meta-analysis

Shorr AF, Chung K, Jackson WL, et al (Washington Hosp Ctr, Potomac, Md; Walter Reed Army Med Ctr, Washington, DC; Washington Univ, St Louis)
Crit Care Med 33:1928-1935, 2005 4–14

Objective.—To evaluate the impact of fluconazole prophylaxis on the incidence of fungal infections and on mortality among critically ill surgical patients.

Design.—Meta-analysis of randomized, placebo-controlled trials of fluconazole prophylaxis.

Patients.—Subjects participating in the clinical trials in this area.

Measurements and Main Results.—We identified four randomized studies comparing fluconazole to placebo for prevention of fungal infections in the surgical intensive care unit (SICU). The studies enrolled 626 patients and used differing dosing regimens of fluconazole. All trials were double-blind and two were multicenter studies. Fluconazole administration significantly reduced the incidence of fungal infections (pooled odds ratio, 0.44; 95% confidence interval, 0.27-0.72; $p < .001$). However, fluconazole prophylaxis was not associated with a survival advantage (pooled OR for mortality, 0.87; 95% confidence interval, 0.59-1.28; p = NS). Fluconazole did not statistically alter the rate of candidemia, as this was low across the studies and developed in only 2.2% of all participants. Performing a sensitivity analysis and including two additional studies that indirectly examined fluconazole prophylaxis in the critically ill did not change our observations. Data from the reports reviewed were insufficient to allow comment on the impact of fluconazole prophylaxis on resource utilization, the distribution of nonalbicans species of *Candida*, and the emergence of antifungal resistance. Generally, fluconazole appeared to be safe for SICU patients.

Conclusions.—Prophylactic fluconazole administration for prevention of mycoses in SICU patients appears to successfully decrease the rate of these infections, but this strategy does not improve survival. The absence of a survival advantage may reflect the few studies in this area and the possibility that this issue has not been adequately studied. Because of the potential for both resistance and emergence of nonalbicans isolates, clinicians must consider these issues when evaluating fluconazole prophylaxis in the SICU. Future trials should focus on more precisely identifying patients at high risk for fungal infections and on determining if broader use of fluconazole alters the distribution of candidal species seen in the SICU and impacts measures of resource utilization such as length of stay and duration of mechanical ventilation.

► Candidal isolates account for a rising proportion of nosocomial bloodstream infections and are a common cause of catheter-related infection. The incidence of these infections has increased during the past 20 years, and they represent a particular problem in surgical patients. Mortality is increased in SICU patients with candidemia, though attributing the increase in mortality to this infection remains controversial. This meta-analysis evaluated 4 randomized studies that compared fluconazole prophylaxis with placebo for fungal infections in SICUs. The authors were able to conclude that fluconazole administration successfully decreased the rates of candidal infections, but no effect on survival was identified. Further research should be directed at identifying a high-risk patient population using end points of mortality and hospital stay before adopting the routine use of fluconazole prophylaxis in surgical patients.

D. W. Mozingo, MD

Systemic Coagulation Changes Caused by Pulmonary Artery Catheters: Laboratory Findings and Clinical Correlation

King DR, Cohn SM, Feinstein AJ, et al (Univ of Miami, Fla)

J Trauma 59:853-859, 2005 4–15

Background.—A higher rate of pulmonary embolism has been associated with pulmonary artery (PA) catheters; however, no mechanism has been described. Conventional tests of coagulation reveal no changes related to PA catheterization. The purpose of this study was to determine whether PA catheterization resulted in a hypercoagulable state detectable by thrombelastography (TEG).

Methods.—*Animal:* Healthy, anesthetized swine (n = 19) underwent PA catheterization. Samples were drawn from 7F femoral arterial catheters before and two hours after PA catheterization, at 5 mL/min, and analyzed (native whole blood, n = 15, kaolin activated blood, n = 4) by TEG (Hemoscope, Niles, IL) at precisely two minutes. *Human:* An IRB-approved prospective, observational trial was conducted in critically ill patients (n =

19). Samples were drawn from 22-gauge radial artery catheters, before and three hours after PA catheterization. Kaolin-activated TEG samples were analyzed at precisely five minutes. Data are mean ± SE; Groups were compared with analysis of variance and significance was assessed at the 95% confidence interval.

Results.—In both animals and patients, PA catheterization truncated R times (time to initial fibrin formation). In swine, the R times were 17.6 ± 1.3 minutes (native) and 3.8 ± 0.4 (kaolin) before PA catheterization, and decreased to 6.3 ± 1.0 minutes ($p = 0.002$) and 1.9 ± 0.5 minutes ($p = 0.010$) afterward. There were no changes in pH or temperature during the experiment. In patients, 4 of 19 were excluded for protocol violations. The R time was 6.3 ± 1.0 minutes (kaolin) before and 3.0 ± 0.3 minutes after catheterization ($p = 0.003$). No changes were observed in conventional coagulation parameters, temperature or pH.

Conclusion.—In healthy swine, and critically ill patients, PA catheters may enhance thrombin formation and fibrin polymerization, indicating a systemic hypercoagulable state. This may explain why PA catheters are associated with an increased risk of pulmonary emboli.

► The use of PA catheters in the management of critically ill patients has been repeatedly questioned and remains controversial. The use of PA catheters has been associated with a higher rate of embolic events, although the mechanism for this complication is unclear. In this selection, the investigators studied, both in animals and patients, the effect of PA catheterization on coagulation parameters as detected by TEG. In both animals and patients, PA catheterization decreased the time to initial fibrin formation. This suggests that the catheter's contact with the circulation may in itself induce a relative hypercoagulable state. This, in part, may explain the association of PA catheters with an increased risk of pulmonary embolism.

D. W. Mozingo, MD

5 Transplantation

Introduction

The number of people awaiting organ transplantation continues to increase more rapidly than the number of transplants performed. At the end of 2005, more than 90,000 people were awaiting organ transplants in the United States. However, only 17,757 people received organs from deceased donors, and 5,763 living donations occurred (UNOS database). The continuing disparity between supply and societal need has been a major focus for the transplant community, interest groups, and regulatory agencies. The waitlist represents "hard" numbers, but there remains uncertainty regarding the penetrance of transplantation therapy for the management of people with endstage organ failure. Kidney transplantation is the one form of therapy where information about potential numbers of recipients is obtainable. 2003 USRDS data note almost 325,000 people on dialysis in the United States, of whom only 65,000 were awaiting kidney transplantation. Abstract 5–1 discusses the heterogeneity in transplant rates as a function of patient autonomy. It suggests that the more people are "empowered" with deciding the type of impending renal support therapy, the greater the percentage of patients choosing renal transplantation will be. Even in the most "mature" existing transplant field, kidney transplantation, the penetration of the transplantation therapy "benefit" may not yet be optimized for the targeted service population. How transplantation will eventually fit into the overall healthcare commerce remains to be determined.

However, a substantial disparity exists between need and availability which has taken on significant proportions and has led to the use of organs from donors that previously would have not been used because they were thought not to be "adequate" for transplantation. In the United States, to acknowledge the variability in the quality of organs from deceased donors, organs are stratified as coming from 3 groups: standard criteria donor, expanded criteria donor, and donation after cardiac death. The standard criteria donor is a brain-dead, younger individual commonly thought of as the "typical" organ donor. The expanded criteria donor has been defined upon the suitability of recovered organs for kidney transplantation (donor>60 yrs or donor 50-59 with at least 2 of terminal creatinine > 1.5 mg/dL, history of hypertension or death by cerebrovascular accident). The recovering of organs after cardiac death occurs after a decision has been made to withdraw life-sustaining therapy for a person not meeting the criteria for brain death. Although such organs suffer from warm ischemia and hypoperfusion injury, they represent a significant source of transplantable organs that would otherwise be totally lost. A myriad of issues surround the ethical identification and management of this sort of donor and the subsequent use of the organs. Some of the major issues were addressed at a national conference, and a summary of the report is found in Abstract 5–2.

Organs procured from these 3 groups would not be expected to have identical short- and long-term outcomes, leading to quite a heterogeneous national allocation and acceptance of such organs for specific patients. Abstract 5–3 describes the beneficial effect of a modification of the current kidney allocation system to one based on waiting time alone in order to match extended criteria kidneys with patients that transplant centers have listed as appropriate candidates for such kidneys. Abstract 5–4 is a report about kidney outcomes from non–heart-beating donors (donation after cardiac death). Early graft failure was more frequent in recipients of this type of organ, especially in those instances with protracted warm ischemia times, although long-term function appears to be quite satisfactory. The long-term organ function from either the older donor with comorbid conditions or the donor with morbidities that lead to withdrawal of life support and death after cessation of cardiac activity is quite heterogeneous. The future will require an increased standardization of allocation policy for organs to specific individual recipients based upon accurate prediction of function of an organ and recipient acceptance of that potential function. In addition, the function of the extrarenal organs from these donors can be quite heterogeneous, and simple allocation guidelines are not readily apparent. Assignment of these organs to specific individuals on the waiting list raises a host of policy issues pertaining to the fundamental principles regarding which recipient is given which organ. Whether the current US allocation policy (giving organs to the "sickest first") will continue to optimize use and long-term function of these organs remains to be seen.

In the United States, over the past few years, the number of living donors has exceeded the number of deceased donors. Live organ (kidney) donation started with family members and remained the cornerstone of organ donation until recently. However, biologically unrelated donors have become increasingly common. Abstract 5–5 reports from the UNOS database that kidney graft survival rates from biologically unrelated living donors surpass those from parental kidney donors (and are significantly better than kidneys from deceased donors). This finding is giving impetus to a variety of novel approaches for increasing the numbers of kidney transplants performed using live donors, including Internet outsourcing, soliciting organ donors, and transplant center–sponsored sharing/matching of kidneys from live donors who cannot donate to a specific individual. Abstract 5–6 discusses the preliminary experience using paired kidney donation from a single institution and gives an optimistic assessment about the utility of this technique to gain survival and financial advantage for individuals with endstage renal disease. Subjecting a healthy individual to the risks of major surgery for the sake of removing an organ without providing any medical benefit is a significant endeavor. Because of the international concerns around commerce in human organs and adverse outcomes in donors, the need to standardize the process of live donor care has been recognized as a worldwide issue. Abstract 5–7 is from a consensus statement from a conference in Amsterdam with representatives from more than 40 countries performing living donor kidney transplants. The statement delineates 6 elements that the international transplant community feels should be included in the care of the live kidney donor. The clinical success of live kidney transplantation has increased the pressures to increase organ availability. The need for more information pertaining to donor outcomes is necessary for the informed consent process. It is unclear the degree of responsibility that will be conferred upon the transplant center, but it will certainly not be lessened. Live donors are used to a lesser extent in the United States for other types of organ transplants, but as needs increase, one can expect increased utilization of live donors for extrarenal transplantation (liver, lung, pancreas, intestine) with associated procedural, legal, and ethical issues.

From a transplant outcomes perspective, the search for good organ function with minimal side effects of immunosuppressive agents remains an acknowledged goal. In 2005, most approaches attempting to maintain excellent long-term graft function with minimal side effects from maintenance immunosuppression focus upon elimination of the responder cell, the T lymphocyte. Abstract 5–8 is a summary of an experience with protracted thymoglobulin or alemtuzumab (anti-CD52 mAb, Campath 1-H) in which most kidney transplant recipients were able to decrease maintenance immunosuppression to single agents given in a spaced manner. Although a predictive algorithm for weaning of immunosuppression was not able to be precisely defined, the promise of steroid-free and exceedingly low-dose immunosuppression was realized in more than half the patients. However, other approaches strive to modify the host immune response to the donor before transplantation. Many years ago, routine use of blood transfusions was employed to decrease the risk of kidney loss from rejection. The notion of pretransplant manipulation of the donor is still an attractive approach to dealing with minimization of immunosuppression. In Abstract 5–9, a primate kidney transplant model was used to show that rejection could be prevented by adoptive transfer of ex vivo created anergic allospecific T cells. The prospect of generating immunologic acceptance of a specific transplanted organ while maintaining immunocompetence towards other nonself antigens (such as infectious agents and cancers) continues to be one of the major goals of transplantation biology.

However, there is still much that is unknown within the transplant field, and before routine clinical use of these techniques is used, the scope of our models will have to be expanded to account for observations that do not fit our current models of alloimmunity. One such observation is discussed in Abstract 5–10. The existence of circulating antibodies towards HLA antigens has long been known to increase the risk for graft loss in transplant recipients. It has been thought that through "perfect" matching of histocompatibility antigens, we would be able to circumvent the risk for increased risk of rejection. However, the experience from the European Collaborative Transplant Study analyzing results from HLA-identical sibling transplants found that the presence of pre-existing alloantibodies in the recipient led to an increased risk of late graft loss of the HLA-identical kidney. In transplantation, a renewed interest in the innate (pattern recognition) arm of the immune response is beginning to resurface. Although innate immunity is often thought to relate primarily to infectious diseases and oncology, Abstract 5–11 reports that blockade of the chemokine receptor, CXCR6, on NK cells resulted in accelerated rejection of a graft in a mouse tolerance model. While clinical transplantation has become routinely successful, the many arms of human immune responses complicate finding the "perfect" balance between exogenous immunosuppressive drugs and inducing an immune unresponsive state to the transplanted organ.

The clinical success of organ transplantation has affected the manner in which the medical community approaches endstage organ disease. Each of the major organs that are clinically transplanted continues to impact the way the medical community addresses problems. In kidney transplantation, while much attention has been placed upon transplanting people with preexisting immunity against antigens on a specific kidney, an increasing interest is in long-term associated health issues. Abstract 5–12 presents the outcomes in kidney recipients with chronic HBV and HCV at the time of kidney transplantation. Although long-term, 12-year survival was good, liver disease was the most common cause of death in the HBV+ patients. With the advent of extensive antiviral therapies, it is important to have baseline comparative outcomes to determine best strategies in treating these individuals. Abstract 5–13 discusses the site of squamous cell carcinomas in Swedish transplant recipients. Gender and age differences were found, suggesting that the level of sun exposure played a significant role in the generation of the condition. Again, with the availability of potential therapies, it is important to have long-term outcomes in the kidney population. Selection of potential transplant recipients and management strategies for transplant patients will continue to have to account for underlying co-morbidities, whether infectious, atherosclerosis, endocrine, oncologic, etc. Understanding the effect of immunosuppression upon predisposition for disease progression is important for optimal patient outcomes. In the liver transplantation field, aside from problems associated with viral hepatitis infection of the transplanted liver, one of the most vexing issues is the evolving role that transplantation plays in the management of hepatocellular carcinoma. Although there is a remarkable survival benefit after transplantation accrued to individuals with small cancers, the optimal role of liver transplantation compared with conventional resectional or other ablation therapies and local or systemic chemotherapy/irradiation in the short- and long-term management of hepatocellular carcinoma continues to be explored (Abstract 5–14). The limited number of livers for transplantation available to manage diseases with such variable benefit continues expansion of the HCCa indication for liver transplantation—a major policy issue. Lung transplantation has moved from being a novelty in the management of chronic pulmonary diseases to a normative therapy. Abstract 13–23 in Chapter 13 summarizes a 15-year experience and the management and selection strategies in a single large center. This paper discusses evolutionary changes to the problems of primary graft dysfunction/failure, airway complications, and the immunosuppressive management strategies that have evolved over the past 15 years. Technology evolution greatly impacts upon the indications for transplantation. Indications to transplant the heart have been dramatically impacted by the development of ventricular assist devices (VADs). While in the United States, patients with such devices are given priority for the receipt of a donor heart, an analysis of the literature (Abstract 5–15) for the British National Health Service concluded that VADs are not cost-effective as a bridge to transplantation, and their role as long-term chronic support remains to be assessed. Many interesting public policy issues are raised regarding the number of suitable hearts available for transplantation compared with the clinical needs, the evolution and cost of the VADs and the need for the development of a healthcare infrastructure as a prerequisite to provide optimal therapy for the individual with endstage heart failure. Type 1 diabetes mellitus is often treated with whole-organ pancreas transplantation, either simultaneously at the time of kidney transplantation, after a prior kidney transplant, or sometimes as a pancreas alone. Islet cell transplantation has demonstrated many advances over the past several years and is often touted as a potentially superior form of therapy due to the supposition that cellular transplantation is superior and has less morbidity and mortality than pancreas transplantation. Although this contention is probably true, cellular transplantation is not without its pitfalls. Abstract 5–16 describes complications in 26 islet recipients. Although there were no deaths, no CMV disease, no graft-vs-host disease, and no posttransplant lymphoma, there were significant requirements for treatment of neutropenia, hyperlipidemia, and even the need to withdraw immunosuppression therapy. Most patients manifested some variation of transient elevation of liver enzymes, most in association with portal infusion of the islets. Given enough numbers, it should be expected that there will be a consistent and predictable mortality associated with islet transplantation. A major goal will be to improve the quality and quantity of the islets available for transplantation through ex vivo manipulation. Abstract 5–17 describes how human islets (with acinar tissue) cultured with epidermal growth factor and gastrin increased the β-cell numbers after culture. It is possible that the efficacy of cellular transplantation may significantly improve with an increased understanding of culture techniques and environmental conditions. An ultimate goal would be to go through ex vivo manipulation to have progenitor cells from an ill individual to differentiate into the needed effector cells or even an organ that would function in the patient without needing immunosuppression. Abstract 5–18 discusses the techniques by which human monocytes can be made into "neohepatocytes" with the prospect of autologous cell therapy.

A discussion of the "solutions" to the supply-demand disparity is incomplete without mentioning the prospect of using animal organs in humans. One of the major hurdles to xenotransplantation continues to be the fear of transmission of one species' chronic infections to the human recipient. Abstract 5–19 reports an experience with pig-to-baboon xenotransplantation and the fact that neither porcine retrovirus nor antibody to retrovirus was detected in the serum of baboons transplanted with porcine organs. However, many readers of this report will be concerned about the short duration of the baboon survival (all groups survived <60 days) and that porcine retrovirus DNA was detected in the PBMC of the baboons.

Enormous strides have been made in the field of organ transplantation. The application of organ replacement therapies can be successfully made for increasing numbers of diseases. However, despite its successes, significant obstacles pertaining to numbers of organs and immunologic barriers persist, which will require new insights and therapies.

Timothy L. Pruett, MD

Association of Patient Autonomy With Increased Transplantation and Survival Among New Dialysis Patients in the United States

Stack AG, Martin DR (Letterkenny Gen Hosp, Ireland; Univ of Texas, Houston)

Am J Kidney Dis 45:730-742, 2005 5–1

Background.—It is unclear whether patients with chronic kidney disease who are more autonomous in medical decision making have better outcomes than those who are not. We examined the contribution of patient autonomy to treatment selection (peritoneal dialysis versus hemodialysis) and subsequent association with transplantation and survival.

Methods.—Data were obtained from the Dialysis Morbidity and Mortality Study Wave 2, a national random sample of 4,025 new dialysis patients enrolled during 1996 and 1997 and followed up until October 31, 2001. Responders were asked to quantify their contribution to treatment selection and were grouped based on perceived degree of participation as patient led, team led, or patient and team led. Groups were compared and subsequent outcomes were evaluated by using Cox regression.

Results.—Six hundred thirty-six patients (26.3%) reported a patient-led decision, 860 patients (35.6%) reported a team-led decision, and 922 patients (38.1%) reported a patient-and-team–led decision in treatment assignment. Unadjusted death rates were significantly lower (127 versus 159 versus 207 deaths/1,000 patient-years at risk; $P < 0.0001$), and transplantation rates were significantly higher (103 versus 88 versus 41 transplantations/1,000 patient-years at risk; $P < 0.0001$) for patients reporting the greatest contribution to modality selection. With adjustment for case mix, mortality risks were lowest (relative risk [RR], 0.84; 95% confidence interval [CI], 0.71 to 0.99) and transplantation rates were highest (RR, 1.44; 95% CI, 1.07 to 1.93) for the patient-led group.

Conclusion.—Although the contribution of patient selection factors cannot be completely ignored, this analysis supports an association of patient autonomy with transplantation and survival. Greater efforts to empower patients with chronic kidney disease during the period before end-stage renal disease may improve clinical outcomes.

▶ The length of the waiting list for kidney transplantation is staggering. It is always assumed that it is a fixed number and that the optimal number of people benefiting from kidney transplantation has been recognized. There are several reasons to doubt this assumption. Several years ago it was demonstrated that patients from not-for-profit dialysis units had better access to transplantation than patients in for-profit dialysis units. The current study comprised a random sample of over 4000 dialysis patients who were enrolled between 1996 and 1997. The individuals were asked to quantify their contribution to treatment selection and were grouped according to their perceived degree of participation. The results demonstrated that 26% thought they had a patient-led decision, 36% thought there was a team-led decision, and 38% reported a joint patient and team decision for treatment assignment. There was a direct correlation with the likelihood of survival at the end of the follow-up period based on the patients' perception of their participation in selecting the treatment modality. There was also a higher correlation with transplantation when the patients were actively involved in the decision-making process.

There are many methodological problems with this study, but it underscores the notion that we have probably not maximized the role of transplantation within the various at-risk populations. The number of patients who would seek transplantation as a mode of therapy can and probably should be increased.

T. L. Pruett, MD

Report of a National Conference on Donation After Cardiac Death

Bernat JL, D'Alessandro AM, Port FK, et al (Dartmouth-Hitchcock Med Ctr; Univ of Virginia; Loma Linda Univ; et al)

Am J Transplant 5:1-11, 2005 5–2

Background.—A national conference on organ donation after cardiac death (DCD) was convened in Philadelphia in 2005. The purpose of this conference was to address the increasing incidence of DCD and to affirm the ethical propriety of transplanting organs from these donors as not violating the dead-donor rule. Among the participants were neuroscientists, critical care professionals, distinguished bioethicists, and others in the medical community. Within this conference, 6 work groups were assembled to address specific DCD issues and fulfill the conference objectives. The conference's views on many of the issues involved in the use of organs obtained from persons after cardiac death were presented in this report.

Overview.—The ethical propriety of DCD as not violating the dead-donor rule was affirmed in this report. In addition, thanks to new developments not previously reported, the conference was able to resolve the controversy surrounding the period of circulatory cessation that determines death and allows administration of prerecovery pharmaceuticals. In addition, the report established conditions of DCD eligibility and presented current data regarding the successful transplantation of organs from DCD. A new framework regarding the reporting of ischemic events was proposed, specific recommendations were made regarding the removal of barriers to DCD, and guidelines were presented regarding organ allocation and the process of informed consent. In addition, an action plan was set to address media issues. In the setting of a consensual decision by the attending physician and patient or family member or surrogate to withdraw life support, a routine opportunity for DCD should be available to honor the deceased donor's wishes in every donor service area in the United States.

Conclusions.—A national conference on organ donation after cardiac death has affirmed DCD as an ethically acceptable practice of end-of-life care. DCD has the potential to increase the number of deceased-donor organs available for transplantation.

▶ The increasing gap between the number of people awaiting transplantation and the available organs has been quite discouraging. The need to increase the number of available organs for transplantation has recently resulted in a reexamination of the use of organs obtained from individuals after cardiac death. This article addresses many of the issues surrounding the routine utilization of the donor who has sustained cardiac death. Issues regarding definition of death assessment of medical criteria to predict candidacy for donation after cardiac death, trying to find protocols to optimize successful transplantation with organs retrieved from such donors, and other issues are all addressed within this article. The difficulty associated with expansion to these types of donors are real, and the article addresses many of the potential problems.

T. L. Pruett, MD

Impact of the Expanded Criteria Donor Allocation System on the Use of Expanded Criteria Donor Kidneys

Sung RS, Guidinger MK, Lake CD, et al (Univ of Michigan, Ann Arbor; Univ Renal Research and Education Assoc, Ann Arbor, Mich; United Network for Organ Sharing, Richmond, Va; et al)

Transplantation 79:1257-1261, 2005 5–3

Background.—The U.S. Organ Procurement and Transplantation Network recently implemented a policy allocating expanded criteria donor (ECD) kidneys by waiting time alone. ECD kidneys were defined as having a risk of graft failure ≥1.7 times that of ideal donors. ECDs include any donor ≥60 years old and donors 50 to 59 years old with at least two of the following: terminal creatinine >1.5 mg/dL, history of hypertension, or death by cerebrovascular accident. The impact of this policy on use of ECD kidneys is assessed.

Methods.—The authors compared use of ECD kidneys recovered in the 18 months immediately before and after policy implementation. Differences were tested using *t* test and χ^2 analyses.

Results.—There was an 18.3% increase in ECD kidney recoveries and a 15.0% increase in ECD kidney transplants in the first 18 months after policy implementation. ECD kidneys made up 22.1% of all recovered kidneys and 16.8% of all transplants, compared with 18.8% (P<0.001) and 14.5% (P<0.001), respectively, in the prior period. The discard rate was unchanged. The median relative risk (RR) for graft failure for transplanted ECD kidneys was 2.07 versus 1.99 in the prepolicy period (P=not significant); the median

RR for procured ECD kidneys was unchanged at 2.16. The percentage of transplanted ECD kidneys with cold ischemia times (CIT) <12 hr increased significantly; the corresponding percentage for CIT ≥24 hr decreased significantly.

Conclusions.—The recent increase in ECD kidney recoveries and transplants appears to be related to implementation of the ECD allocation system.

▶ Part of the issue relating to maximize the potential organs for transplantation has been one in which the donor organ and recipient are well matched. Because kidneys from older donors are often thought not to be suitable for younger recipients, placement has sometimes been awkward. The US allocation system does not intrinsically assume that organs have differential function. It is only through transplant center modification and assignment of given patients to willingness to accept a certain quality of organs that the organs are subsequently used. The current article has demonstrated an increased utilization of organs from ECDs through a simplification process of allocation. In this setting, the individuals who expressed interest in receiving an allocated either, standard or ECD kidney. The ECD kidneys were allocated solely on the basis of waiting time, irrespective of HLA mismatching, to simplify the allocation process. With this format, the number of ECD kidneys recovered increased by 18%, and the number transplanted increased by 15%. There was no significant change in the percentage of discarded organs.

The article highlights many of the issues concerning the use of organs from donors who would traditionally be considered as having organs not worthy of being transplanted. A binary decision for ECD versus standard criteria donor is probably not in the best interest of patients or in the best interest of optimal utilization of organs. Other potential discrimination mechanisms may be useful to better match recipients with a potential function of organs.

T. L. Pruett, MD

Non–Heart-Beating Donor Kidneys in The Netherlands: Allocation and Outcome of Transplantation

Keizer KM, de Fijter JW, Haase-Kromwijk BJJM, et al (Dutch Transplantation Found, Leiden, The Netherlands)

Transplantation 79:1195-1199, 2005 5–4

Background.—Since February 1, 2001, kidneys from both heart-beating (HB) and non–heart-beating (NHB) donors in The Netherlands have been indiscriminately allocated through the standard renal-allocation system.

Methods.—Renal function and allograft-survival rate for kidneys from NHB and HB donors were compared at 3 and 12 months.

Results.—The outcomes of 276 renal transplants, 176 from HB donors and 100 from NHB III donors, allocated through the standard renal allocation system, Eurotransplant Kidney Allocation System, and performed between February 1, 2001 and March 1, 2002 were compared. Three months after transplantation, graft survival was 93.7% for HB kidneys and 85.0% for NHB kidneys ($P<0.05$). At 12 months, graft survival was 92.0% and 83.0%, respectively ($P<0.03$). Serum creatinine levels in the two groups were comparable at both 3 and 12 months. Multivariate analysis identified previous kidney transplantation (relative risk [RR] 3.33; $P<0.005$), donor creatinine (RR 1.01; $P<0.005$), and NHB (RR 2.38; $P<0.05$) as independent risk factors for transplant failure within 12 months. In multivariate analysis of NHB data, a warm ischemia time (WIT) of 30 minutes or longer ($P<0.005$; RR 6.16, 95% confidence interval 2.11-18.00) was associated with early graft failure. No difference in 12-month graft survival was seen between HB and NHB kidneys after excluding the kidneys that failed in the first 3 months.

Conclusion.—Early graft failure was significantly more likely in recipients of kidneys from NHB donors. A prolonged WIT was strongly associated with this failure. Standard allocation procedures do not have a negative effect on outcome, and there is no reason to allocate NHB kidneys differently from HB kidneys.

▶ There has been great enthusiasm for attempting to use organs from NHB donors. Many of the earlier US studies with NHB donors tend to be populated with younger donors rather than with brain-dead organ donors. In this study from The Netherlands, the median age of HB donors was 48 years versus 46 years in NHB donors, significant, again for a younger donor in the NHB donation after cardiac death. Early graft failure was higher with organs procured after cardiac death. The standard allocation procedures, however, did not appear to have a significant long-term negative impact upon outcomes, and the authors have concluded that the standard allocation procedures should be applied to such kidneys. It is still not known whether organs from DCD donors will have long-term function comparable to that of organs from donors who do not undergo the cardiac event. As the age of the donors increases, one would not be totally surprised to see a differential in long-term graft function.

T. L. Pruett, MD

Living-Unrelated Donors Yield Higher Graft Survival Rates Than Parental Donors

Futagawa Y, Waki K, Gjertson DW, et al (Terasaki Found Lab, Los Angeles; Univ of California, Los Angeles)

Transplantation 79:1169-1174, 2005 5–5

Background.—Living-unrelated donors (LURD) have been shown to yield kidney graft survival rates equivalent to that of related donors. Here, we show that in three diseases, LURDs supply grafts that survive at a higher rate than parental or offspring donors.

Methods.—We analyzed 111,643 first adult kidney transplants from the United Network for Organ Sharing database performed between 1991 and

2003 by Kaplan-Meier curves, log-rank tests, and Cox proportional hazard tests.

Results.—Five-year kidney graft survival rates in patients receiving grafts from LURD, parental, and offspring donors were 75.4%, 74.3%, and 75.7% among patients with typical original diseases excluding three diseases. In focal glomerulosclerosis (FGS), the corresponding results were 87.4%, 70.1%, and 81.6%. In polycystic kidney disease (PC) rates were 86.4%, 78.6%, and 85.3%, and in diabetes mellitus (type 1 DM) rates were 75.9%, 69.8%, and 70.5%. Parental donors yielded significantly lower graft survival rates than LURDs in all three diseases. Although statistically significant differences were lost in the Cox tests, functional graft survival showed significantly lower graft survival rates from parental donors compared with LURDs, suggesting that donor age was a significant factor.

Conclusions.—If living donors are considered for kidney transplantation into patients with FGS, PC, or type 1 DM, grafts from LURD are preferred over parental and offspring donors. Although genetic susceptibility of parental and offspring donor grafts may be a factor, the simple donor age factor probably results in lower survival of parental donor grafts. Lower survival of offspring donor grafts may suggest genetic susceptibility because such donors were, in general, younger than in LURD grafts.

▶ The gap between the waitlist and available organs has led to an increasing pressure to use organs from living donors. It has long been thought that the closer the genetic match, the more likely the graft would survive. The advent of the use of LURDs has been met with some concern that function would be different. In the report from the United Network for Organ Sharing database, 5-year survival rates were determined between a variety of living donor and deceased donor kidney transplants. Interestingly, with respect to long-term graft function, LURDs had superior graft survival when compared with parents donating to children. The striking difference in the populations was age, with parental donors being significantly older than either sibling donors or LURDs. This article again stresses the importance of organ quality in determining long-term graft survival. The living donor has, by far, the optimal preservation of organ function with minimal ischemia time and maximal perfusion optimization during retrieval. The fact that there is a discernable difference in graft survival based on age of the donor makes one suspect that the organs from deceased donors will have amplified differential in short- and long-term function based on management and death variance.

T. L. Pruett, MD

Clinical Results From Transplanting Incompatible Live Kidney Donor/ Recipient Pairs Using Kidney Paired Donation

Montgomery RA, Zachary AA, Ratner LE, et al (Johns Hopkins Univ, Baltimore, Md; Columbia Univ, New York)

JAMA 294:1655-1663, 2005 5–6

Context.—First proposed 2 decades ago, live kidney paired donation (KPD) was considered a promising new approach to addressing the shortage of organs for transplantation. Ethical, administrative, and logistical barriers initially proved formidable and prevented the implementation of KPD programs in the United States.

Objective.—To determine the feasibility and effectiveness of KPD for the management of patients with incompatible donors.

Design, Setting, and Patients.—Prospective series of paired donations matched and transplanted from a pool of blood type or crossmatch incompatible donors and recipients with end-stage renal disease (6 conventional and 4 unconventional KPD transplants) at a US tertiary referral center (between June 2001 and November 2004) with expertise in performing transplants in patients with high immunologic risk.

Intervention.—Kidney paired donation and live donor renal transplantation.

Main Outcome Measures.—Patient survival, graft survival, serum creatinine levels, rejection episodes.

Results.—A total of 22 patients received transplants through 10 paired donations including 2 triple exchanges at Johns Hopkins Hospital. At a median follow-up of 13 months (range, 1-42 months), the patient survival rate was 100% and the graft survival rate was 95.5%. Twenty-one of the 22 patients have functioning grafts with a median 6-month serum creatinine level of 1.2 mg/dL (range, 0.8-1.8 mg/dL) (106.1 μmol/L [range, 70.7-159.1 μmol/L]). There were no instances of antibody-mediated rejection despite the inclusion of 5 patients who were highly sensitized to HLA antigens due to previous exposure to foreign tissue. Four patients developed acute cellular rejection (18%).

Conclusions.—This series of patients who received transplants from a single-center KPD pool provides evidence that recipients with incompatible live donors, even those with rare blood type combinations or high degrees of HLA antigen sensitization, can receive transplants through KPD with graft survival rates that appear to be equivalent to directed, compatible live donor transplants. If these results can be generalized, broader availability of KPD to the estimated 6000 patients with incompatible donors could result in a large expansion of the donor pool.

▶ The goal of increasing access of patients to live donors has led to transplanting incompatible live kidney donor/recipient pairs using KPD. There are many reasons to consider KPD, from financial to patient satisfaction–related issues. The initial reports are quite favorable. Difficulties are perceived to arise when procedures are not done at a single institution, such as when adverse events occur and it is not clear as to which center is responsible for aftercare or for the screening of transmissible disease. It has yet to be determined how these more difficult side effect issues will be addressed in the KPD swaps.

T. L. Pruett, MD

The Consensus Statement of the Amsterdam Forum on the Care of the Live Kidney Donor

The Ethics Committee of the Transplantation Society (Montreal)

Transplantation 78:491-492, 2004 5–7

Background.—The International Forum on the Care of the Live Kidney Donor was held in Amsterdam in 2004. More than 100 kidney transplant physicians and surgeons from 40 countries met to develop an international standard of care with a position statement of the Transplantation Society regarding the responsibility of the community for the live kidney donor. The position statement was subsequently adopted by the Council of the Transplantation Society and is presented in this report.

Overview.—The forum expressed the recognition of the international transplant community that the use of kidneys from the living donor must be performed in a manner that will minimize the physical, psychological, and social risk to the individual donor and will not jeopardize the public trust of the health care community. The potential donor must be allowed to make the donation decision in an autonomous manner. The increased need for transplantable kidneys has resulted in consideration of potential donors with conditions that may increase the health risks for the donor and/or recipient. It is recommended that the acceptance of such persons as kidney donors be conducted in an ethical manner, accounting for the autonomy and safety of the donor and with rigorous attention to clinical outcomes. The 6 major tenets of the consensus statement are as follows. First, prior to a live kidney donation to a potential recipient, the donor must receive a complete medical and psychosocial evaluation. Second, prior to donor nephrectomy, the potential donor must be informed of the nature of the evaluation process, the results and potential adverse consequences of testing, the risks of the procedure, the responsibility of the individual and the health and social system in the management of discovered conditions, and expected outcomes of transplant, and the disclosure of recipient specific information. Third, the potential donor should be informed of alternative renal replacement therapies available to the potential recipient. Fourth, the potential donor should be capable of understanding the information presented in the consent process. Fifth, the decision to donate should be voluntary. Sixth, the transplant center has specific postdonation responsibilities, including overseeing postoperative recovery, facilitating long-term follow-up and treatment of the donor, identifying and tracking complications, and working with the general health care community to provide optimal care and surveillance of the donor.

Conclusions.—The international transplant community has come together to present a consensus statement on the responsibilities of the transplant center toward the live kidney donor.

▶ The increased use of organs from live donors and from a variety to different types of donors has led the international transplant community to come to some form of consensus regarding the care of the live kidney donor. A conference was held through the Ethics Committee of the Transplantation Society in an attempt to find international consensus on what the transplant center's responsibility should be toward the live kidney donor with respect to medical and psychosocial evaluation, the amount of information that should be given to the potential donor, alternative therapies that are available to the recipient, and other related issues. The cornerstone of live organ donation is a voluntary decision with the capacity and the ability to withdraw from the donation process at any time.

T. L. Pruett, MD

Kidney Transplantation Under Minimal Immunosuppression After Pretransplant Lymphoid Depletion With Thymoglobulin or Campath
Shapiro R, Basu A, Tan H, et al (Univ of Pittsburgh, Pa)
J Am Coll Surg 200:505-515, 2005 5–8

Background.—Multiple drug immunosuppression has allowed the near elimination of rejection, but without commensurate improvements in longterm graft survival and at the cost of quality of life. We have suggested that transplantation outcomes can be improved by modifying the timing and dosage of immunosuppression to facilitate natural mechanisms of alloengraftment and acquired tolerance.

Study Design.—Two therapeutic principles were applied for kidney transplantation: pretransplant recipient conditioning with antilymphoid antibody preparations (Thymoglobulin [Sangstat] or Campath [ILEX Pharmaceuticals]), and minimal posttransplant immunosuppression with tacrolimus monotherapy including "spaced weaning" of maintenance doses when possible. The results in Thymoglobulin- (n = 101) and Campath-pretreated renal transplantation recipients (n = 90) were compared with those in 152 conventionally immunosuppressed recipients in the immediately preceding era.

Results.—Spaced weaning was attempted in more than 90% of the kidney transplant recipients after pretreatment with both lymphoid-depleting agents, and is currently in effect in two-thirds of the survivors. Although there was a much higher rate of acute rejection in the Thymoglobulin-pretreated recipients than in either the Campath-pretreated or historic control recipients, patient and graft survival in both lymphoid depletion groups is at least equivalent to that of historic control patients. In the Thymoglobulin-conditioned patients for whom followups are now 24 to 40 months, chronic allograft nephropathy (CAN) progressed at the same rate as in historic control patients. Selected patients on weaning developed donor-specific nonreactivity.

Conclusions.—After lymphoid depletion, kidney transplantation can be readily accomplished under minimal immunosuppression with less dependence on late maintenance immunosuppression and a better quality of life. Campath was the more effective agent for pretreatment. Guidelines for spaced weaning need additional refinement.

▶ A continued goal in transplantation is to provide excellent graft function with minimum sequela of chronic immunosuppression. One of the mechanisms to provide such function has been to provide pretransplant lymphoid depletion with subsequent minimal immunosuppression. In this report, the majority of kidney transplant recipients were able to be successfully maintained on immunosuppression administered less than once a day. The authors describe a differential in lymphocyte-depleting products and suggest that anti-CD52 (Campath) is more effective than polyclonal rabbit antithymocyte globulin. Irrespective of what is, in fact, optimal at this time, this article stresses the approach the transplantation community is taking to modulate the immune response at the time of transplantation in an attempt to decrease some of the long-term morbidities associated with chronic drug administration.

T. L. Pruett, MD

Renal Allograft Rejection Is Prevented by Adoptive Transfer of Anergic T Cells in Nonhuman Primates

Bashuda H, Kimikawa M, Seino K, et al (Juntendo Univ, Tokyo; Tokyo Women's Med Univ; Inst of Physical and Chemical Research (RIKEN), Kanagawa, Japan; et al)

J Clin Invest 115:1896-1902, 2005 5–9

Introduction.—Anergic T cells generated ex vivo are reported to have immunosuppressive effects in vitro and in vivo. Here, we tested this concept in nonhuman primates. Alloreactive T cells were rendered anergic ex vivo by coculture with donor alloantigen in the presence of anti-CD80/CD86 mAbs before adoptive transfer via renal allograft to rhesus monkey recipients. The recipients were briefly treated with cyclophosphamide and cyclosporine A during the preparation of the anergic cells. Thirteen days after renal transplantation, the anergic T cells were transferred to the recipient, after which no further immunosuppressive agents were administered. Rejection-free survival was prolonged in all treated recipients, and 3 of 6 animals survived long term (410-880 days at study's end). In the long-surviving recipients, proliferative responses against alloantigen were inhibited in a donor-specific manner, and donor-type, but not third-party, skin allografts were also accepted, which demonstrated that antigen-specific tolerance had been induced. We conclude that anergic T cells generated ex vivo by blocking CD28/B7 costimulation can suppress renal allograft rejection after adoptive transfer in nonhuman primates. This strategy may be applicable to the design of safe clinical trials in humans.

Non-HLA Transplantation Immunity Revealed by Lymphocytotoxic Antibodies

Opelz G, for the Collaborative Transplant Study (Univ of Heidelberg, Germany; et al)
Lancet 365:1570-1576, 2005 5–10

Background.—The presence of panel-reactive antibodies (PRA) against HLA antigens before transplantation is associated with early rejection of kidney grafts from cadaver donors. Transplants from HLA-identical sibling donors do not provide a target for antibodies to HLA antigens and should therefore not be affected by PRA.

Methods.—Data from the Collaborative Transplant Study were used to examine the influence of PRA on graft survival. Uncensored graft survival and death-censored graft survival were calculated, and the data were analysed by multivariate Cox's regression methods.

Findings.—Among recipients of HLA-identical sibling transplants, 3001 patients with no PRA had significantly higher 10-year graft survival (72.4% [SE 1.1]) than 803 patients with 1-50% PRA (63.3% [2.5]; $p=0.0006$) or 244 patients with more than 50% PRA (55.5% [4.0]; $p<0.0001$). The effect of PRA became apparent after the first post-transplant year and was, therefore, strikingly different from the early steep decline in graft survival during the first year associated with PRA in recipients of cadaver kidneys. We could not discern whether graft loss was a direct effect of non-HLA humoral sensitisation or whether PRA served as an indicator of heightened immunity against non-HLA transplantation antigens.

Interpretation.—PRA reactivity is strongly associated with long-term graft loss in kidney transplants from HLA-identical sibling donors.

Relevance to Practice.—Our findings suggest that non-HLA immunity has a much stronger role in clinical transplantation than previously thought. In contrast to immunity against HLA mediated by antibodies present before transplantation, which leads to early acute graft rejection, non-HLA immunity is associated with chronic graft loss. The possibility of identifying recipients at increased risk of late graft loss before transplantation could be used to devise specific immunosuppressive strategies for these patients.

Cutting Edge: Critical Role of CXCL16/CXCR6 in NKT Cell Trafficking in Allograft Tolerance

Jiang X, Shimaoka T, Kojo S, et al (RIKEN Research Ctr for Allergy and Immunology, Kanagawa, Japan; Univ of Tsukuba, Ibaraki, Japan; Kyoto Univ, Japan)

J Immunol 175:2051-2055, 2005 5–11

Introduction.—It is well-documented that certain chemokines or their receptors play important roles in the graft rejection. However, the roles of chemokines and their receptors in the maintenance of transplantation tolerance remain unclear. In this study, we demonstrate that blocking of the interaction between the chemokine receptor, CXCR6, highly expressed on $V\alpha14^+$ NKT cells and its ligand, CXCL16, resulted in the failure to maintain graft tolerance and thus in the induction of acceleration of graft rejection. In a mouse transplant tolerance model, the expression of CXCL16 was up-regulated in the tolerated allografts, and anti-CXCL16 mAb inhibited intragraft accumulation of NKT cells. In vitro experiments further showed that blocking of CXCL16/CXCR6 interaction significantly affected not only chemotaxis but also cell adhesion of NKT cells. These results demonstrate the unique role of CXCL16 and CXCR6 molecules in the maintenance of cardiac allograft tolerance mediated by NKT cells.

► An intriguing method of recipient modulation is through in vitro manipulation of the recipient's immune cells. In the article by Bashuda et al (Abstract 5–9), alloreactive T cells were rendered anergic ex vivo by coculture with donor alloantigen in the presence of monoclonal antibodies and then adoptively transferred in a primate model. Graft function without immunosuppression was maintained for over a year in the donor-specific alloantigen model. This was an interesting study demonstrating that ex vivo–generated anergic cells can allow for long-term renal allograft function in a nonhuman primate model. Donor-specific unresponsiveness was not transferred to third-party alloantigens, however. The prospect of developing graft-specific hyporesponsive conditions is an exciting venue in an attempt to minimize or avoid long-term immunosuppressive regimens.

Immunity to HLA antigens has been the backbone of transplant-related research. There are, however, many other non-MHC immunologic mechanisms that may be important in long-term function. One such finding was described from the European experience with HLA-identical siblings (Abstract 5–10). In a large database, 3000 patients with no antibodies against human alloantigens had a 10-year graft survival of 72%. In 800 patients who had 1% to 50% panel-reactive antibodies, the 10-year graft function was present in 63%, and in those patients with greater than 50% panel-reactive antibodies, the graft function was only 55%. The adverse effect of elevated alloantibodies only became apparent after the first year of transplantation, as the 1-year graft function was identical in all groups. This is strikingly different from the very steep decline that is seen in graft function during the first year of recipients of deceased donor kidneys as stratified by alloreactive antibodies. This is a very interesting article stressing the heterogeneity of the immune response to transplanted organs and the avenues that will need to be explored for maintenance of long-term function.

In keeping with the role of non-MHC antigen recognition and mechanisms for transplant alloimmunity, there are a variety of immune responses that are dependent upon nonspecific chemokines or pattern recognition receptors that appear to impact allo-unresponsiveness. In the study by Jiang et al (Abstract 5–11), it was demonstrated that blocking the interaction between the chemokine receptors CXCR6 (expressed on NKT cells) and its ligand, CXCL16, resulted in failure to maintain graft tolerance. This was performed in a murine transplant tolerance model where CXCL16 was upregulated in the tolerated allografts, and monoclonal antibody was used to inhibit intragraft accumulation of NKT cells. The role of chemokine expression and regulation of its receptors is very nonspecific. A variety of autoimmune and inflammatory processes have been shown to modulate these receptors, making one query as to the durability of attempted tolerance in the clinical setting. It is well recognized that extrapolation from a mouse model to humans is uncertain at best; however, the importance of such a fundamental immune response such as chemokines and their receptors in the subsequent breaking of tolerance needs to be acknowledged as studies move forward in clinical practice.

T. L. Pruett, MD

Natural History of Hepatitis B and C in Renal Allograft Recipients

Aroldi A, Lampertico P, Montagnino G, et al (Ospedale Maggiore IRCCS, Milano, Italy; IRCCS Istituto Auxologico, Milano, Italy)

Transplantation 79:1132-1136, 2005 5–12

Background.—In renal allograft recipients, most cases of liver dysfunction are caused by hepatitis B virus and hepatitis C virus (HCV). The natural history of hepatitis C and B was studied in 286 renal allograft recipients who received a kidney allograft between 1972 and 1989 when tests for anti-HCV became available.

Methods.—In all patients, hepatitis B (HB) surface (s) antigen (Ag) was tested before and anti-HCV (by enzyme-linked immunosorbent assay II) after transplantation.

Results.—At enrollment in 1989 (5.5±4 years after transplantation), 209 patients were anti-HCV positive (C+), 42 patients were HBsAg-positive (B+), and 35 patients were both B+ and C+ (C+B+). One hundred four patients were receiving azathioprine (AZA) and 182 were on cyclosporine A (CsA). Since transplantation, the median follow-up was 18 years in AZA-treated and 13 years in CsA-treated patients. Liver biopsy showed chronic hepatitis in 73 patients, cirrhosis in 20 patients, and fibrosing cholestatic hepatitis in 2 patients. In 34 patients, liver biopsy was repeated, and progression of fibrosis was observed in 24 patients. Thc 12-year patient survival rate was similar in B+, C+, and B+C+ patients (67%, 78%, and 71%, respectively; *P*=not significant). Liver-related death was the first cause of death in B+ and B+C+ infected patients (58% and 72%, respectively), whereas cardiovascular disease was the leading cause of death in C+ patients (40%). Multivariate analysis showed that older age (>40 years) (relative risk [RR], 2.8), B+ status (RR, 2.36), and C+ status (RR, 1.65) were independently associated with a worse patient survival.

Conclusions.—In the long term, B+ patients had a higher risk of death related to liver disease than C+ patients, and co-infection did not worsen patient survival.

▶ Patients with chronic hepatitis have often been considered poor candidates for organ transplantation. As both hepatitis B and C are endemic in many parts of the world, excluding such people is oftentimes difficult. In the current study, patients with hepatitis B, hepatitis C, both hepatitis B and C, and without hepatitis (controls) were followed up for a mean in excess of 10 years. Compared with the patients without hepatitis (B−C−), the individuals with chronic viral hepatitis had an increased risk of death but a fairly comparable graft function. Death associated with liver failure was seen in both hepatitis B and C patients, but was more prevalent in patients with hepatitis B virus infection. The significance of the study speaks to the importance of management of these chronic viral diseases. Newer agents to control both hepatitis B and C are available. Their ultimate utility in allowing patients to access the transplant cure successfully remains to be seen.

T. L. Pruett, MD

Cutaneous Squamous Cell Carcinoma in Organ Transplant Recipients: A Study of the Swedish Cohort With Regard to Tumor Site

Lindelof B, Dal H, Wolk K, et al (Karolinska Inst, Stockholm; Ctr of Public Health, Stockholm)

Arch Dermatol 141:447-451, 2005 5–13

Objective.—To establish the anatomical site distribution of cutaneous squamous cell carcinoma (SCC) in organ transplant recipients (OTRs) with regard to age and sex.

Design.—Retrospective population-based cohort study of OTRs.

Setting.—Patients who underwent organ transplantation in Sweden from January 1, 1970, to December 31, 1997, registered in the Swedish In-patient Registry and national Swedish Cancer Registry.

Patients.—From the cohort of 5931 OTRs, we could include 179 patients with 475 cutaneous SCCs. Information on the sites was received from the cancer registry and from the histopathological reports.

Results.—The site of each SCC was registered in a computer program displaying the results on a 3-dimensional human figure. The head and neck were the predominant sites in male patients, and the trunk was the predominant site in female patients. The most common site in younger patients (born in 1940 or after) was the chest; and in older patients, the face. The ear was a common site in male patients, but, in contrast, no tumors were located there in female patients. Overall, the OTRs were younger compared with the overall Swedish population with cutaneous SCC.

Conclusions.—There are differences in the anatomical site distribution of cutaneous SCCs in OTRs with regard to sex and age, and with regard to the general distribution in Swedish patients. The level of sun exposure is considered the most important factor in explaining those differences, and highlights the importance of sun avoidance in this group of patients.

▶ Another form of long-term morbidity has been the evolution of SCC. There is an estimated 100-fold increased risk of the development of this cancer after organ transplantation. The reasons are probably multifactorial, including immunosuppression, local infection, and UV radiation. In this Swedish study, differences in site distribution with regard to age and sex were highly suggestive of the level of sun exposure as being the most important factor explaining the differences. This only goes to reconfirm the importance of educating transplant recipients regarding skin care and protection. Reduction of long-term morbidity is a major issue for the transplantation community.

T. L. Pruett, MD

Liver Transplantation for Hepatocellular Carcinoma

Befeler AS, Hayashi PH, di Bisceglie AM (St Louis Univ)

Gastroenterology 128:1752-1764, 2005 5–14

Background.—The therapeutic options for hepatocellular carcinoma (HCC) patients have changed significantly in the last decade, and liver transplantation has emerged as the preferred option for patients with early-stage HCC. Transplantation offers a potential for cure, and it also decreases the recurrence risk and eliminates other complications of cirrhosis. However, the use of transplantation for the treatment of HCC has increased at the same time that there is an increasing incidence of HCC and a persistent shortage of organs. It is therefore vital that the transplant community understands both the benefits of transplantation and the adjunctive therapies for the treatment of HCC. The status of liver transportation in the management of patients with HCC was reviewed.

Overview.—HCC is the fifth most common malignancy in men and the ninth most common malignancy in women throughout the world. The incidence of HCC is expected to continue to increase through the next decade. Cirrhosis of any etiology can lead to HCC, but the risk varies with the etiology. In the United States, most cases of HCC are related to hepatitis C virus (HCV) infection with or without alcohol. In addition to transplantation, several nontransplantation treatments are available, particularly for patients in the early stages of disease. Surgical resection and ablation are potentially curative in patients with early stage HCC; however, advanced tumor stage in conjunction with advanced cirrhosis will significantly limit therapeutic options. Unfortunately, most patients present in the late stages of disease. Staging systems for HCC should both direct the treatment options and help predict overall survival within staging groups. Biopsies are generally not required for staging if a patient meets the European Association for the Study of the Liver (EASL) noninvasive criteria for HCC. Accurate diagnosis and staging and optimal pretransplantation care are key components in the prioritization of HCC patients to optimize both the efficacy and the just allocation of organs. Among the remaining controversies facing the transplant community are the roles of living donation, tumor downstaging, and rescue transplantation.

Conclusions.—Liver transplantation can offer prolonged disease-free and overall survival for carefully selected patients with small HCCs. However, many patients have HCC that is not treatable with transplantation, and transplantation is not widely available in many countries in which HCC is common. The scarcity of donor organs has magnified the importance of settling the controversies that remain regarding some aspects of transplantation for HCC.

► The extraordinary increase in cirrhosis in the United States with the combination of viral hepatitis and nonalcoholic steatohepatitis has led to a marked increase in the prevalence of hepatocellular carcinoma. As these tumors often arise in the face of cirrhosis, the therapy is often limited by the functional reserve of the liver. Transplantation has been remarkably successful in caring for patients with small-stage T1 and T2 lesions. Its role in the larger tumors or more numerous tumors has been limited, and with reduced numbers of organs available for transplantation, it has fallen out of favor as a form of treatment. The importance of understanding both the potential benefit of transplantation and the adjunctive therapies is exceedingly important to the practicing surgeon. The current article reviews the status of the role of liver transplantation and the management of patients with hepatocellular carcinoma.

T. L. Pruett, MD

The Clinical and Cost-Effectiveness of Left Ventricular Assist Devices for End-Stage Heart Failure: A Systematic Review and Economic Evaluation

Clegg AJ, Scott DA, Loveman E, et al (Univ of Southampton, England; Fourth Hurdle Consulting Ltd, London; Univ of Aberdeen, England)

Health Technol Assess 9:1-148, 2005 5–15

Background.—The incidence and prevalence of heart failure are increasing in England and Wales, leading to frequent admissions to hospital and long-term drug costs. Concern regarding the effects of heart failure and its attendant costs on the quality of life of patients and the costs to the National Health Service has prompted several government initiatives in the United Kingdom. Heart transplantation has become the accepted treatment for patients with end-stage heart failure (ESHF); however, organ donation in England and Wales has been declining, and transplantation is a viable option for relatively few patients. Mechanical circulatory support through left–ventricular-assist devices (LVADs) has attracted increased interest as an option for patients with ESHF either as a bridge to transplantation or myocardial recovery or as a long-term chronic support. The clinical and cost-effectiveness of LVADs in persons with ESHF were reviewed.

Methods.—A systematic review was conducted of 18 electronic databases from inception through October 2003. The inclusion criteria included studies that evaluated currently available LVADs used for the following purposes: (1) as a bridge to transplantation, myocardial recovery, or chronic support; (2) for subjects, 16 years or older, with ESHF and considered suitable for receipt of an LVAD; (3) for assessing survival, functional capacity, and quality of life; and (4) for conducting systematic reviews, controlled clinical trials, cohort studies, case series, case studies, economic evaluations, or cost studies.

Results.—A systematic review of the clinical effectiveness of LVADs showed that, while they are clinically effective as a bridge to transplantation in patients with ESHF, they are not cost effective. In light of the limited and declining availability of donor hearts for transplantation, the future of this technology is in its use as long-term chronic support. However, at present the evidence of clinical and cost effectiveness of LVADs as long-term chronic support for ESHF patients is limited, and there is a need for further study. There is also a need for a systematic review of the epidemiology of ESHF to determine its potential impact.

► In heart transplantation, the advent of ventricular-assist devices has dramatically altered the urgency and need for heart transplantation. In the United States, the placement of a ventricular assist device (albeit with some fine tuning) is 1 of the primary driving factors for allocation of a heart for transplantation. This article discusses the clinical and cost effectiveness of LVADs as either bridged transplantation, bridged myocardial recovery or as a long-term chronic support for people with cardiac dysfunction. In a study for the National Health Service in England and Wales, it was demonstrated that LVADs, although clinically effective as a bridge for transplantation, were not shown to be cost effective in an economic evaluation. It was concluded that with the limited and declining availability of donor hearts for transplantation that the future of the technology was going to be as a long-term support. The study is limited by the generation of LVADs that were available for review, but the overall societal impact of cost and benefit is one that has to be taken seriously for the allocation of resources for given populations. Each society will have to discern what resources will be allocated for given individuals.

T. L. Pruett, MD

Immunosuppression and Procedure-related Complications in 26 Patients With Type 1 Diabetes Mellitus Receiving Allogeneic Islet Cell Transplantation

Hafiz MM, Faradji RN, Froud T, et al (Univ of Miami, Fla)

Transplantation 80:1718-1728, 2005 5–16

Background.—The success of sirolimus and low-dose tacrolimus in islet cell transplantation has influenced many transplant centers to utilize this novel regimen. The long-term safety and tolerability of this steroid-free immunosuppressive protocol for allogeneic islet transplantation has yet to be determined.

Methods.—We transplanted 26 adult patients with long standing type 1 diabetes mellitus between April 2000 and June 2004. Immunosuppression consisted of induction with daclizumab and maintenance therapy with tacrolimus and sirolimus. Adverse events (AEs) in patients were followed and graded using the Common Terminology Criteria for Adverse Events, version 3.0 (National Cancer Institute).

Results.—To date, the majority of patients were able to remain on the immunosuppression combination for up to 22±11 months. Four patients were successfully converted to Mycophenolate Mofetil due to tacrolimus-related toxicity. Withdrawal from immunosuppression was decided in four patients due to hypereosinophilic syndrome, parvovirus infection, aspiration pneumonia, and severe depression, respectively. Six patients required filgrastim therapy for neutropenia. Transient elevation of liver enzymes was observed in most patients early after islet infusion. Increased LDL in 20 patients required medical treatment.

Conclusion.—There was a varying range of AEs, most of them mild and self-limiting; however, some required urgent medical attention. The majority of patients were able to tolerate and remain on this effective regimen. To date, no deaths, cytomegalovirus disease, graft-versus-host disease, or post-transplant lymphoproliferative disease has been observed.

▶ It is often assumed that islet cell transplantation will have minimal complications. Although this is undoubtedly true, the results of the procedure-related complications of 26 islet cell transplants are reported here. The majority of complications appear to be related to immunosuppression, but it is significant that 15% to 16% of AEs were procedure-related. Bleeding is not unexpected with portal vein manipulation using a transhepatic route. The complication of transiently elevated serum levels of aspartate aminotransferase and alanine aminotransferase is also not unexpected, but needs to be further followed up. The majority of complications related to long-term immunosuppression will also vary, depending upon the optimal dose of the agents chosen. Because nothing is free, one has to strike a good balance between risk and benefit. The list of complications reported in this article is quite thorough and reasonably presented.

T. L. Pruett, MD

Combination Therapy With Epidermal Growth Factor and Gastrin Induces Neogenesis of Human Islet β-Cells From Pancreatic Duct Cells and an Increase in Functional β-Cell Mass

Suarez-Pinzon WL, Lakey JRT, Brand SJ, et al (Univ of Alberta, Edmonton, Canada; Waratah Pharmaceuticals, Woburn, Mass)

J Clin Endocrinol Metab 90:3401-3409, 2005 5–17

Introduction.—Pancreatic islet transplantation is a viable treatment for type 1 diabetes, but is limited by human donor tissue availability. The combination of epidermal growth factor (EGF) and gastrin induces islet β-cell neogenesis from pancreatic exocrine duct cells in rodents. In this study we investigated whether EGF and gastrin could expand the β-cell mass in adult human isolated islets that contain duct as well as endocrine cells. Human islet cells were cultured for 4 wk in serum-free medium (control) or in medium with EGF (0.3 μg/ml), gastrin (1.0 μg/ml), or the combination of EGF and gastrin. β-Cell numbers were increased in cultures with EGF plus gastrin (+118%) and with EGF (+81%), but not in cultures with gastrin (−3%) or control medium (−62%). After withdrawal of EGF and gastrin and an additional 4 wk in control medium, β-cell numbers continued to increase only in cultures previously incubated with both EGF and gastrin (+232%). EGF plus gastrin also significantly increased cytokeratin 19–positive duct cells (+678%) in the cultures. Gastrin, alone or in combination with EGF, but not EGF alone, increased the expression of pancreatic and duodenal homeobox factor-1 as well as insulin and C peptide in the cytokeratin 19–positive duct cells. Also, EGF plus gastrin significantly increased β-cells and insulin content in human islets implanted in immunodeficient nonobese diabetic-severe combined immune deficiency mice as well as insulin secretory responses of the human islet grafts to glucose challenge. In conclusion, combination therapy with EGF and gastrin increases β-cell mass in adult human pancreatic islets in vitro and in vivo, and this appears to result from the induction of β-cell neogenesis from pancreatic exocrine duct cells.

► Certainly, one of the limitations in transplantation of cells has been adequate generation of functioning cells and maintenance of such in vitro. The experimentation with growth factors is an important adjunct to increase functional activity in cells. This article describes the use of EGF and gastrin to increase the functional β-cell mass in isolated human islets. It was hypothesized that EGF and gastrin induce neogenesis of human islet β-cells from pancreatic ductal cells, resulting in an increased number of β-cells. While this is a very exciting concept, the durability of this form of therapy, with subsequent dedifferentiation back to ductal cells when the stressed events abate, remains to be seen. The notion of ex vivo modulation of tissue to achieve such a desired goal is still an active area of investigation.

T. L. Pruett, MD

Human Monocyte-Derived Neohepatocytes: A Promising Alternative to Primary Human Hepatocytes for Autologous Cell Therapy

Ruhnke M, Nussler AK, Ungefroren H, et al (Univ Hosp of Schleswig-Holstein, Kiel, Germany; Humboldt Univ, Berlin; Univ of Leipzig, Germany; et al)

Transplantation 79:1097-1103, 2005 5–18

Background.—There is growing interest in new therapeutic options for the treatment of end-stage liver diseases. In addition to mechanical devices supporting liver function, such as bioreactors, the transplantation of hepatocyte-like cells derived from (adult) stem cells offer great perspectives. We have generated hepatocyte-like (NeoHep) cells from terminally differentiated peripheral blood monocytes and, in this study, have evaluated these cells as a possible tool for autologous cell therapy.

Methods.—Peripheral blood monocytes were cultured under conditions that promote hepatocyte-like differentiation and were characterized for hepatocyte marker expression by reverse-transcriptase polymerase chain reaction, immunohistochemistry, and immunoblotting and for specific secretory and metabolic functions with the appropriate biochemical assays.

Results.—NeoHep cells resembled primary human hepatocytes with respect to morphology, expression of hepatocyte markers (albumin, cytochrome P450 isoenzymes, asialoglycoprotein receptor, coagulation factor VII), various secretory and metabolic functions (albumin secretion, urea production, lactate formation, and lactate dehydrogenase and aspartate transaminase release), and drug detoxification activities (phase I metabolization of ethoxycoumarin into 7OH-coumarin after stimulation with 3-methylcholanthren, induction of CYP3A4 activity, and phase II metabolization through UDP-glucuronidation of 4-methyl-umbelliferone).

Conclusions.—These data convincingly show that NeoHep cells display a phenotype and specific in vitro metabolic functions that are quantitatively and qualitatively comparable in part with those of primary human hepatocytes. These cells could thus be clinically applied in an autologous setting for the treatment of end-stage liver diseases or for improving liver function in patients who have undergone critical liver-mass resection.

► The use of nondifferentiated cells to move into a differentiated cell function is also an area of great interest. Stem cell research has been the major emphasis in this regard; however, other cell lines are potentially possible to derive differential function. This article describes cells appearing to have significant hepatotcyte function that came from circulating human mononuclear cells. Cells were treated for 6 days in culture with β-mercaptoethanol, macrophage–colony-stimulating factor, and human interleukin-3. They were then cultured an additional 2 weeks with fibroblast growth factor. These cells were subsequently able to express a variety of different hepatocyte markers such as albumin, cytochrome P450 isoenzymes, asialoglycoprotein receptor, and coagulation factors. They also had various secretory and metabolic functions, such as albumin secretion, urea production, and lactate formation, and drug detoxification activities, including phase I metabolism of ethoxycoumarin into 7-hydroxycoumarin after stimulation as well as induction of CYP3A4 activity. These differential functions portend the possibility of patients with organ dysfunction having their own cells removed in significant quantity to produce functioning cells. With an autotransplant, the need for immunosuppression and other drug utilization clearly is obviated. Again, the issues relating to whether the cell lines will be stable or whether they will differentiate back to their original cells remain to be discerned, but the initial experimentation with phenotypic changes induced by culture techniques is very exciting.

T. L. Pruett, MD

Lack of Cross-Species Transmission of Porcine Endogenous Retrovirus in Pig-to-Baboon Xenotransplantation With Sustained Depletion of Anti-αGal Antibodies

Moscoso I, Hermida-Prieto M, Mañez R, et al (CHU Juan Canalejo, La Coruña, Spain; Universidad de la Coruña, Spain; Universitario de Bellvitge, Spain)

Transplantation 79:777-782, 2005 5–19

Background.—Nonhuman primates are potential permissive animals for studying the risk of in vivo infection with porcine endogenous retrovirus (PERV). Anti-αGal natural antibodies are considered one of the barriers for preventing PERV infection, and it has been postulated that reduction of these antibodies could increase the risk of this infection. The aim of this study was to investigate the role of GAS 914, which depletes anti-αGal antibodies, in the potential in vivo transfer of PERV after pig-to-baboon organ xenotransplantation.

Methods.—Twenty-seven baboons underwent xenotransplantation with hDAF or hMCP/hDAF transgenic pig organs, including heterotopic heart (n = 14) and kidney (n = 13) transplants. All of them received GAS 914 along with different immunosuppression protocols. PERV sequences were investigated by reverse-transcriptase polymerase chain reaction and by polymerase chain reaction assays in samples obtained at autopsy. The presence of PERV-specific antibodies and/or pig xenomicrochimerism was also evaluated.

Results.—PERV RNA was not detected in any baboon plasma sample. In addition, all plasma samples were negative for PERV antibodies. However, PERV DNA sequences were detected in peripheral blood mononuclear cells from 6 of 14 (43%) animals investigated. Porcine mitochondrial DNA was also found in all of these positive samples and in six of the eight (75%) samples with negative PERV DNA, indicating that the detection of PERV sequences was attributable to xenochimerism. PERV-positive cells as a result of xenochimerism were also found in eight of nine (89%) spleen and lymph node tissue samples tested.

Conclusions.—Sustained depletion of anti-alphaGal antibodies does not augment the risk of PERV infection in pig-to-baboon organ transplantation.

► Part of the Holy Grail of transplantation has been the use of organs from other species. One of the major limiting factors has been the concern regarding retroviral transmission past species as well as the generation of xenoproteins that will potentially illicit antibodies and immune complex diseases. This article describes a series of baboons who underwent xenotransplantation with transgenic pig organs. The model to be tested under this experiment was the role of depletion of the anti-αGal antibodies. The authors were quite encouraged by the fact that no PERV was detected in the baboon plasma sample. In addition, all the plasma samples were negative for PERV antibodies. The authors, however, could detect DNA sequences of PERV in the peripheral blood mononuclear cells from 43% of the animals. Porcine mitochondrial DNA was found in the positive samples, suggesting that the detection of the retroviruses was in the chimeric condition from the donor organs. The authors were quite enthused that there was no evidence of retroviral activation. Concerns about this study are mainly the short duration of the experimentation; the longest time any of the organs was functioning was 60 days, and the shortest was 4 days. Although it is reassuring to observe that there is no retroviral activation during this time, a longer observation period is necessary. There are many hurdles to overcome in xenotransplantation, of which infection is only one of many.

T. L. Pruett, MD

6 Surgical Infections

Introduction

Infection remains one of the costly and often preventable complications of surgery. Decreasing the frequency of surgical site infections (SSI) is an initiative that is being undertaken by governmental and medical bodies. Abstract 6–1 discusses the 1-year demonstration project of the National Surgical Infection Prevention Collaborative. Factors that have been shown to alter the risk of SSI were tracked in 56 hospitals. These included timeliness and duration of antibiotics, as well as the appropriate spectrum of antimicrobial activity for the contaminating flora; prevention of hyperglycemia; maintenance of normothermia; optimized oxygen tension, and avoidance of shaving of the surgical site. In the collaborative facilities, the reported SSI rate fell 27%. While there are significant methodologic issues with this study, the overall contention is sound. If one does the things that have been associated with decreasing the risk of infection in a timely and efficient manner, it is likely that the rate of SSI will decrease. Interestingly, not all of the sentinel methods had been conclusively demonstrated to reduce the risk of SSI. In fact, another report supporting the use of supplemental oxygen to decrease the risk of SSI was published in 2005. This was necessary because the 2 published prior clinical studies had opposite conclusions regarding the benefit of exogenous oxygen. In the current report (Abstract 6–2), patients undergoing colorectal surgery were randomized to FiO_2 of 30% or 80% intraoperatively and for 6 hours after surgery. In the higher oxygen tension group, the risk of SSI was 39% lower. In the discussion of the findings, the authors discuss their findings in light of the prior studies regarding oxygen tension and risk for SSI. The rationale for the perioperative maintenance of high blood oxygen tension is sound and the risks are minimal, and now with 2 of 3 studies demonstrating reduction in SSI, the practice should be routine.

Better granularity of patient risk for adverse outcome would certainly be helpful. Abstract 6–3 discusses risk factors for the prediction of SSI in clean surgical procedures. Through multivariate logistic regression analysis, the combination of cirrhosis, preoperative indwelling urinary catheter, and other disease was found to be predictive of a group of patients that benefited from routine use of antibiotic prophylaxis. In patients not meeting the threshold score, antibiotics did not prove to be useful in altering the rate of SSI. Indeed, other variables can be found to be significant as one delves more into the practice at individual centers. Abstract 6–4 discusses the 11-fold increase in SSI associated with the use of spinal anesthesia in an outpatient surgical center. In this report, where more than 95% of patients had an ASA score of 1, the risk of SSI was drastically increased with spinal anesthesia. In delving for explanations for this unexpected finding, a selection bias was identified where spinal anesthesia was preferentially offered to individuals with extensive tobacco use and those thought to be at pulmonary risk. Nonetheless, these series illustrate the heterogeneity of variables associated with the development of SSI and the importance of methodologic consistency.

It has been commonly observed that the majority of clean surgical infections come from the flora colonizing the skin and mucous membranes of the patient (although the operating theater environment and personnel also contribute to a differing degree). While resistance to antimicrobial agents is common in bacteria that are isolated from the hospital, bacteria from the community have typically been sensitive to a broad spectrum of agents. One of the most common organisms that both colonizes people in the community and also results in serious wound infectious complications is undergoing a major change in susceptibility to antimicrobial agents. *Staphylococcus aureus* isolated from community-acquired infections is commonly found to be methicillin resistant. Abstract 6–5 summarizes MRSA infections in 3 areas of the United States and concludes that community-associated MRSA infections are now a common and serious problem. Although these infections usually involve the skin and often lead to hospitalization, the finding has not been extrapolated yet to SSI. No changes in recommendations for routine prophylactic antimicrobial agents have been made, but the day may soon arrive when cephalosporins and penicillins will not be effective anti-*Staphylococcus* prophylaxis for common operations.

To further expand on this issue, in the setting of prosthetic material implantation, prevention of infection becomes critical. Pasteur demonstrated that spontaneous generation of the species does not occur and in logical consequence, the bacteria that cause SSI during clean procedures either get into the wound through direct contamination at the time of surgery or hematogenously during or after the procedure. Infection of implantable devices/materials often leads to either the need for device removal or significant intervention to attempt to salvage the device or graft. In either case, there is significant morbidity and risk for the patient. The cost of *Staphylococcus aureus* bacteremia in individuals with prosthetic devices is discussed in Abstract 6–6. Although the device was not the culprit in all cases, 58% of individuals underwent surgery as a consequence of the infection, with the generation of significant morbidity and cost. In the cases of *Staphylococcus* bacteremia, the device was infected in about 40% of cardiac and orthopedic devices, 93% of long-term catheters, and 34% of other devices. MRSA accounted for 53% of the isolates. Twelve-week mortality was in excess of 20% in the patient population. If this complication can be prevented, it surely should be. It is interesting in this article that the authors do not address the issue of anti-*Staphylococcus* prophylaxis at the time of device implantation. In a study to determine whether antibiotics were "beneficial" when mesh herniorrhaphy was performed (Abstract 6–7), 360 patients were randomly assigned to receive either a placebo or a first-generation cephalosporin. Three patients in the antibiotic arm and 6 patients in the placebo arm developed SSI, and 1 patient in each arm developed a deep infection necessitating mesh removal. The authors concluded that anti-*Staphylococcus* antibiotics were not necessary in mesh herniorrhaphy as the incidence of SSI, 1.7% (antibiotics) versus 3.3% (placebo), was not statistically different (p=0.5). The data demonstrated that *Staphylococcus* species were was present in all instances of the SSI, with *S aureus* being present in 9 of 11 infections. The study was powered to show differences assuming a high infection rate in the placebo arm (7% is a high SSI rate for clean surgery) and an optimistic beneficial effect from antibiotics (decrease SSI infection to 1%). The observed benefit of 50% reduction in SSI with antibiotics is about right, but would need many more patients to prove statistically what most physicians and surgeons already know. The authors did not address the issue of whether MRSA was present in any of the wounds, and the prospect that cefazolin prophylaxis may have given the same protection as the placbo agent.

Although infection of the surgically implanted device usually requires removal for "cure," sometimes complete cure is not necessary, or the removal of the device is not feasible. Management of device/graft infection usually requires some form of surgical intervention, but the goals of therapy need to be aligned with clinical needs. A variety of creative management approaches are being developed to deal with infected surgically implanted devices. Chronic exit-site infections with double-cuffed peritoneal dialysis catheters can frequently be managed through unroofing of the exit-site tract and shaving of the superficial cuff (Abstract 6–8). Although the more proximal/deep cuff would sometimes get infected and the catheter removed, many months of functional dialysis were salvaged through a relatively simple technique. Cases of infected mesh associated with large abdominal wall defects can prove especially challenging. In these instances, removal of prosthetic materials is the first line of therapy and then reconstruction with a combination of advancement flaps and relaxing incisions, but sometimes there is a need for more synthetic materials. Abstract 6–9 discusses many issues relating to the management of the large contaminated abdominal wall defect. One of the exceedingly complicated issues is an infected prosthetic graft of large vessels. Conservative therapy with debridement and antibiotics routinely fails, and mortality is significant. The obliteration of dead space and wrapping of the infected prosthetic material with vascularized muscle pedicle grafts has been suggested, to encouraging results (Abstract 6–10). The difficulty that prosthetic infection presents to the surgeon and patient warrants attempts of refinement. A primary goal in the implantation of prosthetic materials should be to prevent prosthetic device infections through careful management of the surgical site and judicious use of antimicrobial therapies. In the event that the graft does become infected, careful weighing of the risks of device removal or debility associated with attempted definitive therapy versus the risk of persistent infection needs to be balanced.

There are some infections where surgical therapy is essential for adequate management. This is particularly true of necrotizing soft tissue infections.

Abstract 6–11 summarizes the bacteria isolated from debridement specimens from 113 patients. The reported findings are a bit surprising in that no instance of clostridial infection was noted. The series was also a bit unusual in that more than two thirds of the infections were monomicrobial, whereas in the United States with a considerable number of necrotizing soft tissue infections arising from the perineal area, a polymicrobial flora is more common. This report is useful to emphasize again that inoculum source determines the flora and outcome. In this series, 11% of patients required an amputation for adequate infection source control. The variables that are associated with the need for amputation to control necrotizing soft tissue infections are examined in Abstract 6–12, in which an overall mortality of 17% was reported, and loss of limb occurred in 26% of patients with extremity involvement. The authors observed that clostridial infection was an independent predictor of both limb loss and death and was associated with IV drug use and leukocytosis. Surgical management of the wounds created by the necessary debridement that occurs with the management of necrotizing soft tissue infections can be quite complex. In many cases, reconstruction and management of soft tissue defects require the skills of wound care and critical care experts most commonly found in burn centers (Abstract 6–13). In a small series of 65 patients, the authors describe multiple instances of debridement and skin grafting, but are silent about amputations. In the microbiology section, there is no mention of treating any patient with clostridial infection. One could speculate that the burn surgeon/staff is well equipped to manage the complex soft tissue infection with an eye towards maintenance of function; however, the described resources can certainly be found in other venues, such as many trauma services. An often discussed adjunct to the management of necrotizing soft tissue infections is hyperbaric oxygen. In a review (Abstract 6–14) of the effect of hyperbaric oxygen upon resolution of necrotizing fasciitis found in the published English language literature, the authors state that resuscitation, radical debridement, and broad-spectrum antibiotics form the cornerstones of management of necrotizing fasciitis, but were interested in any potential incremental benefit associated with hyperbaric oxygen. As with previous publications, the results are inconclusive. The theoretic reasons for benefit are solid; it is just that the observed events belie the benefit of hyperbaric oxygen therapy. It would be nice if it were demonstrated that the extent of radical debridement could be minimized through hyperbaric oxygen, but such a study has not been designed (nor is it likely to be done). The use of such therapy will continue as a source of controversy within the surgical community.

Traditional surgical wisdom states that intra-abdominal abscesses mandate surgical drainage. This dictum has undergone some modification with improvements in abdominal imaging capacity and alternative drainage modalities. An experience (Abstract 6–15) with mesocolic and pelvic abscesses associated with diverticular disease demonstrates the current heterogeneity of therapies employed in the care of people with intra-abdominal abscesses. Initial diagnosis was made radiographically after clinical presentation. In order to effect a one-stage therapy, the initial management of infected intra-abdominal fluid/abscess is typically drainage through a percutaneously placed catheter. Although usually quite successful, instances exist where the utility is less than optimal. More than 20 years ago, conditions were identified that were associated with less-than-optimal outcomes with catheter drainage. These included abscesses associated with carcinoma, enteric fistula, and infections that were predominantly fungus or yeast. Abstract 6–16 reviews the results of a current series of fungus-containing abdominal infections. Clinical success in this setting is still low and behooves the surgeon to consider different approaches to these difficult-to-treat infections. Radiographic placement of catheters is not the only "minimally invasive" format for dealing with cavitary-contained infections; the endoscopists are competing heavily with minimalist approaches to drainage of fluid collections. The management of 20 patients with paraesophageal mediastinal abscesses is described in Abstract 6–17. The authors describe successful drainage and debridement with subsequent successful control of the esophageal defect. Although this is an overly optimistic assessment of therapy, these series illustrate the options confronting the surgeon. When in the management of intra-abdominal infection does the surgeon deliver the primary or definitive therapy in the patient with intra-abdominal infection? It is clear that endoscopic, particularly with ultrasound and radiographic, techniques are definitive and useful in many circumstances. It is just as clear that conditions exist that reduce the likelihood of success of a minimalist approach to infection. It will be incumbent on the practicing surgeon to know the limitations of the various techniques in order to maximize therapeutic benefit. In this setting, the consequences of a surgical procedure, even if nothing is done, must be weighed. The notion that a negative second-look laparotomy in the face of peritonitis was of minimal consequence is challenged in Abstract 6–18. In a review of patients with peritonitis associated with acute mesenteric ischemia, survival was highest in a group of patients, who after their definitive procedure and response proved to be "adequate" such that the attending surgeon chose to observe the patient. The routine reexploration (second look) was associated with a higher mortality than judicious observation.

In the era of increasing antibiotic-resistant microorganisms, it is incumbent that new therapies be evolved to serve the patients with surgical infections. The use of bacteriophages has been postulated as an effective agent for the treatment of surgical infections. Lysis-deficient bacteriophage therapy was associated with an improvement of mouse survival in a peritonitis model. Interestingly, this form of therapy was associated with diminished amounts of endotoxin and proinflammatory cytokines. There is considerable promise that some of the biologic agents will afford new therapies for the pathogens that afflict our patients. In addition, the debate as to whether a gender and race difference exists for the susceptibility to infection persists. There are considerable experimental and animal arguments on both sides. In a group of 25 Japanese patients, it was found that men's preoperative cytokine release pattern from mononuclear cells was significantly different from women's. The men had more TNF-α and IFN-γ production of PBMC as well as decreased amounts of class II MHC.

Surgical infection still serves as a source of significant morbidity and mortality. There is much to be learned and implemented in the prevention and optimal treatment of infections in the surgical patient. It is disappointing that we have not made significant strides in the past few years. Technology has changed the manner in which we look at infections, but the basic problems remain the same. Much of the current literature appears to attempt to answer questions that had been thought to be answered.

Timothy L. Pruett, MD

Hospitals Collaborate to Decrease Surgical Site Infections

Dellinger EP, Hausmann SM, Bratzler DW, et al (Univ of Washington, Seattle; Qualis Health, Seattle; Oklahoma Found for Med Quality, Inc, Oklahoma City)

Am J Surg 190:9-15, 2005 6–1

Background.—Despite a large body of evidence describing care processes known to reduce the incidence of surgical site infections, many are underutilized in practice.

Methods.—Fifty-six hospitals volunteered to redesign their systems as part of the National Surgical Infection Prevention Collaborative, a 1-year demonstration project sponsored by the Centers for Medicare & Medicaid Services. Each facility selected quality improvement objectives for a select group of surgical procedures and reported monthly clinical process measure data.

Results.—Forty-four hospitals reported data on 35,543 surgical cases. Hospitals improved in measures related to appropriate antimicrobial agent selection, timing, and duration; normothermia; oxygenation; euglycemia; and appropriate hair removal. The infection rate decreased 27%, from 2.3% to 1.7% in the first versus last 3 months.

Conclusions.—The Collaborative demonstrated improvement in processes known to be associated with reduced risk of surgical site infections. Quality improvement organizations can be effective resources for quality improvement in the surgical arena.

► Much work has been done to understand why surgical site infections occur. Despite the abundance of information regarding risk factors associated with surgical site infections, few reports have consistently demonstrated the beneficial effects of standardized procedures. In this article, an initiative through the Institute for Healthcare Improvement established a collaborative among hospitals. Forty-four hospitals reported on over 35,000 surgical cases and demonstrated that, through attention to appropriate antimicrobial agent selection timing and duration, normothermia, oxygenation, euglycemia, and appropriate hair removal, the infection rate could be reduced 27%. Interestingly, performance improved dramatically as hospitals chose to follow these various parameters. The importance of these observations will be in the durability of the results. The individual variables have been known for a long time; the will to continue monitoring them has been highly variable.

T. L. Pruett, MD

Supplemental Perioperative Oxygen and the Risk of Surgical Wound Infection: A Randomized Controlled Trial

Belda FJ, for the Spanish Reduccion de la Tasa de Infeccion Quirurgica Group (Hosp Clínico Universitario, Valencia, Spain; Hosp de Galdakao, Bizkaia, Spain; Hosp Universitario de La Princesa, Madrid; et al)

JAMA 294:2035-2042, 2005 6–2

Context.—Supplemental perioperative oxygen has been variously reported to halve or double the risk of surgical wound infection.

Objective.—To test the hypothesis that supplemental oxygen reduces infection risk in patients following colorectal surgery.

Design, Setting, and Patients.—A double-blind, randomized controlled trial of 300 patients aged 18 to 80 years who underwent elective colorectal surgery in 14 Spanish hospitals from March 1, 2003, to October 31, 2004. Wound infections were diagnosed by blinded investigators using Centers for Disease Control and Prevention criteria. Baseline patient characteristics, anesthetic treatment, and potential confounding factors were recorded.

Interventions.—Patients were randomly assigned to either 30% or 80% fraction of inspired oxygen (FIO_2) intraoperatively and for 6 hours after surgery. Anesthetic treatment and antibiotic administration were standardized.

Main Outcome Measures.—Any surgical site infection (SSI); secondary outcomes included return of bowel function and ability to tolerate solid food, ambulation, suture removal, and duration of hospitalization.

Results.—A total of 143 patients received 30% perioperative oxygen and 148 received 80% perioperative oxygen. Surgical site infection occurred in 35 patients (24.4%) administered 30% FIO_2 and in 22 patients (14.9%) administered 80% FIO_2 (P=.04). The risk of SSI was 39% lower in the 80% FIO_2 group (relative risk [RR], 0.61; 95% confidence interval [CI], 0.38-0.98) vs the 30% FIO_2 group. After adjustment for important covariates, the RR of infection in patients administered supplemental oxygen was 0.46 (95% CI, 0.22-0.95; P=.04). None of the secondary outcomes varied significantly between the 2 treatment groups.

Conclusions.—Patients receiving supplemental inspired oxygen had a significant reduction in the risk of wound infection. Supplemental oxygen appears to be an effective intervention to reduce SSI in patients undergoing colon or rectal surgery.

▶ Even though oxygenation was one of the variables controlled in the prior article (Abstract 6–1), its role in SSIs has not been without controversy. Two prior studies on the effectiveness of perioperative oxygen in reducing the incidence of SSIs reached different conclusions, with one study demonstrating a decreased risk of infection and the other study showing an increased risk. This study was intended to be the tiebreaker and demonstrated that, in patients undergoing colon or rectal surgery, supplemental oxygen (80% FIO_2 in the perioperative period) significantly reduced the risk of SSI. The authors of this study included only SSIs that occurred within the first 14 days, a decision that would decrease the total number of SSIs but probably not affect the overall results. The incidence of SSI was reduced by approximately 10%, and the RR of SSI in patients who received 80% FIO_2 was 0.46. This study does not entirely put to rest the question about the relative value of supplemental perioperative oxygen, but the science regarding increased oxygen tension and making a wound more resistant to infection is well established, giving credibility to the notion that perioperative oxygen administration is, in fact, beneficial to patients after significant contamination.

T. L. Pruett, MD

Risk Factors for Prediction of Surgical Site Infections in "Clean Surgery"

Pessaux P, for The French Associations for Surgical Research (Universitaire Angers, France; et al)

Am J Infect Control 33:292-298, 2005 6–3

Background.—The aim of this study was to determine the risk factors of surgical site infections (SSI) in clean surgery and to identify high- and low-risk patients from whom efficacy of the antibiotic prophylaxis was analyzed.

Methods.—From June 1982 to September 1996, a database was established from 3 prospective multicenter randomized studies, containing information of 5798 patients who underwent abdominal noncolorectal surgery. Multivariate analysis was performed using nonconditional logistic regression expressed as an odds ratio (OR).

Results.—A total of 2374 patients underwent a clean surgery. An antibiotic prophylaxis was administered to 1943 patients (81.8%). A multivariate analysis was performed including only preoperative factors and disclosed 3 independent factors: cirrhosis (OR, 2.8; 95% CI: 1.6-12.8), other disease (OR, 2.7; 95% CI: 1.3-5.8), and preoperative urinary catheter (OR, 2.1; 95% CI: 1.1-4.6). A risk score for SSI was constructed: −4.9 + (1.5 × cirrhosis†) + (other disease†) + (0.8 × preoperative urinary catheter†) († = 0 if absent or 1 if present). The study included 1 group of patients having no risk factors for SSI with a score below −4.5 (S1R−) and 1 group of patients having 1 or more risk factors for SSI with a score over −4.5 (S1R+). Antibiotic prophylaxis did not reduce the infectious complication rate in the S1R− group, whereas, in the S1R+ group, it reduced significantly the rate of SSI and of parietal infectious complications by 58% and 69%, respectively.

Conclusions.—Antibiotic prophylaxis in clean abdominal surgery was effective in high-risk patients. Urinary catheter must be avoided.

► In many surgical procedures, there is no obvious exogenous contamination of the wound. These are called "clean" surgical procedures. The utility of antibiotics in these circumstances has never been entirely clear. In this study, over 5000 patients who underwent abdominal nonenteric surgical procedures were analyzed for the risk of SSI. After multivariant analysis, the authors concluded that the presence of preoperative urinary catheterization, cirrhosis, and other disease were the only variables associated with an increased risk of SSI.

The conclusions were arrived at from information from a 3-institution database. Specifically, the authors do not state how the information was obtained and put into the database and how SSIs were identified. Of specific note, inguinal hernias comprised approximately two thirds of all procedures performed.

There are many methodologic issues relating to this report. However, the importance of stratification by underlying systemic risk is very important. The finding that patients with cirrhosis and other diseases such as diabetes, heart failure, chronic respiratory failure, and renal failure influences the rate of clean surgical procedures is not surprising. In light of the previous studies (Abstracts 6–2 and 6–3), it would be very helpful to know the compliance rates of administration of antimicrobial therapy and integrity of the present outcomes. Although this article is interesting, its main value is in the observation that not all patients are the same. The specific use of antimicrobial agents in other preoperative variables (such as blood replacement, glucose control, body temperature, and others) to minimize the risk of SSIs in these patients was not addressed.

T. L. Pruett, MD

Risk Factors for Surgical Site Infections in a Free-standing Outpatient Setting

Hirsemann S, Sohr D, Gastmeier K, et al (Brandenburg Community Hosp, Germany; Charité -Univ Medicine, Berlin; Outpatient Clinic, Potsdam, Germany; et al)

Am J Infect Control 33:6-10, 2005 6–4

Background.—More information about risk factors for surgical site infections in outpatient settings is necessary for creation of surveillance systems in this field.

Objective.—The aim of this study was to determine the incidence of surgical site infections (SSI) in an outpatient setting and to investigate whether the risk index of the National Nosocomial Infections Surveillance (NNIS) System is appropriate for outpatient settings.

Methods.—A retrospective cohort design was used to investigate SSI following all hernia repairs and varicose veins operations over a 9-year period in a freestanding outpatient setting. The exposure variables studied were age, sex, and American Society of Anesthesiologists (ASA) score of the patient; duration of operation; performing surgeon's name; type of operation; type of anesthesia; and follow-up period. An univariable and a multivariable analysis was performed to determine risk factors for SSI.

Results.—A total of 1095 operations were performed: 714 on varicose veins and 381 on hernia repairs. The median follow-up period was 43 days. The crude SSI rate was 1.2% (varicose veins operations, 1.5%; hernia repair operations, 0.5%). According to the results of the logistic regression model, only 1 factor remained significant: Patients with spinal anesthesia were 11 times as likely to develop a SSI as patients with any other type of anesthesia (95% CI, 2.15-200.5).

Conclusion.—The NNIS risk index was not suitable for assessing SSI rates in this outpatient setting and for these specific procedures.

▶ This study attempts to determine the risks for SSIs in 2 clean procedures (hernia repair and varicose vein operations) in an outpatient setting. It demonstrated that only the use of spinal anesthesia was associated with an increased risk of SSI. This is certainly an outlier with respect to other procedures. Subsequently, the authors determined that the variables which determined the use of spinal anesthesia was not clear. After this finding, the authors surveyed the anesthesiologists and found that spinal anesthesia was the preferred type of anesthesia for anyone with pulmonary disease or a significant smoking history. It is conceivable that this selection process identified a population of patients at high risk for SSIs than those with poor tissue oxygenation and the establishment of increased risk.

T. L. Pruett, MD

Methicillin-Resistant *Staphylococcus aureus* Disease in Three Communities

Fridkin SK, for the Active Bacterial Core Surveillance Program of the Emerging Infections Program Network (Ctrs for Disease Control and Prevention, Atlanta, Ga; et al)

N Engl J Med 352:1436-1444, 2005 6–5

Background.—Methicillin-resistant *Staphylococcus aureus* (MRSA) infection has emerged in patients who do not have the established risk factors. The national burden and clinical effect of this novel presentation of MRSA disease are unclear.

Methods.—We evaluated MRSA infections in patients identified from population-based surveillance in Baltimore and Atlanta and from hospital-laboratory–based sentinel surveillance of 12 hospitals in Minnesota. Information was obtained by interviewing patients and by reviewing their medical records. Infections were classified as community-associated [correction] MRSA disease if no established risk factors were identified.

Results.—From 2001 through 2002, 1647 cases of community-associated [correction] MRSA infection were reported, representing between 8 and 20 percent of all MRSA isolates. The annual disease incidence varied according to site (25.7 cases per 100,000 population in Atlanta vs. 18.0 per 100,000 in Baltimore) and was significantly higher among persons less than two years old than among those who were two years of age or older (relative risk, 1.51; 95 percent confidence interval, 1.19 to 1.92) and among blacks than among whites in Atlanta (age-adjusted relative risk, 2.74; 95 percent confidence interval, 2.44 to 3.07). Six percent of cases were invasive, and 77 percent involved skin and soft tissue. The infecting strain of MRSA was often (73 percent) resistant to prescribed antimicrobial agents. Among patients with skin or soft-tissue infections, therapy to which the infecting strain was resistant did not appear to be associated with adverse patient-reported outcomes. Overall, 23 percent of patients were hospitalized for the MRSA infection.

Conclusions.—Community-associated MRSA infections are now a common and serious problem. These infections usually involve the skin, especially among children, and hospitalization is common.

► Surgeons are often called upon to assess and treat soft tissue infections. *S aureus* is one of the major pathogens associated with skin furuncles and other soft tissue infections. It has commonly been assumed that staphylococcal infections within the community are methicillin sensitive and that first-generation cephalosporins or methicillin-type penicillins are effective adjunct agents. MRSA is becoming a very common hospital-associated pathogen, but it has been slow to penetrate into the general population. This article, however, describes MRSA infections from 3 widely disparate geographic areas within the United States. In 2001 and 2002, 8% to 20% of all MRSA isolates came from community-acquired infections. Over 75% of these infections were skin and soft tissue infections, but 6% were invasive infections. This report is important for the practicing surgeon in that one cannot assume that community-acquired soft tissue infections are associated with antimicrobial-sensitive agents. It stresses the importance of adequate surgical management, since adjunctive antimicrobial agent prescription often is inadequate to effectively treat these organisms (73% in this particular series).

T. L. Pruett, MD

Staphylococcus aureus **Bacteremia in Patients With Prosthetic Devices: Costs and Outcomes**

Chu VH, Crosslin DR, Friedman JY, et al (Duke Univ, Durham, NC; Health Economics Consulting, Craftsbury, Vt)
Am J Med 118:1416, 2005 6–6

Background.—A marked increase has been observed in the rate of prosthetic device implantation in the last decade. The prosthetic devices provide life-saving interventions and improve the quality of life of many patients, but they also place these patients at risk for device-related infections. Although only a fraction of patients will develop a prosthetic device infection, each infection is associated with a high rate of morbidity and mortality. *Staphylococcus aureus* is a leading cause of nosocomial infection, but little is known of the effect of *S aureus* bacteremia in patients with prosthetic devices. The clinical outcome, health care resource use, and infection-associated costs of *S aureus* bacteremia in patients with prosthetic devices were determined.

Methods.—All patients hospitalized at 1 university-affiliated hospital with a prosthetic device and *S aureus* bacteremia for 96 months were identified prospectively. Clinical data were collected at the time of hospitalization. Data regarding infection-related resource use and infection-related costs within 12 weeks of the initial bacteremia were also recorded.

Results.—A total of 298 patients with 1 prosthesis or more and *S aureus* bacteremia were identified. Overall, 58% of patients underwent surgery as a consequence of the infection. Infection-related complications occurred in 41% of patients, and the overall 12-week mortality rate was 27%. The mean infection-related cost was $67,439 for patients with hospital-acquired *S aureus* bacteremia and $37,868 for community-acquired *S aureus* bacteremia. The rates of device infection, complications, 12-week mortality, and mean cost varied by type of prosthesis.

Conclusions.—*S aureus* bacteremia in patients with prosthetic devices is associated with frequent complications, considerable costs, and a high level of health care resource utilization.

▶ *S aureus* is a common problem for any surgeon making an incision. This becomes particularly problematic when a device is inserted with the risk of device-associated infection. In this article, the risk and costs associated with *Staphylococcus* bacteremia in patients with prosthetic devices was assessed. The authors looked at 298 patients with prostheses in *S aureus* bacteremia. The majority of these devices were cardiovascular in origin or orthopedic. In general *S aureus* bacteremia in a patient with a prosthetic device was associated with infection of that device in more than 40% of the cases. It was important to note that although it was a common association, it was by no means a universal association. It would have been much more helpful had the authors noted the time association from insertion of the device to the time of *S aureus* bacteremia. One would assume that if the *S aureus* bacteremia had occurred within several weeks of the insertion of the device, the incidence of infection of the device would have been much higher. The importance of this article, however, is to state the seriousness of the finding with the all-cause 12-week mortality rate of 25% in the orthopedic device group and 35% in the cardiac device group. A significant percentage of the patients had MRSA with a higher 12-week mortality rate also. The importance of preventing *S aureus* bacteremia and, particularly, infection of implantable devices is considerable. The combination of appropriate antimicrobial therapy and good intraoperative and perioperative management should minimize these problems.

T. L. Pruett, MD

A Randomized, Double-blind, Placebo-controlled Trial to Determine Effectiveness of Antibiotic Prophylaxis for Tension-free Mesh Herniorrhaphy

Perez AR, Roxas MF, Hilvano SS (Univ of the Philippines, Manila)
J Am Coll Surg 200:393-398, 2005 6–7

Background.—In recent years, use of prosthetic material for inguinal hernia repair has increased dramatically. Tension-free repairs have gained popularity not only for recurrent or complicated hernias, but for primary hernia repairs as well. Although routine use of prophylactic antibiotics is not recommended in the Philippines for open nonimplant herniorrhaphy, there is little direct clinical evidence on which to base recommendations when implantable mesh is used.

Study Design.—We conducted a prospective, randomized, double-blind, placebo-controlled trial comparing wound infection rates in 360 patients (180 received prophylactic antibiotics, 180 received a placebo) undergoing primary inguinal hernia repair electively using polypropylene mesh. Age, gender, American Society of Anesthesiologists class, type of hernia, type of anesthesia, and duration of operation were recorded. Infections were evaluated 1 week, 2 weeks, and 1 month after operation by an independent surgeon. All complications were recorded. Results were assessed using chi-square, Fisher's exact test, and Student's *t*-tests as appropriate.

Results.—Groups were well matched for all preoperative variables studied, including comorbid conditions. Six patients from the antibiotic group and four from the placebo group failed to followup after the second week. Superficial surgical site infection developed in 3 patients (1.7%) from the antibiotic group and 6 (3.3%) from the placebo group ($p = 0.50$). One from each group developed deep surgical site infection. Both patients were readmitted and underwent repeated debridement, which eventually resulted in graft loss.

Conclusions.—Preoperative administration of single-dose antibiotic for tension-free inguinal mesh herniorrhaphy did not markedly decrease risk of wound infection in this patient population. Our results do not support use of antibiotic prophylaxis for tension-free mesh herniorrhaphy.

▶ This article attempts to describe the role of antibiotic prophylaxis for tension-free mesh herniorrhaphy. In this setting, the patients were repaired with polypropylene mesh. Patients were randomly given either cefazolin or saline. One inspection occurred up to 4 weeks after discharge and then by phone interviews. The authors concluded that antibiotics were not useful in the prevention of surgical site infections after mesh herniorrhaphy. The incidence of surgical site infections was 1.7% in the antibiotic group and 3.3% in the placebo group, with a *P* value of 0.50. Only 360 patients underwent randomization, with the power calculations initially being chosen based on a 7% wound infection rate in the no-antibiotic group and a reduction to 1% in the antimicrobial group. Both of these assumptions proved to be wrong. In the placebo group, the infection rate was only 3.3%, not 7%, and the efficacy of antibiotics would not be expected to reduce surgical site infections as much as the authors assumed. Yet interestingly, all the infections that occurred, both in the antibiotic and placebo groups, were caused by *Staphylococcus* species, with the vast majority being caused by *Staphylococcus aureus*. Patients with deep polymicrobial infections that included *Pseudomonas* species had to have their grafts removed. The authors concluded that antibiotics were not beneficial in this patient population. However, I do not believe that the methods justify that conclusion, and the results actually suggest that had the subject population been larger, the antibiotics would have been beneficial and led to decreased morbidity.

T. L. Pruett, MD

Surgical Salvage of Peritoneal Dialysis Catheters From Chronic Exit-Site and Tunnel Infections

Crabtree JH, Burchette RJ (Kaiser Permanente Bellflower Med Ctr, Calif; Kaiser Permanente Southern California, Pasadena)

Am J Surg 190:4-8, 2005 6–8

Background.—Chronic exit-site and tunnel infections of the peritoneal dialysis catheter are significant causes of catheter loss. Surgical salvage procedures that can effectively resolve the infection and preserve dialysis are of major importance.

Methods.—Thirteen patients with chronic exit-site and tunnel infections underwent surgical salvage consisting of unroofing the tunnel tract and shaving of the superficial catheter cuff. A control group of 138 patients implanted during the same time span as the study group was used for infection rate and survival comparisons.

Results.—The salvage procedure cured the infection in all patients. No dialysate leaks occurred. Peritoneal dialysis was not interrupted. Surgical salvage provided successful long-term peritoneal dialysis that was equivalent to the cohort dialysis population.

Conclusion.—Surgical salvage by unroofing/cuff shaving is an effective long-term solution for chronic exit-site and tunnel infection.

► There are a variety of different approaches to dealing with the infected prosthetic material. Typically, the consulting services state that the only way to cure and to maintain infection-free status is to remove the foreign material. While this is certainly a truism in ultimate control of infections, a variety of different techniques have been developed to maintain the functionality of surgical devices without their removal. One such manuscript is cited here describing many of the technical issues relating to the management of devices that cross the skin.

T. L. Pruett, MD

Surgical Treatment of Large Contaminated Abdominal Wall Defects

van Geffen HJAA, Simmermacher RKJ, van Vroonhoven TJMV, et al (Univ Med Centre, Utrecht, The Netherlands)

J Am Coll Surg 201:206-212, 2005 6–9

Background.—Repair of a large, severely contaminated abdominal wall defect is a challenging problem. Most patients are currently treated with a multistaged procedure, which is time consuming, carries a high complication rate, and is often not finalized.

Study Design.—In this study, our experience with a one-stage repair of contaminated abdominal wall defects using the Components Separation Method was evaluated with respect to morbidity and recurrence. Medical records of patients with contaminated abdominal wall defects, treated with the Components Separation Method from 1996 to 2000, were studied. Patients were invited to visit the outpatient clinic for a physical examination.

Results.—Twenty-six patients with a median age of 49 years and a mean defect size of 267 cm^2 were treated. Intraoperative contamination, graded according to the National Research Council (NRC), showed 22 National Research Council III patients and 4 National Research Council IV patients. Postoperatively, five superficial wound infections, three cases of pneumonia, three instances of recurrent enterocutaneous fistulation, and two cases of sepsis were observed. One of the patients with sepsis died after anastomotic disruption led to peritonitis and multiple organ failure. Two asymptomatic recurrences were diagnosed (8%) after a median followup of 27 months.

Conclusions.—Large contaminated abdominal wall hernias can be closed by the Components Separation Method, with a low recurrence rate but considerable morbidity.

▶ The management of the large open wound from intra-abdominal infection has proven to be particularly challenging. The article by van Geffen et al discusses many of the technical issues relating to closure techniques of these wounds. Of particular note is the issue of the chronic fistula within the operative site. The recurrence of fistulas after repair is always problematic, and these patients represent a significant challenge. The components separation method as described can be quite successful, but leads to significant morbidity and some mortality.

T. L. Pruett, MD

Salvage of Infected Prosthetic Grafts of the Great Vessels via Muscle Flap Reconstruction

Mitra A, Spears J, Perrotta V, et al (Temple Univ, Philadelphia)

Chest 128:1040-1043, 2005 6–10

Objective.—The infection of an aortic prosthetic graft presents a difficult challenge for surgeons. Conservative treatments such as debridement and antibiotic irrigation routinely fail, and patient survival rates are low. Literature has indicated that flap procedures often provide better treatment. In the present article, we report our experience utilizing pectoralis major muscle flaps, occasionally coupled with latissimus dorsi, rectus abdominis, and/or serratus anterior flaps, to wrap infected grafts and fill dead space.

Patients.—Between 1990 and 2004, 10 patients were brought to our attention with infections of prosthetic grafts of the great vessels (7 men and 3 women; mean age, 53 years). Infections in nine patients involved an ascending aortic graft, while one patient had an infected pulmonary artery graft.

Design.—Following diagnosis and exploration, an initial debridement is performed, followed by 48 h of antibiotic irrigation. A definitive muscle flap procedure is then utilized to fill dead space and clear the infection, followed by an appropriate antibiotic regimen.

Results.—The infections in all 10 patients were cleared using the muscle flap procedure. Two patients required a tapered-dose regimen of oral steroids, one of whom also required a secondary flap procedure due to the advanced stage of infection. Two other patients later died due to unrelated complications; however, autopsies revealed that operative sites had healed successfully. Patients were followed up for a period of 2 months to 2 years, and recurrence was not found.

Conclusions.—Our outcomes suggest that muscle flap procedures, specifically utilizing the pectoralis major and regional muscles, should be kept in mind in the management of life-threatening infections of aortic grafts. Due to the limited number of patients in this study, we feel more research with a larger volume of cases is warranted.

► Management of the infected prosthetic graft is exceptionally challenging. The current series consists of 10 patients in whom salvage of infected prosthetic grafts of the great vessels was accomplished by using primarily pectoralis major muscle flaps. The importance of adequate drainage and obliteration of dead space with replacement of well-vascularized material is a well-documented technique in the literature. These infected vascular grafts in the great vessels are particularly challenging, as there is often no alternative to removal. Of considerable concern in all of these techniques is the eventual disruption of anastomotic sites between the native vessel and the graft over time. The duration of appropriate antimicrobial therapy, although unknown, is quite protracted. The management is a combination of excellent surgical technique as well as appropriate antimicrobial therapy. The observation in this series that no patients died of exsanguination is probably related to too short of a duration of follow-up; however, the early results are quite encouraging.

T. L. Pruett, MD

Microbiology and Factors Affecting Mortality in Necrotizing Fasciitis

Liu Y-M, Chi C-Y, Ho M-W, et al (St Joseph Hosp, Yulin, Taiwan; China Med Univ, Taichung, Taiwan)

J Microbiol Immunol Infect 38:430-435, 2005 6–11

Introduction.—Necrotizing fasciitis is a life-threatening soft-tissue infection primarily involving the superficial fascia. This study investigated the microbiologic characteristics and determinants of mortality of this disease. The medical records of 87 consecutive patients with a diagnosis of necrotizing fasciitis from 1999 to 2004 were retrospectively reviewed. A single pathogen was identified as the infectious agent in 59 patients (67.8%), multiple pathogens were identified in 17 patients (19.6%), and no organism was identified in 11 patients (12.6%). *Klebsiella pneumoniae*, identified in 17 patients, was the most commonly isolated species. The most common comorbidity was diabetes mellitus (41 patients; 53.2%). Multivariate logistic regression analysis showed that more than 1 comorbidity, thrombocytopenia, anemia, more than 24 h delay from onset of symptoms to surgery and age greater than 60 were independently associated with mortality. This study found that *K. pneumoniae* was the most common cause of necrotizing fasciitis. Early operative debridement was independently associated with lower mortality.

► Treatment of necrotizing fasciitis is typically within the purview of the surgeon. An intriguing portion of the medical literature is written by our nonsurgical colleagues. In this article, the authors describe the importance of comorbidities and ultimate survival is stressed. Patients with cirrhosis, immunosuppression, and malignancy had a significantly higher mortality rate with necrotizing fasciitis. The authors, however, did not describe, other than amputation, the surgical techniques and the timing to adequate debridement. The current series has a high rate of water-associated organisms, consistent with the island setting of the study. The management strategy, however, of necrotizing soft tissue infections is increasingly becoming an important issue for the practicing surgeon. Strategies to manage necrotizing infections arising in the perineum and buttocks or truncal area are certainly different from those to manage infections originating from the extremities.

T. L. Pruett, MD

Predictors of Mortality and Limb Loss in Necrotizing Soft Tissue Infections

Anaya DA, McMahon K, Nathens AB, et al (Harborview Med Ctr, Seattle; Univ of Washington, Seattle)

Arch Surg 140:151-157, 2005 6–12

Hypothesis.—Necrotizing soft tissue infections are associated with a high mortality rate. We hypothesize that specific predictors of limb loss and mortality in patients with necrotizing soft tissue infection can be identified on hospital admission.

Design.—A retrospective cohort study.

Setting.—A tertiary care center.

Patients.—Patients with a diagnosis of necrotizing soft tissue infection during a 5-year period (1996-2001) were included. Patients were identified with *International Classification of Diseases, Ninth Revision* hospital discharge diagnosis codes, and diagnosis was confirmed by medical record review.

Interventions.—Standard current treatment including early and scheduled repeated debridement, broad-spectrum antibiotics, and physiologic and nutritional support was given to all patients.

Main Outcome Measures.—Limb loss and mortality.

Results.—One hundred sixty-six patients were identified and included in the study. The overall mortality rate was 16.9%, and limb loss occurred in 26% of patients with extremity involvement. Independent predictors of mortality included white blood cell count greater than $30{,}000 \times 10^3/\mu L$, creatinine level greater than 2 mg/dL (176.8 µmol/L), and heart disease at hospital admission. Independent predictors of limb loss included heart disease and shock (systolic blood pressure <90 mm Hg) at hospital admission. Clostridial infection was an independent predictor for both limb loss (odds ratio, 3.9 [95% confidence interval, 1.1-12.8]) and mortality (odds ratio, 4.1 [95% confidence interval, 1.3-12.3]) and was highly associated with intravenous drug use and a high rate of leukocytosis on hospital admission. The latter was found to be a good variable in estimating the probability of death.

Conclusions.—Clostridial infection is consistently associated with poor outcome. This together with the independent predictors mentioned earlier should aid in identifying patients on hospital admission who may benefit from more aggressive and novel therapeutic approaches.

The Evolving Characteristics and Care of Necrotizing Soft-Tissue Infections

Endorf FW, Supple KG, Gamelli RL (Loyola Univ, Maywood, Ill)

Burns 31:269-273, 2005 6–13

Background.—Necrotizing soft-tissue infections such as necrotizing fasciitis and Fournier's gangrene are a source of high morbidity and mortality. These difficult cases are increasingly being referred to burn centers for specialized wound and critical care issues. In this study, we examine our institution's recent experience with a large series of necrotizing soft-tissue infections.

Study Design.—A retrospective chart review was performed of 65 consecutive patients over a 5-year period with necrotizing soft-tissue infections that required radical surgical debridement.

Results.—Overall survival was 83%, with an average length of stay of 32.4 ± 3.32 days for survivors and for the entire group of 29.5 ± 3 days. Time from onset of symptoms to initial presentation to our institution averaged 6.9 ± 1.19 days. Patients averaged 2.9 ± 0.22 surgical procedures, and 46% of patients required skin grafting with an average graft area of 1554 ± 248 cm^2. Of the survivors, only 54% were able to return home, with 46% needing further hospitalization or transfer to an inpatient rehabilitation facility.

Conclusions.—There were frequent delays in diagnosis and referrals to and from within our institution, and progress can be made in educating the medical community to identify these patients. Advancements in wound care and critical care have made inroads into the treatment of patients with necrotizing soft-tissue infections. However, these infections continue to be a source of high morbidity and mortality and significant healthcare resource consumption. These challenging patients are best served with prompt diagnosis, immediate radical surgical debridement, and aggressive critical care management. Referral to a major burn center may help provide optimal surgical intervention, wound care, and critical care management.

► The group from the University of Washington describes its experience with 166 patients seen over a 5-year period (Abstract 6–12). The majority of these infections arose in the extremities and were associated with IV drug use. The need for amputation to control infection was associated predominately with clostridial myonecrosis. Most infections were polymicrobial. The authors do not describe in their "Results" section a time to surgical debridement; however, in their "Discussion" section it is a general premise that all patients undergo an early resection after resuscitation. In this setting, the majority of patients underwent debridement within the first 24 hours after presentation. The summary that sick people die is intuitively correct; however, the delineation of the number of variables associated with the definition of "sick people" is quite useful.

The management of necrotizing soft tissue infections can be quite complex, with the need for multiple debridements and then rehabilitation. As a consequence, the notion of a dedicated team to care for not only the medical but rehabilitation components associated with these advanced wounds is discussed in the article by Endorf et al (Abstract 6–13). In this setting, the average number of procedures performed was 2.9, with a high of 10 procedures, before definitive control was gained. The use of vacuum-assisted wound closure was shown to be quite useful in many of these individuals. In comparison with the prior articles on necrotizing soft tissue infections (Abstracts 6–11 and 6–12), in this series streptococcal species were the most common organisms. The diversity of infections and laboratory isolates emphasizes the diversity of the disease and the need for consistent surgical management and culture assessment of the causative organisms. It is quite clear, however, that this is not just a debridement procedure but also one in which it is necessary to establish rehabilitation functional goals.

T. L. Pruett, MD

Hyperbaric Oxygen as Adjuvant Therapy in the Management of Necrotizing Fasciitis

Jallali N, Withey S, Butler PE (Royal Free Hosp, London)
Am J Surg 189:462-466, 2005 6–14

Background.—Necrotizing fasciitis (NF) is an uncommon but serious infection of fascia and skin associated with considerable morbidity and mortality. One modality proposed for improving the outcome of this condition is hyperbaric oxygen (HBO) therapy. This is a form of medical treatment that involves intermittent inhalation of 100% oxygen under pressures exceeding the atmosphere. The aim of this article is to review current practice and evidence for the use of HBO as adjunctive therapy in the management of NF.

Methods.—A survey of published English literature through searches of Medline and PubMed was carried out using the following key words: "necrotizing fasciitis," "Fournier's gangrene," "necrotizing soft tissue infections," "hyperbaric oxygen therapy," and "hyperbaric oxygen chambers."

Results.—The results of studies on the use of HBO therapy in NF are inconsistent. Some studies have demonstrated that HBO can improve patient survival and decrease the number of debridements required to achieve wound control, whereas others have failed to show any beneficial effect.

Conclusions.—Encouraging results have been achieved with the addition of HBO therapy to standard treatment regimes, thus justifying further research in this field. More robust evidence by way of a prospective randomized trial is necessary before widespread and routine use of HBO in the management of NF can be recommended.

► One of the more discussed adjuncts to the management of NF has been the use of HBO. The current article reviews the existing English-language literature for efficacy of HBO in necrotizing infection. "There is general consensus that resuscitation, radical debridement, and broad-spectrum antibiotics form the corner stones of management of NF. HBO must compliment and not substitute these interventions." This statement within the "Clinical Evidence" section summarizes the remaining portion of the article. There are believers and nonbelievers. The rationale for the use of HBO is considerable, but the clinical evidence of it efficacy is lacking. The evidence stresses that resuscitation and surgical debridement should be the primary goals to maintain adequate results in managing NF.

T. L. Pruett, MD

Long-term Outcome of Mesocolic and Pelvic Diverticular Abscesses of the Left Colon: A Prospective Study of 73 Cases

Ambrosetti P, Chautems R, Soravia C, et al (Univ Hosp of Geneva)

Dis Colon Rectum 48:787-791, 2005 6–15

Purpose.—The aim of this study was to evaluate prospectively the long-term outcome of mesocolic and pelvic diverticular abscesses of the left colon.

Methods.—Between October 1986 and October 1997, a total of 465 patients urgently admitted to our hospital with a suspected diagnosis of acute left-sided colonic diverticulitis had a CT scan. Of 76 patients (17 percent) who had an associated mesocolic or pelvic abscess, 3 were lost to follow-up. The remaining 73 patients (45 with a mesocolic abscess and 28 with a pelvic abscess) were followed for a median of 43 months.

Results.—Of the 45 patients with a mesocolic abscess, 7 (15 percent) required surgery during their first hospitalization versus 11 (39 percent) of the 28 patients with a pelvic abscess ($P = 0.04$). At the end of follow-up, 22 (58 percent) of the 38 patients with a mesocolic abscess who had successful conservative treatment during their first hospitalization did not need surgical treatment *vs.* 8 (47 percent) of the 17 who had a pelvic abscess. Altogether, 51 percent of the patients with a mesocolic abscess had surgical treatment versus 71 percent of those with a pelvic abscess ($P = 0.09$).

Conclusions.—Considering the poor outcome of pelvic abscess associated with acute left-sided colonic diverticulitis, percutaneous drainage followed by secondary colectomy seems justified. Mesocolic abscess by itself is not an absolute indication for colectomy.

► The management of intra-abdominal abscesses has changed considerably during the past decade. There are many proponents of minimally invasive source control procedures. The problem with most studies has been the inability to stratify patients appropriately or with enough granularity to discern optimal treatments predicated upon the etiology of the disease. This study is an attempt to prospectively assess the management of abscesses associated with diverticular disease of the left colon. It attempts to stratify entry criteria but necessarily allows all the subjective criteria as to indications for operation, percutaneous drainage, success or failure of such procedures, and types of antimicrobial therapy. In general, an attempt was made to allow for a single-stage procedure with percutaneous drainage and resolution of an abscess and then determination of whether definitive therapy was required. The findings were that patients with pelvic abscesses were more likely to require surgery than those with colic abscesses. Drainage was commonly necessary for abscesses greater than 5 cm, making conservative management with antimicrobial therapy unpalatable. This is a useful article in trying to stratify diseases. However, many variables are left out, such as previous courses of antibiotics, types of organisms found, complexity and duration of symptoms, and time to resolution. Despite all of these factors, this is still a useful article.

T. L. Pruett, MD

Fungus-Infected Fluid Collections in Thorax or Abdomen: Effectiveness of Percutaneous Catheter Drainage

Varghese JC, Hahn PF, Harisinghani MG, et al (Massachusetts Gen Hosp, Boston)

Radiology 236:730-738, 2005 6–16

Purpose.—To retrospectively evaluate the effectiveness of percutaneous catheter drainage in the treatment of fungus-infected fluid collections in the thorax or abdomen and to identify any factor that may be predictive of a poor clinical outcome.

Materials and Methods.—Approval for this study was obtained from the hospital ethics subcommittee on human studies. Because the study was retrospective, patient informed consent was not required. This study was compliant with the Health Insurance Portability and Accountability Act. Retrospective analysis was performed of cases of fungus-infected fluid collections in the thorax or abdomen treated by using percutaneous catheter drainage in 60 patients (36 male and 24 female patients; mean age, 57 years; range, 2 months to 91 years) during 5 years. The patient medical records were reviewed to identify recognized factors for predisposition to fungal infection. The details of percutaneous catheter drainage and microbiologic findings were recorded. The technical success (ability of catheters placed to drain collections treated) and the clinical success (ability of patients to recover fully without surgery) of percutaneous catheter drainage were determined. A multifactor logistic regression analysis was performed to identify any clinical or microbiologic factor predictive of a poor clinical outcome.

Results.—Seventy-three fungus-infected fluid collections were drained in 60 patients. The collections originated from the pleura ($n = 6$), mediastinum ($n = 2$), liver ($n = 3$), pancreas ($n = 5$), obstructed biliary or urinary tract ($n = 9$), gallbladder ($n = 1$), and abdominopelvic area ($n = 47$). The technical success rate for catheter drainage was 79% (41 of 52 patients); the clinical success rate, 57% (34 of 60 patients). Twenty (33%) patients died from all causes during hospital admission. Multifactor logistic regression analysis was used to identify predictors of a poor clinical outcome; complexity of collection, history of malignancy, and admission to intensive care unit were significant ($P < .03$) and independent predictors.

Conclusion.—Despite a moderately high technical success rate with percutaneous catheter drainage of fungus-infected fluid collections, clinical success rate was much lower. Both imaging appearance (complexity of collection) and clinical factors (history of malignancy, admission to intensive care unit) influenced prognosis.

► The issue of how to manage patients with difficult fluid infections has always been controversial. Initial early studies in the 1980s with percutaneous drainage suggested a high failure rate with abscesses predominately contaminated with fungus because of their consistency and failure to evacuate through a catheter tube. The current series looks at the success of percutaneous catheter drainage with fungus-infected fluid collections. There were 60 cases reviewed from a variety of sources. The clinical success rate was about 60%; about one third of the patients died of various causes during the hospital admission. This report, being primarily a radiology article, notes the relatively higher success rate than that found in previous surgical series, but still notes the modestly inferior rate compared with routine bacterial-type infections. For the clinician, the importance is not so much the identification of the specific organism, but rather whether the catheter is effectively able to do what is desired—that is, source control. Allowing for obliteration of the abscess cavity is key to resolution of any space infection. Sometimes fungal infections do not portend adequate removal of infected material.

T. L. Pruett, MD

Endoscopic Debridement of Paraesophageal, Mediastinal Abscesses: A Prospective Case Series

Wehrmann T, Stergiou N, Vogel B, et al (Klinikum Hannover-Siloah, Germany; Klinikum Hannover-Heidehaus, Germany)
Gastrointest Endosc 62:344-349, 2005 6–17

Background.—Mediastinal abscesses after esophageal perforation or postoperative leakage nearly always require surgical intervention.

Methods.—Patients with paraesophageal abscesses were treated with EUS-guided or endoscopic mediastinal puncture if the abscess was >2 cm and sepsis was present. Abscess cavities were entered with a 9.5-mm endoscope after balloon dilation to allow irrigation and drainage. Debris was removed with a Dormia basket. Concomitant pleural effusions were treated with transthoracic drains. Patients received intravenous antibiotics and enteral/parenteral nutrition.

Results.—Twenty patients fulfilled the entry criteria. Simple drainage was sufficient in 4 cases, and puncture was impossible in one case. Of the 15 treated patients (age 39-76 years, 5 women) the etiology of perforation was Boerhaave's syndrome (n = 8), anastomotic leak (n = 3), and iatrogenic perforation (n = 4). Debridement was successful in all cases and required a median of 5 daily sessions (range 3-10). All patients became apyrexial, with a C-reactive protein < 5 mg/L within a median of 4 days (range 2-8 days). Esophageal defects were closed with endoclips (n = 7), fibrin glue (n = 4), metal stents (n = 1), or spontaneously healed (n = 3). One patient died from a massive pulmonary embolism one day after successful debridement (mortality 7%). No other complications were seen. Median follow-up was 12 months (range 3-40 months).

Conclusions.—Nonoperative endoscopic transesophageal debridement of mediastinal abscesses appears safe and effective.

► In keeping with the minimal and invasive approach to the management of infections, this article describes the endoscopic debridement of paraesophageal mediastinal abscesses. In these settings, paraesophageal abscesses were initially treated and identified through endoscopic US and mediastinal puncture of the abscess. A combination of techniques was obtained to generate adequate evacuation of the contents, and resolution was frequent. It does not appear to matter how one approaches an infection, whether it is through a tube or a minimally invasive procedure. The importance resides in the adequacy and adherence to surgical principles of evacuation allowing of collapse and ensuring the absence of foreign bodies, tumors, fistulas, etc, within the infected bed. The technique tricks, to adequately accomplish drainage, are important. More such studies are needed to find the optimal way to manage infections with the least amount of morbidity.

T. L. Pruett, MD

Does a Second-Look Operation Improve Survival in Patients With Peritonitis Due to Acute Mesenteric Ischemia? A Five-Year Retrospective Experience

Kaminsky O, Yampolski I, Aranovich D, et al (Rabin Med Ctr, Petah Tiqva, Israel; Tel Aviv Univ, Israel)

World J Surg 29:645-648, 2005 6–18

Introduction.—Second-look laparotomy is one of the mainstays of surgical treatment of acute mesenteric ischemia (AMI). The aim of this study was to analyze its role in the survival of patients with infarcted gangrenous bowel resulting from AMI. A retrospective chart review of all patients admitted over the study period was undertaken. The study population consisted of 41 patients with clinical evidence of peritonitis and gangrenous, perforated bowel on surgical exploration. Outcome was compared among patients who underwent second-look laparotomy and those who did not. Fifteen patients with an American Society of Anesthesiologists (ASA) score of less than

4 underwent second-look laparotomy. Six patients had residual necrotic bowel that required additional resection. Only one (17%) of them survived. Of the nine remaining patients, who had no evidence of necrosis, only two survived (22%). Overall survival in this group was 20%. Twenty-six patients were managed without second-look laparotomy. Nine of them, with an ASA score of 4-5, died soon after the operation. The decision not to operate on the remaining 17 patients with an ASA score < 4 was made by an experienced surgeon. Eleven of those patients (65%) survived. Overall survival in the non–second-look group was 42%. Excluding the early deaths, the survival in the non re-explored group was significantly higher than in the second-look group (65% vs. 20%, $p = 0.011$). A selective approach to the surgical treatment of acute mesenteric ischemia based on the sound clinical judgment of an experienced surgeon may be as appropriate as its universal application.

► One of the mainstays of the treatment of peritonitis associated with AMI has been routine second-look procedures to ensure control of infected fluid pockets as well as to verify that there are no missed ischemic lesions with subsequent necrosis. This concept is challenged in this article, in which clinical judgment was used to determine whether patients would be returned for a second look. Forty-one patients who had peritonitis and gangrenous perforated bowel on initial surgical exploration were studied. Outcomes were compared among patients who underwent a second-look operation and those who did not. Fifteen of the patients who had an ASA score of less than 4 underwent second-look laparotomies. Six of these 15 had residual necrotic bowel, and only 1 of the 6 survived. Of the 9 additional patients who had no evidence of necrosis, only 2 survived. Therefore, the overall survival of patients who had a second-look procedure was a paltry 20%. Of the 26 patients who were managed without second-look procedures, 9 with a very high ASA score died soon after the laparotomy. The decision not to operate on the remaining 17 patients with an ASA score of less than 4 was made by clinical judgment, and 65% of these patients survived. The authors recommend a selective approach to the surgical treatment of AMI based on the "sound" clinical judgment of an experienced surgeon.

The pitfall of this article is that it is difficult to quantify what sound judgment consists of. Indeed, if it could be quantified and used as a metric, much of our surgical training would take on an entirely new effort. It is not clear in those patients who died, what the etiologies of death were. One would presume it was a combination of acute renal insufficiency requiring dialysis and subsequent hospital-associated infections. Mechanisms to minimize these complications are optimal for good patient care but are not explicitly described within this article. Further reports describing judgment need to incorporate at least the key components of decision making that are considered to be important to outcomes.

T. L. Pruett, MD

Lysis-Deficient Bacteriophage Therapy Decreases Endotoxin and Inflammatory Mediator Release and Improves Survival in a Murine Peritonitis Model

Matsuda T, Freeman TA, Hilbert DW, et al (Cornell Univ, New York; Temple Univ, Philadelphia)

Surgery 137:639-646, 2005 6–19

Background.—Lysis-deficient (LyD) bacteriophages (phages) kill bacteria without endotoxin (Et) release. This may minimize systemic cytokine responses and limit inflammation in bacterial sepsis. We determined the effects of t amber A3 T4 LyD and virulent wild-type (WT) phages on mouse bacterial peritonitis.

Methods.—Balb/c mice were injected with B40sul *Escherichia coli*, treated intraperitoneally with LyD, WT, or a β-lactam antibiotic [latamoxef sodium (LMOX)], and followed for survival. We measured Et release, tumor necrosis factor (TNF)-α and interleukin (IL)-6, as well as bacterial counts and peritoneal exudative cells (PECs) in peritoneal lavage fluid at 6 and 12 hours after infection.

Results.—LyD mice showed significantly greater survival compared with other groups. Et levels were significantly lower in the LyD mice at 6 and 12 hours after infection. TNF-α and IL-6 levels were lower in LyD mice compared with control (untreated) mice at 12 hours. Compared with controls, bacteria counts in peritoneal lavage fluid were lower in all treatment groups (LyD, WT, or LMOX) at 6 and 12 hours. PEC counts were highest in LyD mice at 6 hours but significantly lower than that in WT phage- and LMOX-treated mice at 12 hours.

Conclusions.—LyD phage therapy significantly improves survival and attenuates the systemic effects of bacterial sepsis by minimizing Et release and pro-inflammatory mediators in murine bacterial peritonitis. Further studies may find phage therapy useful in treating peritonitis and multidrug-resistant bacterial infections.

► On the laboratory side of surgical infection, it is clear that different approaches to control the inflammatory response after contamination that requires surgical intervention need to be undertaken. This article describes the role of LyD bacteriophage therapy in the treatment of a murine peritonitis model. The authors describe that such therapy decreased the Et inflammatory mediator release and allowed for improved survival in an *E coli* peritonitis infection model. There are many potential options to modify bacterial infections that do not involve the use of antimicrobial agents. The possibility that bacteriophages may be useful in the treatment of human disease has been around for some time. There are many limitations to these forms of treatment specifically related to the specificity of the phage-bacteria interaction. Despite these limitations, the prospect of non–antibiotic-based adjuncts in the management of surgical infections is going to be essential as the breadth of antibiotic resistance continues to expand.

T. L. Pruett, MD

Sex Differences in Cytokine Production and Surface Antigen Expression of Peripheral Blood Mononuclear Cells After Surgery

Ono S, Tsujimoto H, Hiraki S-i, et al (Natl Defense Med College, Saitama, Japan)

Am J Surg 190:439-444, 2005 6–20

Background.—Several clinical and epidemiological studies have observed a better outcome after sepsis in women than in men. The purpose of this study was to determine if these sex differences are observed in cytokine responses and the surface antigen expression of monocytes. In addition, the clinical courses of male and female patients after gastrointestinal surgery were compared.

Methods.—A total of 25 patients with gastric carcinoma who underwent gastrectomy were enrolled in this study. Tumor necrosis factor-α (TNF-α), interleukin-10, and interferon-γ (IFN-γ) production by lipopolysaccharide-stimulated peripheral blood mononuclear cells (PBMCs) as well as the expression of Toll-like receptor-4 (TLR-4), TLR-2, human leukocyte antigen–D related (HLA-DR), and CD16 on monocytes in 16 men and 9 women on the day before surgery were compared with measurements on postoperative day (POD) 1. Furthermore, postoperative infectious complications, the development of systemic inflammatory response syndrome, and serum C-reactive protein levels on POD3 were compared.

Results.—TNF-α production of PBMCs and TLR-2 and CD16 expression on monocytes were significantly higher in women than in men before surgery. IFN-γ production of PBMCs and HLA-DR expression on monocytes were significantly lower in men than in women on POD1. Furthermore, TNF-γ production of PBMCs on POD1 was significantly increased, and both IFN-γ production and HLA-DR expression were significantly decreased compared with that observed before surgery in men, but no corresponding significant changes were observed in women. In addition, C-reactive protein levels on POD3 were significantly higher in men than in women.

Conclusions.—Both TNF-α and interleukin-10 production of PBMCs and both TLR-2 and CD16 expression on monocytes were significantly higher in women than in men on the day before surgery. Excessive TNF-α and suppressive IFN-γ production of PBMCs, as well as a decrease in HLA-DR expression on monocytes, occurred more often in men than in women after surgery, suggesting that these factors all contribute to an increased susceptibility of men to develop systemic inflammatory response syndrome or postoperative infectious complications.

► Several clinical and epidemiologic studies have observed better outcomes in women than in men after sustaining infectious insults. A variety of different laboratory attempts have been made to study the role of sex hormones and immune responsiveness. In the current study, 25 patients were assessed, and the differences in monocyte response from men and women were compared on POD1. It was discerned that women had significantly higher TNF production, TLR2, and CD16 expression on monocytes. In addition, IFN-γ production and HLA-DR expression were significantly lower in men than in women on POD1. Interestingly, in this study, all the women were premenopausal, and the ages between women and men were reasonably matched. The authors did not include matched older patients for comparison. The clinical complications that occurred in the 2 groups were not significantly different; however, the trends were intriguing. Differences in gender, polymorphisms of cytokine receptors, and secretion patterns may all have an impact on susceptibility for further infection. The exact role of these differences for the development of clinical diseases is unclear, but certainly stresses the heterogeneity of our population's susceptibility to adverse outcomes.

T. L. Pruett, MD

7 Endocrine

Introduction

This year's chapter on endocrine surgery focuses on the continuing advances made in translational studies on thyroid cancer, as well as highlights progress made in other fields of endocrine surgery. As usual, the number of high-impact articles exceeded the space that can be devoted to endocrine surgery.

The first Abstract by Skinner et al (Abstract 7–1) serves as a landmark paper on the benefits of bench to bedside research. This paper documents the beneficial effects of prophylactic thyroidectomy in patients identified to be carriers of ret gene mutations (familial MTC and MEN-2). While in many ways this is an early interim report, it validates the concept of prophylactic thyroidectomy in patients with MEN-2. Dr Skinner and his group should continue to be applauded for their efforts in treating these patients. The second item (Abstract 7–2) included this year is a graph published in the JNCI demonstrating the rise in thyroid cancer cases in the United States over the last 25 years. While it is unclear how many of these cases result from incidentally discovered masses during imaging of the neck for other reasons, it is clear that the prevalence of thyroid cancer will continue to rise in the United States over the next decade, even if the number of new cases levels off. This has important implications regarding long-term management issues as noted below.

The next Abstract is a consensus report regarding the diagnostic workup of thyroid nodules found at ultrasound (Abstract 7–3). While the report does not really set down firm guidelines, it is an excellent review of the utility of thyroid ultrasound in the diagnosis of thyroid nodules. The next several Abstracts also focus on the diagnostic management of thyroid nodules. Abstract 7–4 looks at a 3-gene combination that the authors say can be utilized to discriminate benign and malignant thyroid nodules. Whether this gene combination will be the most predictive, or other similar tests still under development will prove to be more accurate and widely applicable, remains to be seen. However, this Abstract indicates that a molecular approach to the diagnosis of thyroid nodules is coming. Abstract 7–5 examines an area that remains a focus of controversy—the identification of Hurthle cells on thyroid nodule FNA. Hurthle cells remain a cause for significant concern in many endocrinologists' and patients' minds. Alaedeen et al show that the majority of these lesions are benign and advocate a conservative approach. Abstract 7–6 examines the outcomes of routine calcitonin measurement in patients with thyroid nodules. This large study found a similar rate of detection of medullary thyroid carcinoma as previous large European studies and uses the data to support the contention that calcitonin measurement should be a routine part of the diagnostic screen when managing a patient with a thyroid nodule. Whether calcitonin measurement should be a standard test when evaluating a patient with a thyroid nodule remains to be proven.

The next group of Abstracts focuses on the appropriate treatment of differentiated thyroid cancer (DTC). Abstract 7–7 is a consensus report from Europe regarding indications for treatment of DTC with radioactive iodine. It is a useful guide for management and reflects what many, but certainly not all, endocrinologists and endocrine surgeons currently recommend in their own practices. Abstracts 7–8 and 7–9 focus on the ability to predict recurrence (and thus the need for more intensive therapy up front) in DTC using serum thyroglobulin (Tg) measurement. Both groups used Tg measurement before initial postoperative RAI treatment as a marker for tumors more likely to recur. Kloos and Mazzaferri (Abstract 7–8) used thyrogen-stimulated Tg, while Kim et al (Abstract 7–9) employed thyroid hormone withdrawal to stimulate Tg rise.

In Abstract 7–10, Leboulleux et al examine a large series of patients with papillary thyroid cancer and lymph node metastases. They show that extracapsular extension of thyroid cancer in lymph nodes is a significant risk factor for recurrence. While many thyroid cancer specialists have assumed that this is in fact the case, this paper provides excellent support for the contention that extracapsular lymph node extension is an important prognostic indicator for a high-risk tumor, similar to extrathyroidal extension of the primary tumor.

Abstracts 7–11 and 7–12 examine the predictive value of BRAF mutations in thyroid cancer prognosis. Unfortunately, the 2 groups arrive at opposite conclusions. While the Hopkins group (Abstract 7–11) finds that BRAF mutations are an independent prognostic indicator for aggressive tumors in a multicenter study, the group from Portugal, Spain, and Brazil (Abstract 7–12) found that BRAF mutations correlate with age, but no markers of aggressive behavior in a series of over 300 patients. These 2 diametrically opposed results leave the question of whether BRAF mutations will prove to be a prognostic indicator unanswered for the present time. The last Abstract included on thyroid disease (Abstract 7–13) makes the question of prognosis an important one, not just for how aggressively to treat a patient at diagnosis, but also how aggressively to suppress TSH over the ensuing years. The authors clearly demonstrate cardiac consequences of TSH suppression, specifically diastolic dysfunction, which is a specific risk factor for cardiac events. The implications are quite clear—patients who have low-risk DTCs should not have their TSH significantly suppressed, as this leads to quantifiable cardiac dysfunction. Patients with known metastases or substantial risk for recurrence should continue to have aggressive TSH suppression.

Abstracts 7–14 and 7–15 are related to parathyroid disease. The first of these Abstracts is a study reported in the *The New England Journal of Medicine* regarding the efficacy of cinacalcet in the treatment of primary hyperparathyroidism. The authors show that cinacalcet does control the biochemical changes associated with primary hyperparathyroidism and suggest that this is a viable medical option for the treatment of primary hyperparathyroidism. While the data are good in a well-conducted study, it is far too early to conclude that primary hyperparathyroidism is now a medical disease, as the long-term implications of taking cinacalcet regarding management of primary hyperparathyroidism remain unknown at this time. Prospective studies comparing medical treatment with surgery should be conducted to adequately evaluate the two treatments. Abstract 7–15 reports on the incidence of HRPT2 mutations in parathyroid adenomas. The authors find that the incidence of HRPT2 mutations in adenomas is very low (<1%, and possibly lower). Since these mutations are common in parathyroid carcinomas, the authors suggest that this difference could be exploited to differentiate adenomas from carcinomas. This will have to be tested prospectively in cases that are difficult to classify, such as atypical adenomas.

Abstracts 7–16 through 7–18 focus on adrenal disorders. Abstract 7–16 is a very detailed study examining the utility of the plasma aldosterone–to–plasma renin ratio in screening for primary hyperaldosteronism. The authors conclude that the ratio is helpful, and perhaps more importantly, document that the ratio has equal efficacy when used with patients on their antihypertensive regimens as when they are off. This has the possibility of simplifying the evaluation of patients being screened for primary hyperaldosteronism. Abstract 7–17 is a long-term follow-up study on patients with incidentally discovered adrenal masses. The authors followed both size and biochemical function and document that there can be small fluctuations in size and biochemical function that have largely no consequence in the long-term stability of these lesions. Whether these recommendations can be extended to a time period greater than 10 years is uncertain, and probably will require even longer term follow-up for young patients with adrenal nodules. Abstract 7–18 looks at the utility of reporting Hounsfield Units in assessing adrenal nodules. The authors conclude that this is an important variable in assessing whether an adrenal nodule is benign and can be observed, though it must be taken in the context of other factors that can be determined radiographically.

The final group of papers is focused on the management of GI neuroendocrine tumors. Abstract 7–19 is a study of a large number of patients with neuroendocrine tumors metastatic to the liver. The patients were grouped into 3 groups based on their treatment, with those managed surgically or via interventional radiology considered to be aggressively managed, while those managed by observation considered in a nonaggressive group. The authors conclude that aggressive management leads to better survival, a result that many surgeons feel is correct, but that is not proven in this paper. Further study—a prospective study—is still required to answer this question. Abstract 7–20 reports on a novel technique for imaging neuroendocrine tumors, particularly of the GI tract. This is an interesting technique that appears to have great promise and is based on radiolabeled hydroxytryptophan to identify sites of tumor. Whether the technique can be widely applied is in doubt, but it may be useful at major referral centers where many of these most complex and enigmatic patients are seen and treated anyway. Finally, Abstract 7–21 reports on the utilization of radiolabeled octreotide to kill metastatic neuroendocrine tumors. The treatment regimen does hold out some promise and is well tolerated, but the group of patients that the authors suggest to target is also the group that is most likely to be observed in current treatment algorithms. Further study will be needed to directly compare a treatment arm versus observation in these patients to convince us that the treatment is warranted.

Thomas J. Fahey III, MD

Prophylactic Thyroidectomy in Multiple Endocrine Neoplasia Type 2A

Skinner MA, Moley JA, Dilley WG, et al (Duke Univ, Durham, NC; Washington Univ, St Louis)

N Engl J Med 353:1105-1113, 2005 7–1

Background.—Medullary thyroid carcinoma is the most common cause of death in patients with multiple endocrine neoplasia (MEN) type 2A (MEN-2A) or type 2B or familial medullary thyroid carcinoma. We sought to determine whether total thyroidectomy in asymptomatic young members of kindreds with MEN-2A who had a mutated allele of the *RET* proto-oncogene could prevent or cure medullary thyroid carcinoma.

Methods.—A total of 50 patients 19 years of age or younger who were consecutively identified through a genetic screening program as carriers of a *RET* mutation characteristic of MEN-2A underwent total thyroidectomy. Five to 10 years after the surgery, each patient was evaluated by physical examination and by determination of plasma calcitonin levels after stimulation with provocative agents.

Results.—In 44 of the 50 patients, basal and stimulated plasma calcitonin levels were at or below the limits of detection of the assay (proportion, 0.88; 95 percent confidence interval, 0.76 to 0.95). Two patients had basal and stimulated plasma calcitonin levels above the normal range. Stimulated plasma calcitonin levels had increased but remained within the normal range in four patients. The data suggest that there was a lower incidence of persistent or recurrent disease in children who underwent total thyroidectomy before eight years of age and in children in whom there were no metastases to cervical lymph nodes.

Conclusions.—In this study, young patients identified by direct DNA analysis as carriers of a *RET* mutation characteristic of MEN-2A had no evidence of persistent or recurrent medullary thyroid carcinoma five or more years after total thyroidectomy. A longer period of evaluation will be necessary to confirm that they are cured.

▶ This is an important article that validates current recommendations to proceed with prophylactic thyroidectomy in patients identified as carriers of *RET* mutations.

T. J. Fahey III, MD

Stat Bite: Incidence of Thyroid Cancer by Sex, 1975-2002
National Cancer Institute (Natl Cancer Inst)
J Natl Cancer Inst 97:1722, 2005 7–2

Overview.—Thyroid cancer is a relatively uncommon disease in the United States. It was estimated that in 2005, 25,690 persons in this country would be diagnosed with thyroid cancer; it was expected that 1490 people would die of the disease. Though relatively uncommon, the incidence of thyroid cancer has been increasing in recent years (Figure). Among the risk fac-

STAT BITE

Incidence of Thyroid Cancer by Sex, 1975–2002

Thyroid cancer is relatively uncommon; in 2005, 25,690 people in the United States will be diagnosed with thyroid cancer, and 1,490 people will die of the disease. The incidence of thyroid cancer has been increasing over the last decade. Risk factors for the disease include a history of radiation administered in infancy and childhood, radiation exposure as a consequence of nuclear fallout, a history of goiter, family history of thyroid disease, female gender, and Asian race.

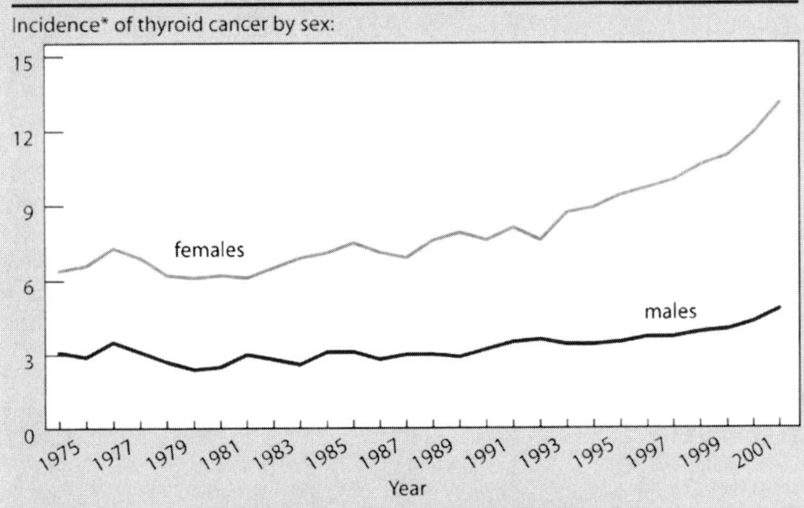

*Incidence rates are per 100,000 and are age-adjusted to the U.S. standard population.

Sources: SEER Cancer Statistics Review, 1975–2002 (NCI 2005), access at http://seer.cancer.gov; Thyroid Cancer (PDQ): Treatment-Health Professionals, access at http://www.cancer.gov.

DOI: 10.1093/jnci/dji426

FIGURE.—Incidence of thyroid cancer by sex, 1975-2002. *Incidence rates are per 100,000 and are age-adjusted to the US standard population. (Courtesy of National Cancer Institute: Stat bite: Incidence of thyroid cancer by sex, 1975-2002. *J Natl Cancer Inst* 97:1722, 2005. Reproduced by permission of Oxford University Press.)

tors for thyroid cancer are a history of radiation administered in infancy and childhood; radiation exposure as a consequence of nuclear fallout; a history of goiter; family history of thyroid disease; female gender; and Asian race.

▶ This graph is included to show the continued rise in thyroid cancer incidence in the United States during the last 10 years. Although the cause of this increase has not been explained, it is important to note that the prevalence of thyroid cancer will also continue to increase, and the long-term management of patients with low-risk thyroid cancers is the focus of several of the following articles.

T. J. Fahey III, MD

Management of Thyroid Nodules Detected at US: Society of Radiologists in Ultrasound Consensus Conference Statement

Frates MC, Benson CB, Charboneau JW, et al (Harvard Med School, Boston; Mayo Clinic, Rochester, Minn; Univ of California at San Francisco; et al)
Radiology 237:794-800, 2005 7–3

Background.—In October 2004, a panel of specialists from a variety of disciplines was convened by The Society of Radiologists in Ultrasound. The purpose of the conference was to reach a consensus about management of thyroid nodules identified at thyroid US. This panel was convened to determine, specifically, which thyroid nodules should undergo US-guided fine needle aspiration (FNA) and which should not undergo aspiration. This statement presented the recommendations of the consensus panel, provided background information and explanations, and suggested topics for future research. The panel consisted of 21 specialists from several disciplines, including radiology, endocrinology, cytopathology, and surgery.

Overview.—Thyroid nodules are very common and are found in 4% to 8% of adults by palpation and in 10% to 41% of adults by means of US (Table 1). In 50% of patients, the nodules are identified by pathologic examination at autopsy. The prevalence of thyroid nodules increases with age. Malignancy is more common in patients younger than 20 years or older than

TABLE 1.—US Features Associated With Thyroid Cancer

US Feature*	Sensitivity (%)	Specificity (%)	Positive Predictive Value (%)	Negative Predictive Value (%)
Microcalcifications (1-5)	26.1-59.1	85.8-95.0	24.3-70.7	41.8-94.2
Hypoechogenicity (2-5)	26.5-87.1	43.4-94.3	11.4-68.4	73.5-93.8
Irregular margins or no halo (2-5)	17.4-77.5	38.9-85.0	9.3-60.0	38.9-97.8
Solid (4-6)	69.0-75.0	52.5-55.9	15.6-27.0	88.0-92.1
Intranodule vascularity (3, 6)	54.3-74.2	78.6-80.8	24.0-41.9	85.7-97.4
More tall than wide (2)	32.7	92.5	66.7	74.8

*Numbers in parentheses are reference numbers. (Courtesy of Frates MC, Benson CB, Charboneau JW, et al: Management of thyroid nodules detected at US: Society of Radiologists in Ultrasound Consensus Conference Statement. *Radiology* 237:794-800, 2005. Reprinted by permission of Radiological Society of North America.)

TABLE 2.—Recommendations for Thyroid Nodules 1 cm or Larger in Maximum Diameter

US Feature	Recommendation
Solitary nodule	
Microcalcifications	Strongly consider US-guided FNA if ≥1 cm
Solid (or almost entirely solid) or coarse calcifications	Strongly consider US-guided FNA if ≥1.5 cm
Mixed solid and cystic or almost entirely cystic with solid mural component	Consider US-guided FNA if ≥2 cm
None of the above but substantial growth since prior US examination	Consider US-guided FNA
Almost entirely cystic and none of the above and no substantial growth (or no prior US)	US-guided FNA probably unnecessary
Multiple nodules	Consider US-guided FNA of one or more nodules, with selection prioritized on basis of criteria (in order listed) for solitary nodule*

Note.— FNA is likely unnecessary in diffusely enlarged gland with multiple nodules of similar US appearance without intervening parenchyma. Presence of abnormal lymph nodes overrides US features of thyroid nodule(s) and should prompt US-guided FNA or biopsy of lymph node and/or ipsilateral nodule.

*Panel had two opinions regarding selection of nodules for FNA. The majority opinion is stated here. (Courtesy of Frates MC, Benson CB, Charboneau JW, et al: Management of thyroid nodules detected at US: Society of Radiologists in Ultrasound Consensus Conference Statement. *Radiology* 237:794-800, 2005. Reprinted by permission of Radiological Society of North America.)

60 years than in persons between the ages of 20 and 60 years. A thyroid nodule was defined in these recommendations as any discrete lesion that is sonographically distinguishable from the adjacent thyroid parenchyma. FNA biopsy should be strongly considered for a nodule 1.0 cm or more in largest diameter when microcalcifications are present and also for a nodule 1.5 cm or more in largest diameter when the nodule is solid or almost entirely solid or when there are coarse calcifications within the nodule (Table 2). FNA should be considered for any nodule 2.0 cm or more in largest diameter when the nodule is mixed solid and cystic or is almost entirely cystic with a solid mural component or when the nodule has shown substantial growth since prior US examination. FNA is probably unnecessary in nodules that are almost entirely cystic with none of the above-mentioned features. For multiple nodules, FNA of 1 or more should be considered, with the selection prioritized on the basis of the above-mentioned criteria. However, FNA is likely unnecessary in diffusely enlarged glands with multiple nodules of similar US appearance without intervening normal parenchyma. FNA may also be appropriate for nodules that do not meet the criteria listed above.

Conclusions.—The recommendations for management of thyroid nodules detected at US contained in this consensus statement are thought to represent a reasonable approach to thyroid nodular disease.

▶ This consensus statement provides guidelines for when thyroid nodule FNA is indicated. The guidelines are intentionally somewhat flexible, and it is apparent that there was a dissenting minority on the panel whose recommendations differed from those ultimately accepted as the guidelines. In addition, how these guidelines extend to subcentimeter thyroid nodules—an increasingly common diagnostic problem—is left to the physician's discretion. Nevertheless, the guidelines are a useful tool. Moreover, the article provides an excellent review of the data pertinent to US evaluation of thyroid nodules and the diagnosis of thyroid cancer, and this may be its greatest benefit.

T. J. Fahey III, MD

Genetic Classification of Benign and Malignant Thyroid Follicular Neoplasia Based on a Three-Gene Combination

Weber F, Shen L, Aldred MA, et al (Ohio State Univ, Columbus; Univ of Essen, Germany; Hosp Bad Oeynhausen, Germany; et al)

J Clin Endocrinol Metab 90:2512-2521, 2005 7–4

Introduction.—Thyroid carcinoma is a common endocrine cancer with a favorable prognosis if subjected to timely treatment. However, the clinical identification of follicular thyroid carcinoma (FTC) among patients with benign thyroid nodules is still a challenge. Preoperative fine needle aspiration-based cytology cannot always differentiate follicular carcinomas from benign follicular neoplasias. Because current methods fail to improve preoperative diagnosis of thyroid nodules, new molecular-based diagnoses should be explored. We conducted a microarray-based study to reveal the genetic profiles unique to FTC and follicular adenomas (FAs), to identify the most parsimonious number of genes that could accurately differentiate between benign and malignant follicular thyroid neoplasia. We confirmed our data by quantitative RT-PCR and immunohistochemistry in two independent validation sets with a total of 114 samples. We were able to identify three genes, cyclin D2 (*CCND2*), protein convertase 2 (*PCSK2*), and prostate differentiation factor (*PLAB*), that allow the accurate molecular classification of FTC and FA. Two independent validation sets revealed that the combination of these three genes could differentiate FTC from FA with a sensitivity of 100%, specificity of 94.7%, and accuracy of 96.7%. In addition, our model allowed the identification of follicular variants of papillary thyroid carcinoma with an accuracy of 85.7%. Three-gene profiling of thyroid nodules can accurately predict the diagnosis of FTC and FA with high sensitivity and specificity, thus identifying promising targets for further investigation to ultimately improve preoperative diagnosis.

► This article provides an important analysis in the effort to refine the molecular diagnosis of thyroid nodules deemed indeterminate on fine-needle aspiration. The authors have defined a 3-gene panel that reliably distinguishes FTC and follicular-variant papillary thyroid carcinoma from FA and hyperplastic nodules. Additionally, the genes identified may provide novel insight into the pathogenesis of FTCs. Further study will be required to analyze a larger group of unknowns, but the results here indicate that molecular diagnosis in broader clinical practice is likely to be a reality.

T. J. Fahey III, MD

Fine-Needle Aspiration Biopsy Specimen With a Predominance of Hürthle Cells: A Dilemma in the Management of Nodular Thyroid Disease

Alaedeen DI, Khiyami A, McHenry CR (Case Western Reserve Univ, Cleveland, Ohio)

Surgery 138:650-657, 2005 7–5

Background.—A fine-needle aspiration biopsy (FNAB) specimen of a thyroid nodule with a predominance of Hürthle cells usually is indicative of a Hürthle cell neoplasm, but it also may occur with nonneoplastic disease.

Methods.—A prospective nodular thyroid disease database was used to identify patients with a FNAB specimen consisting of a predominance of Hürthle cells. Clinical factors were investigated and FNAB specimens were examined in a blinded fashion by a single cytopathologist to determine if there were specific factors that could be used to distinguish nonneoplastic from neoplastic disease.

Results.—Of the 738 patients with nodular thyroid disease, 622 had a FNAB specimen. The FNAB specimen was interpreted as consistent with a Hürthle cell neoplasm in 45 (7%) patients, 7 (16%) with carcinoma, 21 (47%) with adenoma, 12 (27%) with adenomatous hyperplasia, and 5 (11%) with thyroiditis. Extensive cellularity and absent colloid were associated with neoplastic disease ($P < .05$). No cytologic feature reliably excluded neoplastic disease ($P > .05$). No significant differences in age ($\overline{x} \pm SD$) (51 ± 17 vs 54 ± 17 y), sex (female/male ratio, 6/1 vs 15/2), nodule size (3.9 ± 1.9 vs 3.4 ± 2.0 cm), weight of excised thyroid tissue (42 ± 27 vs 33 ± 30 g), or functional status of the thyroid gland was observed between patients with neoplastic (n = 28, 62%) versus nonneoplastic (n = 17, 38%) disease.

Conclusions.—Neoplastic disease accounts for two thirds of the pathology in patients with a predominance of Hürthle cells on FNAB specimen and neither clinical nor cytologic features reliably exclude Hürthle cell adenoma or carcinoma. As a result, thyroidectomy is recommended for all patients with a thyroid nodule and a predominance of Hürthle cells on FNAB specimen.

▶ This article analyzes a cohort of patients who have a predominance of Hürthle cells on FNAB (defined as >50%) and demonstrate that there is no reliable cytologic or clinical feature that permits differentiation of neoplastic and nonneoplastic Hürthle cell lesions. Because only a minority of the patients with Hürthle cell lesions (16%) had carcinoma, the authors advocate a conservative surgical approach.

T. J. Fahey III, MD

Increased Calcitonin Level in Thyroid Nodules Without Medullary Carcinoma

Gibelin H, Essique D, Jones C, et al (Jean Bernard Hosp, Poitiers, France)
Br J Surg 92:574-578, 2005 7–6

Background.—Basal calcitonin measurement is routinely performed in patients with a thyroid nodule to detect medullary carcinoma. However, increased calcitonin does not always correlate with medullary carcinoma. The aim of this study was to analyse increased calcitonin levels in patients without medullary carcinoma and to find out whether absence of this carcinoma can be predicted with certainty.

Methods.—From 1992 to 2003, 5018 patients with thyroid nodules underwent thyroid surgery. A retrospective analysis of preoperative increased calcitonin levels in 67 of these patients was performed.

Results.—Pathology revealed medullary carcinoma in 16 patients (group I), micromedullary carcinoma in 13 (group II) and no medullary carcinoma in 38 (group III). In group III, 30 patients had C-cell hyperplasia. The mean basal calcitonin level was 6250 pg/ml in group I (39-62,500), 109.6 pg/ml in group II (10-728) and 25.5 pg/ml in group III (10.5-145). The mean pentagastrin-stimulated calcitonin level was 1074.1 pg/ml in group II (26-5700) and 67.6 pg/ml in group III (10-205).

Conclusion.—There is an overlap of thyroid C-cell pathology for medullary carcinoma, micromedullary carcinoma and C-cell hyperplasia that occurs when basal calcitonin is between 10 and 145 pg/ml and pentagastrin-stimulated calcitonin between 10 and 205 pg/ml. In these patients, since medullary carcinoma cannot be completely excluded, total thyroidectomy should be recommended.

► This article reports on the utility of routine measurement of calcitonin in the assessment of thyroid nodules. The authors show a similar incidence of medullary thyroid carcinoma as did the report by Elisei[1] included in last year's section on endocrine surgery (0.57%), but also document that more than 50% of the time the elevation in calcitonin proved to be related to C-cell hyperplasia or no C-cell pathology that was detected on final pathology. Though the authors use the data to strongly support their contention that routine measurement of calcitonin essentially saves lives from medullary thyroid cancer, this contention is not adequately supported by the data, and a prospective randomized study is needed before an assay that is unhelpful 99% of the time—and potentially exposes patients to unnecessary increased risk an additional 0.5% of the time—can be advised to be incorporated into routine practice.

T. J. Fahey III, MD

Reference

1. Elisei R, Bottici V, Luchetti F, et al: Impact of routine measurement of serum calcitonin on the diagnosis and outcome of medullary thyroid cancer: Experience in 10,864 patients with nodular thyroid disorders. *J Clin Endocrinol Metab* 89:163-168, 2004.

Post-surgical Use of Radioiodine (^{131}I) in Patients With Papillary and Follicular Thyroid Cancer and the Issue of Remnant Ablation: A Consensus Report

Pacini F, Schlumberger M, Harmer C, et al (Univ of Siena, Italy; Institut Gustave Roussy, Villejuif, France; Royal Marsden Hosp, London; et al)

Eur J Endocrinol 153:651-659, 2005 7–7

Objective.—To determine, based on published literature and expert clinical experience, current indications for the post-surgical administration of a large radioiodine activity in patients with differentiated thyroid cancer.

Design and Methods.—A literature review was performed and was then analyzed and discussed by a panel of experts from 13 European countries.

Results.—There is general agreement that patients with unifocal microcarcinomas = 1 cm in diameter and no node or distant metastases have a <2% recurrence rate after surgery alone, and that post-surgical radioiodine confers recurrence and cause-specific survival benefits in patients, strongly suspected of having persistent disease or known to have tumor in the neck or distant sites. In other patients, there is limited evidence that after complete thyroidectomy and adequate lymph node dissection performed by an expert surgeon, post-surgical radioiodine provides clear benefit. When there is any uncertainty about the completeness of surgery, evidence suggests that radioiodine can reduce recurrences and possibly mortality.

TABLE 2.—Recommended Indications for Post-surgical Radioiodine in Differentiated Thyroid Cancer Patients*

No indication (low risk of relapse or cancer-specific mortality):
- Complete surgery
- Favorable histology
- Unifocal T ≤ 1 cm, N0, M0
- No extra-thyroidal extension

Definite indication (use high activity [≥3.7 GBq (100 mCi)] after thyroid hormone withdrawal):
- Distant metastases
- Incomplete tumor resection
- Complete tumor resection but high risk for recurrence or mortality: tumor extension beyond the thyroid capsule (T3 or T4), extensive lymph node involvement.

Probable indication (use high or low activity [3.7 or 1.1 GBq (100 or 30 mCi)] after withdrawal or rhTSH):
- Less than total thyroidectomy,
- No lymph node dissection
- Age <16 years
- T1 > 1 cm and T2
- Unfavorable histology:
  - papillary: tall-cell, columnar-cell, diffuse sclerosing
  - follicular: widely invasive or poorly differentiated.

*For definite indications, a high activity (≥3.7 GBq) is administered; for probable indications, a lower activity (1.1 GBq) may suffice. (Courtesy of Pacini F, Schlumberger M, Harmer C, et al: Post-surgical use of radioiodine (^{131}I) in patients with papillary and follicular thyroid cancer and the issue of remnant ablation: A consensus report. *Eur J Endocrinol* 153:651-659, 2005. Reproduced by permission of the Society of the European Journal of Endocrinology.)

Conclusion.—This survey confirms that post-surgical radioiodine should be used selectively (Table 2). The modality is definitely indicated in patients with distant metastases, incomplete tumor resection, or complete tumor resection but high risk of recurrence and mortality. Probable indications include patients with tumors >1 cm and with suboptimal surgery (less than total thyroidectomy or no lymph node dissection), with age <16 years, or with unfavorable histology.

▶ This consensus report presents guidelines for the use of postoperative radioiodine (RAI) in patients with differentiated thyroid cancer based on an analysis of the data available in the literature over the past decade or so. The report highlights the fact that current evidence for use of RAI therapy in the vast majority of patients who currently receive RAI remains controversial. The problem is that the number of patients required to complete a randomized prospective study numbers in the thousands and would require follow-up over 20 to 30 years, raising the question of whether it will ever be done.

Table 2 summarizes the consensus of the group and supports the current recommendations of many endocrinologists and endocrine surgeons.

T. J. Fahey III, MD

A Single Recombinant Human Thyrotropin-Stimulated Serum Thyroglobulin Measurement Predicts Differentiated Thyroid Carcinoma Metastases Three to Five Years Later

Kloos RT, Mazzaferri EL (Ohio State Univ, Columbus; Univ of Florida, Gainesville)

J Clin Endocrinol Metab 90:5047-5057, 2005 7–8

Context.—Testing for residual differentiated thyroid carcinoma relies heavily upon recombinant human (rh)TSH-stimulated serum thyroglobulin (Tg) levels, but the positive predictive value is often low.

Objective.—Our objective was to determine the accuracy of a single rhTSH-Tg measurement over time.

Design and Setting.—We conducted a prospective follow-up study at the University referral center.

Patients.—A total of 107 differentiated thyroid carcinoma patients were stratified according to their initial rhTSH-Tg as follows: group 1 with Tg less than 0.5 (n = 68), group 2 with Tg of 0.6-2.0 (n = 19), and group 3 with Tg greater than 2 ng/ml (n = 20).

Intervention.—Clinical evaluations were conducted over 0.9-5.2 yr as follows: Tg during thyroid hormone suppression (n = 27), after rhTSH (n = 59), and/or after thyroid hormone withdrawal (n = 15).

Main Outcome.—Tumor was identified in one patient in each of groups 1 (1.6%) and 2 (5.5%), and 16 in group 3 (80%), comprising 19 tumor locations: 11 locoregional, two mediastinal, five lung, and one brain. Tumor was found in 81% with an initial or follow-up rhTSH-Tg greater than 2 ng/ml. TSH-stimulated Tg fell spontaneously to less than 0.5 ng/ml in 50% of group 2 and 5% of group 3 over 1.7-5.0 yr. The positive predictive value of the initial rhTSH-Tg greater than 2 ng/ml was 80%, and the negative predictive value was 98%. After retreatment, 100% of group 1, 74% of group 2, and 55% of group 3 had no evidence of tumor ($P = 0.0001$).

Conclusions.—1) A single rhTSH-Tg greater than 2 ng/ml predicts persistent tumor, although no value entirely excludes future recurrence. 2) Repeated TSH-stimulated studies are appropriate for patients at risk of recurrence, especially those with an rhTSH-Tg greater than 1 ng/ml. 3) A single rhTSH-Tg less than 0.5 ng/ml without Tg antibody has an approximately 98% likelihood of identifying patients completely free of tumor, a large group in which TSH suppression to less than 0.1 mIU/liter and frequent imaging and TSH-stimulated Tg testing are unnecessary.

► The data presented here confirm the value of rhTSH in Tg testing for follow-up of patients with differentiated thyroid carcinoma. More specifically, a Tg that remains less than 2 ng/mL is associated with a 98% chance of cure from thyroid carcinoma. Given the increased attention directed towards appropriate thyroid hormone dosing and intensity of follow-up, these data are useful in stratifying patients for follow-up regimens and schedules, as well as giving patients reliable prognostic information—which for the majority of thyroid carcinoma patients means being able to reassure them that they don't have to worry about cancer any more.

T. J. Fahey III, MD

Serum Thyroglobulin Levels at the Time of ^{131}I Remnant Ablation Just After Thyroidectomy Are Useful for Early Prediction of Clinical Recurrence in Low-Risk Patients With Differentiated Thyroid Carcinoma

Kim TY, Kim WB, Kim ES, et al (Univ of Ulsan, Seoul, Korea)

J Clin Endocrinol Metab 90:1440-1445, 2005 7–9

Background.—The current treatment for differentiated thyroid carcinoma is total or near-total thyroidectomy followed by ^{131}I remnant ablation and thyroid hormone suppression. During follow-up, serum stimulated-thyroglobulin (Tg) measurement is the best method for detecting the presence of normal and/or malignant thyroid tissue, the only source of Tg. Whether Tg measured at the time of remnant ablation (ablation-Tg) could be a prognostic indicator complementary to serum Tg levels at the time of the first diagnostic whole-body scan (WBS) after thyroid hormone withdrawal (control Tg), prescribed approximately 6 to 12 months after ablation Tg, was investigated. Also investigated was whether ablation-Tg could predict the persistence or recurrence of disease in low-risk patients with differentiated thyroid carcinoma.

Methods.—A series of 268 patients treated with total or near-total thyroidectomy followed by immediate ^{131}I remnant ablation were studied. Two patients who showed remnant uptake on follow-up diagnostic WBS received a second ablation.

Results.—A significant correlation was noted between ablation-Tg and control-Tg levels: 114 (80%) of 143 patients with ablation-Tg greater than 2 μg/L showed detectable (≤1 μg/L) control-Tg, and 70 (56%) of 125 patients with ablation-Tg of 2 μg/L or less showed undetectable (<1 μg/L) control-Tg. When the patients were followed up for a mean of 5.7 years, 13% had recurrences; 27% were classified as Tg positive with no evidence of disease; 60% showed complete remission. Of the 143 patients with ablation-Tg greater than 2 μg/L, recurrence was observed in 23% of cases; 36% of cases were classified as Tg positive with no evidence of disease; and complete remission was noted in 41% of cases. Of the 125 patients with ablation of Tg 2 μg/L or less, 2% of patients showed recurrence during follow up; 17% of patients were classified as Tg positive with no evidence of disease; and 81% showed complete remission. The positive predictive value for recurrence in patients having ablation-Tg greater than 2 μg/L was 23.1% The negative predictive value in these patients was 98.4%.

Conclusions.—Serum Tg levels measured at the time of immediate postoperative ^{131}I remnant ablation correlated well with serum Tg levels at the time of initial diagnostic WBS and played a complementary role in prediction of the persistence or recurrence of disease in the earliest postoperative period.

► This is a large series of patients undergoing routine postoperative radioactive iodine treatment for papillary thyroid cancer. The authors measured serum Tg after thyroid hormone withdrawal and demonstrated that a serum thyroglobulin level greater than 2 μg/L is associated with a higher risk of recurrence and correlates with Tg measured 6 to 8 months after surgery at the time of a diagnostic WBS. It would have been an even more useful study if the authors had also measured serum Tg before hormone withdrawal (or used a thyrogen protocol) to determine whether there was a correlation with unstimulated Tg 4 to 6 weeks after surgery.

T. J. Fahey III, MD

Prognostic Factors for Persistent or Recurrent Disease of Papillary Thyroid Carcinoma With Neck Lymph Node Metastases and/or Tumor Extension Beyond the Thyroid Capsule at Initial Diagnosis

Leboulleux S, Rubino C, Baudin E, et al (Institut Gustave Roussy, Villejuif Cédex, France)

J Clin Endocrinol Metab 90:5723-5729, 2005 7–10

Context.—Reliable prognostic factors are needed in papillary thyroid cancer patients to adapt initial therapy and follow-up schemes to the risks of persistent and recurrent disease.

Objective and Settings.—To evaluate the respective prognostic impact of the extent of lymph node (LN) involvement and tumor extension beyond the thyroid capsule, we studied a group of 148 consecutive papillary thyroid cancer patients with LN metastases and/or extrathyroidal tumor extension.

Initial treatment, performed at the Institut Gustave Roussy between 1987 and 1997, included in all patients a total thyroidectomy with central and ipsilateral en bloc neck dissection followed by radioactive iodine ablation.

Results.—Uptake outside the thyroid bed, demonstrating persistent disease, was found on the postablation total body scan (TBS) in 22% of the patients. With a mean follow-up of 8 yr, eight patients (7%) with a normal postablation TBS experienced a recurrence. Ten-year disease-specific survival rate was 99% (confidence interval, 97-100%). Significant risk factors for persistent disease included the numbers of LN metastases (>10) and LN metastases with extracapsular extension (ECE-LN >3), tumor size (>4 cm), and LN metastases location (central). Significant risk factors for recurrent disease included the numbers of LN metastases (>10), ECE-LN (>3), and thyroglobulin level measured 6-12 months after initial treatment after T_4 withdrawal.

Conclusion.—We highlight an excellent survival rate and suggest risk classifications of persistent and recurrent disease based on the numbers of LN metastases and ECE-LN, LN metastases location, tumor size, and thyroglobulin level.

► This report examines a selected group of patients with papillary thyroid carcinoma and a higher risk of recurrence at baseline. The authors convincingly demonstrate what many already consider to be a marker for high risk of recurrence—LN metastasis with extracapsular extension—as a significant risk factor for recurrence in patients with papillary thyroid carcinoma. Despite this risk for recurrence, fortunately, the risk of death from thyroid cancer in this series remains low. The implications are that these patients should be watched more carefully for recurrence.

T. J. Fahey III, MD

BRAF Mutation Predicts a Poorer Clinical Prognosis for Papillary Thyroid Cancer

Xing M, Westra WH, Tufano RP, et al (Johns Hopkins Univ, Baltimore, Md; Yale Univ, New Haven, Conn; Univ of Bologna, Italy; et al)

J Clin Endocrinol Metab 90:6373-6379, 2005 7–11

Context.—Use of *BRAF* mutation in papillary thyroid cancer (PTC) has the potential to improve risk stratification of this cancer.

Objective.—The objective of the study was to investigate the prognostic value of *BRAF* mutation in patients with PTC.

Design, Setting, and Subjects.—In a multicenter study of 219 PTC patients, data on their clinicopathological characteristics and clinical courses between 1990 and 2004 were retrospectively collected, and their tumor *BRAF* mutation status was determined. Associations of *BRAF* mutation with initial tumor characteristics and subsequent recurrence were analyzed.

Main Outcome Measure.—Relationships between the *BRAF* mutation status and clinicopathological outcomes, including recurrence, were measured.

Results.—We found a significant association between *BRAF* mutation and extrathyroidal invasion ($P < 0.001$), lymph node metastasis ($P < 0.001$), and advanced tumor stage III/IV ($P = 0.007$) at initial surgery. This association remained significant on multivariate analysis, adjusting for conventional clinicopathological predictors of recurrence excluding the histological PTC subtype, but was lost when the tumor subtype was included in the model. *BRAF* mutation was also significantly associated with tumor recurrence, 25 *vs.* 9% with and without mutation, respectively ($P = 0.004$), during a median of 15 (interquartile range, 3-29) months of follow-up. This association remained significant on multivariate analysis adjusting for conventional clinicopathological predictors of recurrence, even including the PTC subtype (odds ratio, 4.0; 95% confidence interval, 1.1-14.1; $P = 0.03$). *BRAF* mutation was even an independent predictor of recurrence in patients with stage I/II disease, 22 *vs.* 5% with and without *BRAF* mutation, respectively ($P = 0.002$). *BRAF* mutation was also more frequently associated with absence of tumor I-131 avidity and treatment failure of recurrent disease.

Conclusions.—In patients with PTC, *BRAF* mutation is associated with poorer clinicopathological outcomes and independently predicts recurrence. Therefore, *BRAF* mutation may be a useful molecular marker to assist in risk stratification for patients with PTC.

▶ This study implicates *BRAF* mutations as one of the factors most associated with aggressive behavior in PTC. The study indicates that *BRAF* mutations are associated with extrathyroidal invasion, lymph node metastases, and more advanced initial stage. The findings in this study are in direct contradiction to the study by Trovisco et al (Abstract 7–12). Although multivariate analysis appears to indicate that *BRAF* mutations are associated with poorer outcome as well, it is unclear if this was due to more aggressive behavior of classic PTC (in which *BRAF* mutations are found more frequently) versus follicular-variant PTC (which typically does not harbor *BRAF* mutations). The authors do note that the significance of their findings was lost when tumor subtype was included in the multivariate analysis.

T. J. Fahey III, MD

Type and Prevalence of *BRAF* Mutations Are Closely Associated With Papillary Thyroid Carcinoma Histotype and Patients' Age But Not With Tumour Aggressiveness

Trovisco V, Soares P, Preto A, et al (Univ of Porto, Portugal; Univ of São Paulo, Brazil; Hosp São João, Porto, Portugal; et al)

Virchows Archiv 446:589-595, 2005 7–12

Introduction.—A high prevalence of the $BRAF^{V600E}$ somatic mutation was recently reported in several series of papillary thyroid carcinomas (PTC). This mutation appears to be particularly prevalent in PTC with a predominantly papillary architecture. Another *BRAF* mutation (K601E) was detected in a follicular adenoma and in some cases of the follicular variant of PTC. The few studies on record provided controversial data on the relationship between the occurrence of *BRAF* mutations and clinicopathologic parameters such as gender, age and tumour staging. In an attempt to clarify such controversies we decided to enlarge our previous series to 315 tumours or tumour-like lesions diagnosed in 280 patients, including a thorough analysis of several clinicopathologic features. The $BRAF^{V600E}$ mutation was exclusively detected in PTC with a papillary or mixed follicular/papillary architecture both of the conventional type (46%) and of other histotypes, such as microcarcinoma (43%), Warthin-like PTC (75%) and oncocytic variant of PTC (55%). The $BRAF^{K601E}$ mutation was detected in four of the 54 cases of the follicular variant of PTC (7%). The mean age of patients with conventional PTC harbouring $BRAF^{V600E}$ (46.7 years) was significantly higher ($P<0.0001$) than that of patients with conventional PTC without $BRAF^{V600E}$ (29.5 years). The *BRAF* ($BRAF^{V600E}$) mutated PTC did not exhibit signs of higher aggressiveness (size, vascular invasion, extra-thyroid extension and nodal metastasis) and were in fact less often multicentric than PTC without the mutation.

► This study, also a large study, finds that *BRAF* mutations are associated with older age at diagnosis, but are not associated with more aggressive features, including extrathyroidal extension, lymph node metastases, vascular invasion, or size of the primary. These findings are virtually diametrically opposed to those of the study by Xing et al (Abstract 7–11). It is difficult to rationalize the findings of the 2 studies, even accounting for the lost significance in the Xing study when tumor subtype is included. Both studies were large, international multicenter studies. The contradictory reports suggest that *BRAF* mutations may predict tumor type, but that further study will be required to determine whether *BRAF* can definitively predict outcome.

T. J. Fahey III, MD

Reversible Diastolic Dysfunction After Long-term Exogenous Subclinical Hyperthyroidism: A Randomized, Placebo-Controlled Study

Smit JWA, Eustatia-Rutten CFA, Corssmit EPM, et al (Leiden Univ, The Netherlands)

J Clin Endocrinol Metab 90:6041-6047, 2005 7–13

Background.—Subclinical hyperthyroidism has been reported to affect systolic and diastolic cardiac function. However, the reversibility of these effects is not well established.

Objective.—Our objective was to investigate the presence and reversibility of cardiac abnormalities in patients with long-term exogenous subclinical hyperthyroidism.

Design.—We conducted a prospective, single-blinded, placebo-controlled randomized trial of 6 months duration with two parallel groups.

Setting.—The study occurred at the Leiden University Medical Center, a tertiary referral center for thyroid carcinoma.

Patients.—As a model for subclinical hyperthyroidism, 25 patients with a history of differentiated thyroid carcinoma with more than 10 yr of TSH suppressive therapy with L-T_4 were studied.

Interventions.—L-T_4 dose was replaced by study medication containing L-T_4 or placebo. Medication was titrated in a single-blinded fashion to establish continuation of TSH suppression (low-TSH group) or euthyroidism (euthyroid group).

Measurements.—We assessed serum levels of free T_4 and TSH and used echo Doppler cardiography including tissue Doppler to establish left ventricular (LV) dimensions and function as well as diastolic function. Baseline echocardiography data were compared with 24 controls.

Results.—There were no differences in baseline cardiac parameters and TSH levels between the two groups. Although mean LV mass index was increased as compared with 24 controls, only four patients had LV hypertrophy at baseline. This was not improved by restoration of euthyroidism. At baseline, diastolic function was impaired in all patients as indicated by abnormal values for the peak flow of the early filling phase (E, 55.3 ± 9.5 mm/sec), the ratio of E and the peak flow of the atrial filling phase (E/A ratio, 0.87 ± 0.13), the early diastolic velocity obtained by tissue Doppler (E', 5.7 ± 1.3 cm/sec), and the peak atrial filling velocity obtained by tissue Doppler (A', 6.8 ± 1.4 cm/sec), prolonged E deceleration time (234 ± 34 msec), and isovolumetric relaxation time (121 ± 15 msec). After 6 months, significant improvements were observed in the euthyroid group in the E/A ratio (+41%; $P < 0.001$), E deceleration time (−18%; $P = 0.006$), isovolumetric relaxation time (−25%; $P < 0.001$), E' (+31%; $P < 0.001$), and the E'/A' ratio (+40%; $P < 0.001$).

Conclusions.—We conclude that prolonged subclinical hyperthyroidism is accompanied by diastolic dysfunction that is at least partly reversible after restoration of euthyroidism. Because isolated diastolic dysfunction may be associated with increased mortality, this finding is of clinical significance.

▶ This study adds to the understanding of the negative cardiac effects of long-standing thyrotropin (TSH) suppression. In a randomized, prospective fashion, the cardiac effects of TSH suppression were documented and demonstrated that diastolic dysfunction was the most striking difference. Although not demonstrated in this study, the authors make the correlation between diastolic dysfunction and premature cardiac death. This study has important implications for defining the proper target TSH range for patients, and especially young patients, with low-risk differentiated thyroid cancers.

T. J. Fahey III, MD

Cinacalcet Hydrochloride Maintains Long-term Normocalcemia in Patients With Primary Hyperparathyroidism

Peacock M, Bilezikian JP, Klassen PS, et al (Indiana Univ, Indianapolis; Columbia Univ, New York; Amgen Inc, Thousand Oaks, Calif; et al)

J Clin Endocrinol Metab 90:135-141, 2005 7–14

Introduction.—Calcimimetics increase the sensitivity of parathyroid calcium-sensing receptors to extracellular calcium, thereby reducing PTH secretion. This multicenter, randomized, double-blind, placebo-controlled study assessed the ability of the oral calcimimetic cinacalcet HCl to achieve long-term reductions in serum calcium and PTH concentrations in patients with primary hyperparathyroidism (HPT). Patients (n = 78) were randomized to cinacalcet or placebo. Cinacalcet was titrated from 30-50 mg twice daily during a 12-wk dose-titration phase. Efficacy was assessed during 12-wk maintenance and 28-wk follow-up phases. The primary endpoint was the achievement of normocalcemia [serum calcium ≤10.3 mg/dl (2.57 mmol/liter)] with at least 0.5 mg/dl (0.12-mmol/liter) reduction from baseline. Plasma PTH, serum and urine biochemistry, biochemical measures of bone turnover, bone mineral density, and safety were also assessed. Seventy-three percent of cinacalcet-treated patients *vs.* only 5% of placebo-treated patients achieved the primary endpoint ($P < 0.001$). Fasting predose plasma PTH decreased 7.6% in cinacalcet patients but increased 7.7% in placebo patients ($P < 0.01$). Bone mineral density was unchanged by cinacalcet, but bone resorption and formation markers increased ($P < 0.05$). Adverse events were mild and similar between treatment groups. Cinacalcet rapidly normalizes serum calcium and reduces PTH in patients with primary HPT, and these effects are maintained with long-term treatment. Cinacalcet may be an effective, nonsurgical approach for management of primary HPT.

▶ Peacock et al convincingly demonstrate that cinacalcet lowers serum calcium and intact parathyroid hormone (PTH) levels over a 1-year treatment course. This is a well-conducted study of the pharmacodynamics and biochemical effects of cinacalcet. It is interesting to note that the effects of cinacalcet are quite cyclical, and the authors suggest that this may be related to the finding that markers of bone turnover are increased over a 1-year period. The authors conclude that cinacalcet may be an effective alternative to parathyroidectomy for the treatment of primary HPT, a conclusion that clearly overstates the findings in this study. Before such a conclusion can be drawn, a study with much longer follow-up and an appropriate control group—a surgery arm—must be done.

T. J. Fahey III, MD

HRPT2 **Mutational Analysis of Typical Sporadic Parathyroid Adenomas**

Krebs LJ, Shattuck TM, Arnold A (Univ of Connecticut, Farmington)
J Clin Endocrinol Metab 90:5015-5017, 2005 7–15

Context.—Mutations of *HRPT2* are frequent in sporadic parathyroid carcinomas and central to their pathogenesis. However, the potential diagnostic utility of *HRPT2* mutation status to distinguish between parathyroid carcinoma and adenoma hinges on the frequency of *HRPT2* mutations in benign adenomas. Even a low rate of *HRPT2* mutation in adenomas would greatly alter diagnostic specificity, because adenomas are far more prevalent than carcinomas. The issue remains open because of the limited number of typical adenomas, not subjected to additional selection criteria, examined in previous studies.

Objective/Design/Patients.—To determine the frequency of *HRPT2* somatic mutations in a substantial series of typical, sporadic parathyroid adenomas, we directly sequenced coding and flanking splice junctional regions of all *HRPT2* exons in solitary adenomas from 60 patients.

Results/Conclusions.—No intragenic *HRPT2* mutations were detected, strengthening the degree of specificity of *HRPT2* mutation as a feature of sporadic parathyroid carcinoma as opposed to sporadic adenomas. Our observations encourage additional study of the diagnostic potential of *HRPT2* in parathyroid neoplasia and support the view that *HRPT2* inactivation is not an important participant in the pathogenesis of typical parathyroid adenomas.

► Mutations in the *HRPT2* gene have been highly associated with parathyroid carcinoma, although the total number of cases examined to date remains small. This series adds to the number of cases of benign solitary adenomas, the group that is most important to differentiate from parathyroid carcinomas (as opposed to hyperplastic glands), and demonstrates that the incidence of *HRPT2* mutations in solitary parathyroid adenomas is very low. There were none detected in this series, and the authors estimate that the overall incidence is probably less than 1%. The suggestion is that screening for *HRPT2* mutations in cases that are difficult to classify as benign or malignant may be useful. While this may be true, it needs testing (atypical adenomas need to be tested), and screening for these mutations will probably only be performed in a research setting for some time to come.

T. J. Fahey III, MD

Screening for Primary Aldosteronism in Essential Hypertension: Diagnostic Accuracy of the Ratio of Plasma Aldosterone Concentration to Plasma Renin Activity

Schwartz GL, Turner ST (Mayo Clinic, Rochester, Minn)

Clin Chem 51:386-394, 2005 7–16

Background.—The ratio of plasma aldosterone concentration to plasma renin activity (PRA) is considered the screening test of choice for primary aldosteronism. Uncertainty exists, however, regarding its diagnostic accuracy and the effects of antihypertensive drugs and dietary sodium balance on test characteristics.

Methods.—We measured PRA and aldosterone in 118 white adults [71 men and 47 women; mean (SD) age, 51 (7) years] with previously diagnosed essential hypertension. Measurements were made while individuals were on antihypertensive drug therapy, after a 2-week drug-free period, after 4 days of dietary sodium loading, and after acute furosemide diuresis. We measured 24-h urine aldosterone excretion and PRA on the 4th day of dietary sodium loading to establish the diagnosis of primary aldosteronism. ROC curves were constructed for ratios measured under each clinical condition, and likelihood ratios were determined for individuals on or off antihypertensive drug therapy.

Results.—Fifteen patients [13%; 95% confidence interval (CI), 7-20%] met the reference standard for primary aldosteronism. The mean (SD) areas under the ROC curves did not differ significantly across conditions of measurement [range, 0.80 (0.10) to 0.85 (0.04); $P = 0.72$]. When measured on and off antihypertensive drug therapy, the 95% CIs for the optimum cutpoint for the ratio overlapped. Point estimates of sensitivity on and off therapy were 73% (95% CI, 50-96%) and 87% (70-100%), respectively, and specificities were 74% (65-83%) and 75% (66-84%). Under either condition, increased ratios were associated with 2.4- to 13-fold increases of posttest odds above pretest odds.

Conclusions.—The aldosterone:PRA ratio provides only fair diagnostic accuracy in screening for primary aldosteronism, but concomitant antihypertensive drug therapy or acute variation in dietary sodium balance does not adversely affect test accuracy. Reporting of likelihood ratios associated with ranges of values of the aldosterone:PRA ratio, rather than use of a single "optimum" cutpoint, may enhance the usefulness of the test.

▶ This study is notable for the excellent attention to detail in the design and execution of the study. Although the authors ultimately give only guidelines as to what ratio of plasma aldosterone to PRA is important in finding patients with possible primary hyperaldosteronism, the finding that the ratio can be effectively applied to patients while on antihypertensive medications is an important contribution that may allow these studies to be done at the initial office visit for evaluation of patients with hypertension and an adrenal mass.

T. J. Fahey III, MD

Long-term Morphological and Hormonal Follow-up in a Single Unit on 115 Patients With Adrenal Incidentalomas

Bernini GP, Moretti A, Orlandini C, et al (Univ of Pisa, Italy)

Br J Cancer 92:1104-1109, 2005 7–17

Introduction.—We investigated the natural course of adrenal incidentalomas in 115 patients by means of a long-term endocrine and morphological (CT) follow-up protocol (median 4 year, range 1-7 year). At entry, we observed 61 subclinical hormonal alterations in 43 patients (mainly concerning the ACTH-cortisol axis), but confirmatory tests always excluded specific endocrine diseases. In all cases radiologic signs of benignity were present. Mean values of the hormones examined at last follow-up did not differ from those recorded at entry. However in individual patients several variations were observed. In particular, 57 endocrine alterations found in 43 patients (37.2%) were no longer confirmed at follow-up, while 35 new alterations in 31 patients (26.9%) appeared de novo. Only four alterations in three patients (2.6%) persisted. Confirmatory tests were always negative for specific endocrine diseases. No variation in mean mass size was found between values at entry (25.4±0.9 mm) and at follow-up (25.7±0.9 mm), although in 32 patients (27.8%) mass size actually increased, while in 24 patients (20.8%) it decreased. In no case were the variations in mass dimension associated with the appearance of radiological criteria of malignancy. Kaplan-Meier curves indicated that the cumulative risk for mass enlargement (65%) and for developing endocrine abnormalities (57%) over time was progressive up to 80 months and independent of haemodynamic and humoral basal characteristics. In conclusion, mass enlargement and the presence or occurrence over time of subclinical endocrine alterations are frequent and not correlated, can appear at any time, are not associated with any basal predictor and, finally, are not necessarily indicative of malignant transformation or of progression toward overt disease.

▶ The authors followed up a large group of patients with incidentally discovered small nonfunctioning adrenal masses considered to be benign by radiologic criteria for a period of up to 7 years. They document that there can be small variations in size (both increases and decreases) as well as endocrine function (in the subclinical range), but that these changes appear to be self-limited and do not portend either evolution into a functioning tumor or growth characteristic of a malignancy. The authors propose a strategy for follow-up that is reasonable for the time period covered by the study, but have few data to support the proposal that no follow-up is required after 10 years.

T. J. Fahey III, MD

Clinical Utility of Noncontrast Computed Tomography Attenuation Value (Hounsfield Units) to Differentiate Adrenal Adenomas/Hyperplasias From Nonadenomas: Cleveland Clinic Experience

Hamrahian AH, Ioachimescu AG, Remer EM, et al (Cleveland Clinic Found, Ohio)

J Clin Endocrinol Metab 90:871-877, 2005 7–18

Introduction.—Radiological characterization of an adrenal tumor as adenoma may decrease the need for follow-up imaging studies, biopsies, and unnecessary adrenalectomies. We retrospectively reviewed 299 adrenalectomies in 290 patients at Cleveland Clinic Foundation over a recent 5-yr period to assess the value of noncontrast Hounsfield units (HU) in characterizing whether an adrenal mass is adenoma or nonadenoma. The mean (±SD) HU value for the adrenocortical adenoma/hyperplasia group was 16.2 ± 13.6 and significantly lower ($P < 0.0001$) than primary adrenocortical cancers (36.9 ± 4.1), metastases (39.2 ± 15.2), and pheochromocytomas (38.6 ± 8.2). The sensitivity and specificity for 10- and 20-HU cutoff values to differentiate adenomas/hyperplasias from nonadenomas were 40.5 and 100% and 58.2 and 96.9%, respectively. The size of the adrenal tumor had less value with only 40.7 and 81.3% sensitivity and 94.7 and 61.4% specificity for 2- and 4-cm cutoff values. A combination of less than or equal to 4-cm adrenal mass size and noncontrast computed tomography HU less than or equal to 20 had 42.1% sensitivity and 100% specificity. Our study, the largest with surgical histopathology as the gold standard for diagnosis, supports a noncontrast computed tomography attenuation value of 10 HU as a safe cutoff value to differentiate adrenal adenomas/hyperplasias from nonadenomas.

► The authors examined a large series of adrenal tumors with pathologic follow-up to determine the utility of HU in the radiographic characterization of adrenal tumors. The findings in this series indicate that a value of 10 HU is a safe cutoff below which a benign lesion can be assumed and safely watched (if nonfunctional). The study verifies and quantifies a finding that many adrenal surgeons already use in determining whether or not to resect an adrenal mass, but does point out that this should not be the only criterion for determining resection. Although HU values are not universally reported by radiologists in the evaluation of adrenal masses, this study should compel radiologists reading a study of an adrenal mass to include the HU value in the report, and surgeons evaluating patients with an adrenal mass to request the HU value if it is not reported.

T. J. Fahey III, MD

Neuroendocrine Hepatic Metastases: Does Aggressive Management Improve Survival?

Touzios JG, Kiely JM, Pitt SC, et al (Med College of Wisconsin, Milwaukee)

Ann Surg 241:776-785, 2005 7–19

Objective.—The aim of this study was to determine whether aggressive management of neuroendocrine hepatic metastases improves survival.

Summary Background Data.—Survival in patients with carcinoid and pancreatic neuroendocrine tumors is significantly better than adenocarcinomas arising from the same organs. However, survival and quality of life are diminished in patients with neuroendocrine hepatic metastases. In recent years, aggressive treatment of hepatic neuroendocrine tumors has been shown to relieve symptoms. Minimal data are available, however, to document improved survival with this approach.

Methods.—The records of patients with carcinoid (n = 84) and pancreatic neuroendocrine tumors (n = 69) managed at our institution from January 1990 through July 2004 were reviewed. Eighty-four patients had malignant tumors, and hepatic metastases were present in 60 of these patients. Of these 60 patients, 23 received no aggressive treatment of their liver metastases, 19 were treated with hepatic resection and/or ablation, and 18 were managed with transarterial chemoembolization (TACE) frequently (n = 11) in addition to resection and/or ablation. These groups did not differ with respect to age, gender, tumor type, or extent of liver involvement.

Results.—Median and 5-year survival were 20 months and 25% for the Nonaggressive group, >96 months and 72% for the Resection/Ablation group, and 50 months and 50% for the TACE group. The survival for the Resection/Ablation and the TACE groups was significantly better (P < 0.05) when compared with the Nonaggressive group. Patients with more than 50% liver involvement had a poor outcome (P < 0.001).

Conclusions.—These data suggest that aggressive management of neuroendocrine hepatic metastases does improve survival, that chemoembolization increases the patient population eligible for this strategy, and that patients with more than 50% liver involvement may not benefit from an aggressive approach.

▶ This is a retrospective study that examines whether surgical or radiologic (chemoembolization) treatment improves survival in patients with neuroendocrine liver metastases over expectant management. The authors find that "aggressive management" (meaning intervention) does improve survival in these patients, a position that most endocrine surgeons believe is correct. Unfortunately, this article will probably do little to convince the nonbelievers, as the patients in the observation arm were far less likely to have their primary tumor resected, at least seemingly biasing the results in favor of the 2 treatment arms. This is a question that desperately needs a randomized prospective study to be conducted to resolve the issue of treat or not treat when managing this disease.

T. J. Fahey III, MD

Whole-Body ^{11}C-5-Hydroxytryptophan Positron Emission Tomography as a Universal Imaging Technique for Neuroendocrine Tumors: Comparison With Somatostatin Receptor Scintigraphy and Computed Tomography

Orlefors H, Sundin A, Garske U, et al (Uppsala Univ, Sweden)

J Clin Endocrinol Metab 90:3392-3400, 2005 7–20

Introduction.—Neuroendocrine tumors (NETs) can be small and situated almost anywhere throughout the body. Our objective was to investigate whether whole-body (WB) positron emission tomography (PET) with ^{11}C-5-hydroxytryptophan (5-HTP) can be used as a universal imaging technique for NETs and to compare this technique with established imaging methods. Forty-two consecutive patients with evidence of NET and a detected lesion on any conventional imaging (six bronchial, two foregut, 16 midgut, and two thymic carcinoids; one ectopic Cushing's syndrome; four gastrinomas; one insulinoma; six nonfunctioning endocrine pancreatic tumors; one gastric carcinoid, one paraganglioma; and two endocrine-differentiated pancreatic carcinomas) were studied. The WB-^{11}C-5-HTP-PET examinations were compared with WB-computed tomography (CT) and somatostatin receptor scintigraphy (SRS). Tumor lesions were imaged with PET in 95% of the patients. In 58% of the patients, PET could detect more lesions than SRS and CT and equal numbers in 34%, whereas in three cases, SRS or CT showed more lesions. In 84% (16 of 19 patients), PET could visualize the primary tumor compared with 47 and 42% for SRS and CT, respectively. The surgically removed PET-positive primary tumor sizes were 6-30 mm. To conclude, this study indicates that WB-^{11}C-5-HTP-PET can be used as a universal imaging method for detection of NETs. This study also shows that WB-^{11}C-HTP-PET is sensitive in imaging small NET lesions, such as primary tumors, and can in a majority of cases image significantly more tumor lesions than SRS and CT.

▶ The authors report a novel technique for imaging gastrointestinal (GI) NETs. The report details the utilization of ^{11}C-5-HT with PET imaging to localize NETs of the GI tract. The technique is sensitive and specific and compares favorably with CT and SRS for the localization of GI neuroendocrine tumors. Whether this technique will become widely applicable remains to be determined, as the compound is expensive, difficult to synthesize, and has a short life that requires a cyclotron for synthesis.

T. J. Fahey III, MD

Radiolabeled Somatostatin Analog [^{177}Lu-DOTA^{0},Tyr^{3}]Octreotate in Patients With Endocrine Gastroenteropancreatic Tumors

Kwekkeboom DJ, Teunissen JJ, Bakker WH, et al (Erasmus Med Ctr, Rotterdam, The Netherlands)

J Clin Oncol 23:2754-2762, 2005 7–21

Purpose.—There are few treatment options for patients with metastasized or inoperable endocrine gastroenteropancreatic (GEP) tumors. Chemotherapy can be effective, but the response is usually less than 1 year. Here, we present the results of treatment with a radiolabeled somatostatin analog, [^{177}Lu-DOTA^{0},Tyr^{3}]octreotate (^{177}Lu-octreotate).

Patients and Methods.—One hundred thirty-one patients with somatostatin receptor–positive tumors were treated with up to a cumulative dose of 600 to 800 mCi (22.2 to 29.6 GBq) of ^{177}Lu-octreotate.

Results.—One patient developed renal insufficiency, and another patient developed hepatorenal syndrome. Creatinine clearance did not change significantly in the other patients. WHO hematologic toxicity grade 3 or 4 occurred after less than 2% of the administrations. We observed complete remission in three patients (2%), partial remission in 32 patients (26%), minor response (tumor diameter decrease of 25% to 50%) in 24 patients (19%), stable disease (SD) in 44 patients (35%), and progressive disease (PD) in 22 patients (18%). Higher remission rates were positively correlated with high uptake on pretherapy somatostatin receptor imaging and a limited number of liver metastases, whereas PD was significantly more frequent in patients with a low performance score and extensive disease. Median time to progression in 103 patients who either had SD or tumor regression was more than 36 months.

Conclusion.—Treatment with ^{177}Lu-octreotate results in tumor remission in a high percentage of patients with GEP tumors. Serious side effects are rare. The median time to progression compares favorably with chemotherapy. Results are better in patients with a limited tumor load. Therefore, early treatment, even in patients who have no PD, may be better.

► This study reports on the treatment of metastatic endocrine gastrointestinal tumors with a novel radiolabeled octreotide compound, ^{177}Lu-octreotate. The report details a favorable response profile with minimal toxicity in a group of patients for whom there exist few other options. A response rate of 47% is reported, based on CT measurement criteria. While this appears to be an excellent response rate in an otherwise untreatable tumor, it must be noted that a significant percentage of these patients were treated without evidence of progression before entry into the study. This makes it very difficult to draw conclusions about the duration of response. Nevertheless, the treatment appears to be well tolerated, and thus, additional trials are warranted to determine its role in the treatment of patients with metastatic neuroendocrine gastrointestinal tumors.

T. J. Fahey III, MD

8 Nutrition

Introduction

This year's selection of papers for review emphasized clinical trials evaluating the use of nutritional support in a variety of circumstances. The focus has shifted away from trials looking at energy balance or protein intake. Vitamin and specific trace metal requirements are less emphasized. Instead, clinical trials have continued to evaluate the method and duration of feeding, the need for nutritional support, and the utilization of such support in special clinical circumstances, such as in infants and children and in patients in the ICU. Particular emphasis has been placed on experimental liver dysfunction. For example, Javid et al (Abstract 8–1) evaluated the role of enteral nutrition in the reversal of parenteral nutrition–associated liver dysfunction in infants. They noted that only after cessation of parenteral nutrition and the use of full enteral nutrition do all signs of liver dysfunction disappear. In circumstances utilizing only parenteral nutrition, there is a high likelihood that infants will develop liver dysfunction. Briassoulis et al (Abstract 8–2) evaluated immune-enhancing nutritional support in pediatric ICU patients. After 5 days of nutritional support, there was a significant decrease in plasma IL-6 levels only in the group receiving immune enhancing nutrition. Many have wished to improve the deposition of nitrogen as skeletal muscle in children receiving nutritional support. Hardin et al (Abstract 8–3) provided growth hormone treatment as a method of enhancing growth of children with cystic fibrosis. These authors noted significant improvement in height, weight, bone mineral content, and lean tissue mass in cystic fibrosis children receiving growth hormone along with enteral nutritional support. Thus, it appears that aggressive treatment of cystic fibrosis with provision of nutrition and growth hormone may dramatically improve these children's lives. Meert et al (Abstract 8–4) evaluated the use of gastric and small bowel feeding in critically ill children. One might have assumed from prior studies that simple placement of the tip of the feeding tube into the small intestine would obviate the possibility of aspiration and pneumonitis. Unfortunately, these authors noted no difference in the proportion of tracheal aspirates positive for pepsin between groups fed either with the tip of the enteral feeding tube in the stomach or with the tip of the enteral feeding tube in the upper small intestine. These authors emphasize that methods to decrease the risk of pulmonary aspiration are essential in all critically ill children being enterally fed. Teitelbaum et al (Abstract 8–5) evaluated the use of cholecystokinin-octapeptide (CCK-OP) to prevent parenteral nutrition–associated cholestasis. In this randomized trial, the use of CCK-OP was not beneficial in reducing cholestasis. Negative trials such as this are extremely important so that one does not continue believing that CCK may help prevent liver dysfunction in patients being partially fed.

In numerous animal studies, administration of glutamine demonstrates trophic function relative to the small intestine. It has been used in a trial by Kalhan et al (Abstract 8–6) as a supplement. They noted substantial decrease in whole-body proteolysis in low birth weight infants. Thus, further clinical trials are indicated to determine the clinical effectiveness of glutamine in this patient population.

Dennis et al (Abstract 8–7) evaluated the timing and method of enteral tube feeding in patients who suffered dysphagic stroke. They noted that if the patient's prognosis is reasonable, nutritional support is one of the many methods of rehabilitation. However, they did not demonstrate an absolute difference in the risk of death in favor of early feeding. Standard administration of nutritional supplementation did not appear to be of benefit. Elia et al (Abstract 8–9) evaluated the use of diabetes-specific formulas in diabetic patients. As expected, the use of these formulas made it easier to maintain blood sugar control in this study in which the authors reviewed 23 papers comprising nearly 800 patients. However, it is unclear whether the use of this formula truly affects morbidity and mortality in this patient group.

In severely burned patients, the use of glutamine supplementation with glutamine granules along with feeding improved protein synthesis in wound healing and appeared to reduce hospital length of stay. In patients with perforation peritonitis, it has for a long time been unclear whether enteral feeding can be conducted safely. Kaur et al (Abstract 8–12) demonstrated that in the presence of perforation peritonitis, early enteral feeding could be carried out. However, the authors note that great care must be observed in patients who get fed in this circumstance to avoid the problems of paralytic ileus, overfeeding, abdominal distention, vomiting, and its adverse sequelae.

Hypocaloric parenteral nutrition is used only sparingly because of the cost and lack of efficacy. Leucine balance has been noted to be positive in the study by Schricker et al (Abstract 8–13), but true clinical benefit remains to be seen. Lucha et al (Abstract 8–14) evaluated the economic impact of earlier parenteral feeding in patients undergoing GI surgery. They did not find an economic benefit. However, these authors only studied approximately 25 patients per group. Thus, this study was severely underpowered to demonstrate clinical effectiveness. Implantable ports that have valves appear to have far fewer complications than nonvalved implantable ports and probably should become the standard of care, particularly to reduce problems with blood clotting and catheter blockage. This is extremely important as patients have only so many sites in which these catheters can be placed, and thus, every effort should be made to maintain patency.

Several studies evaluated immunonutrition. Tsuei et al (Abstract 8–18) noted that supplemental enteral arginine is metabolized to ornithine in injured patients. In a heterogeneous intensive care population, a large randomized trial of nearly 600 patients evaluated the use of either immunonutrition or standard feeding. In this heterogeneous general ICU population, immunonutrition appeared to have no beneficial effect on clinical outcome parameters.

Doig et al (Abstract 8–20) reviewed the literature on methodology in nutritional support trials and felt that these trials were generally quite poor. Reviews such as these are important to allow us to focus on the methodology that is used in clinical research. It would be wonderful if these same authors could help the clinical scientist by performing a rigorous nutritional support trial that could be used so that others could emulate their methodology.

A number of studies evaluated nutritional support in animal models. One by Chen et al (Abstract 8–21) looked at the time course of hepatic adaptation to total parenteral nutrition (TPN) and its relationship to glycogen depletion. The long-term use of TPN has been well known to result in atrophy of the intestinal tract, but the effects of TPN on the enteral nervous system and bowel motility are less well known. However, there were no major changes in the neurotransmitter expression of enteric neurons or in motor activity. Nutritional status does seem to improve the reperfusion injury in the rat fatty liver. However, it is critical that one does not feed to the extent of creation of a fatty liver, which then appears to hold some risk should sepsis or other problems supervene. It is clear that enteral nutrition seems to provide intestinal immune function. Thus, as previous studies have suggested, it is important to provide some enteral nutritional support even while patients are fed primarily using parenteral nutrition. Wherever possible, some enteral nutrients should be infused.

John M. Daly, MD

The Role of Enteral Nutrition in the Reversal of Parenteral Nutrition-associated Liver Dysfunction in Infants

Javid PJ, Collier S, Richardson D, et al (Harvard Med School, Boston)

J Pediatr Surg 40:1015-1018, 2005 8–1

Background.—Liver dysfunction in children dependent on parenteral nutrition (PN) is well established, and the extent of hyperbilirubinemia has been shown to correlate with morbidity and mortality. The aim of this study was to assess whether increasing provisions of enteral nutrition can improve PN-associated hyperbilirubinemia over time.

Methods.—A retrospective review was conducted on infants in our institution's Short Bowel Syndrome Clinic from 1999 to 2004. Inclusion criteria included PN duration more than 1 month, serum direct bilirubin more than 3 mg/dL while on PN, and tolerance of full enteral nutrition with eventual discontinuation of PN. Paired *t* tests were used for statistical analyses.

Results.—Twelve infants were identified with a PN duration of 5 ± 1 months. Five patients underwent liver biopsy while on PN, and histological evidence of cholestasis was found on all specimens. Peak total and direct bilirubin levels were 10.5 ± 1.9 and 7.0 ± 1.6 mg/dL, respectively, and occurred at time of PN discontinuation. Only 2 patients had improvement in serum bilirubin levels before initiation of full enteral nutrition. After initiation of full enteral nutrition and discontinuation of PN, all patients achieved permanent normalization of bilirubin levels by 4 months ($P < .05$) after a 1-month plateau phase. Alkaline phosphatase levels approached reference range within this time but were not significant.

Conclusion.—These data demonstrate for the first time that although PN-dependent infants can achieve normalization of marked hyperbilirubinemia with enteral nutrition, the improvement in liver function usually begins only after full enteral nutrition is tolerated and PN is withdrawn. These findings support the aggressive weaning of PN to enteral nutrition in infants with short bowel syndrome.

► It is well known that infants and adults receiving only PN develop liver dysfunction and fatty liver. This retrospective study evaluated 12 infants receiving PN for an average of 5 months or more. These authors demonstrate that only after cessation of PN and the use of full enteral nutrition do all signs of liver dysfunction disappear. These results support the use of some enteral nutrition during PN, and early weaning from PN to full enteral nutrition to achieve complete normalization of liver function in infants with short bowel syndrome.

J. M. Daly, MD

Comparative Effects of Early Randomized Immune or Non-immune-enhancing Enteral Nutrition on Cytokine Production in Children With Septic Shock

Briassoulis G, Filippou O, Kanariou M, et al (Aghia Sophia Children's Hosp, Athens, Greece; Univ Hosp of Heraklion, Crete, Greece)

Intensive Care Med 31:851-858, 2005 8–2

Objective.—To compare the effect of early enteral feeding using immune-enhancing (IE) vs. non-immune-enhancing (NIE) formulas on cytokines in children with septic shock.

Design and Setting.—A single-center, randomized, blinded controlled trial in a pediatric intensive care unit of a university hospital.

Patients.—We randomized 38 patients with septic shock to either IE or NIE. Feedings were advanced to a target volume of energy intake equal to 1/2, 1, 5/4, 6/4, and 6/4 of the predicted basal metabolic rate on days 1-5, respectively.

Measurements and Results.—Interleukins (IL) 1β, 6, and 8, tumor necrosis factor α, C-reactive protein, Pediatric Risk of Mortality (PRISM) score, survival, secondary infections, length of stay, and mechanical ventilation were compared within and between the two groups. Actual mean energy and protein intakes did not differ between the two groups and the caloric-protein balance was not correlated to cytokine levels. On day 5 IL-6 levels were significantly lower (11.8±2.4 vs. 38.3±3.6) and IL-8 significantly higher in the IE than in the NIE group (65.4±17 vs. 21±2.5). After 5 days of nutritional support a significant decrease in IL-6 levels was recorded only in group IE (mean of paired differences 39.4±3 pg/ml). In multivariate regression analysis the variation in cytokines was independently correlated only to PRISM ($R^2 = -0.50$), but pediatric intensive care unit outcome endpoints did not differ between the two groups.

Conclusions.—Early IE nutrition may modulate cytokines in children with septic shock, but there is no evidence that this immunomodulation has any impact on short-term outcome.

► Briassoulis et al studied 38 children with septic shock who were randomly assigned to receive either an IE or an NIE enteral formula. In those who received the IE formula, plasma IL-6 levels were significantly lower on day 5 and afterwards, compared with those in the NIE diet formula group. The variation in cytokines was related to the risk of mortality. However, pediatric ICU outcome end points were not affected in either of the 2 groups. Thus, IE diets may modulate plasma cytokine levels but do not affect short-term outcome in critically ill children.

J. M. Daly, MD

Growth Hormone Treatment Enhances Nutrition and Growth in Children With Cystic Fibrosis Receiving Enteral Nutrition

Hardin DS, Rice J, Ferkol T, et al (Univ of Texas, Dallas; Univ of Texas-Houston; Indiana Univ, Indianapolis; et al)

J Pediatr 146:324-328, 2005 8–3

Objectives.—Impaired longitudinal growth and poor weight gain are common and important problems in children with cystic fibrosis. This study evaluates the hypothesis that adjunctive growth hormone (GH) therapy augments the growth response to nutritional supplementation.

Study Design.—We recruited 18 prepubertal children who received enteral nutritional supplementation for at least 2 years before enrollment. Nine were randomly assigned to receive no GH for 1 year, followed by 1 year of GH. Nine were randomly assigned to receive 1 year of GH followed by a second year of GH. Measurements included height, weight, pulmonary function, lean tissue mass, bone mineral content, hospitalizations, outpatient antibiotic use, and caloric intake.

Results.—Growth hormone resulted in significant improvement in height, weight, bone mineral content, lean tissue mass, and number of hospitalizations. Pulmonary function was similar at baseline. Absolute forced vital capacity and forced expiratory volume in 1 minute significantly increased in GH treatment, but there was no significant change in percent predicted pulmonary function. Caloric intake was similar in both groups during both years.

Conclusions.—These results suggest that GH is useful for enhancing growth in children with cystic fibrosis receiving enteral nutritional supplementation.

▶ Children with cystic fibrosis commonly suffer from malnutrition and growth retardation. Thus, consensus conferences have documented the need for aggressive nutritional support in these children. This study in 18 children evaluated the use of GH therapy in addition to nutritional supplementation. In children receiving GH, height, weight, bone mineral content, and lean tissue mass were significantly improved, and the number of hospitalizations was significantly reduced. While pulmonary function was similar at baseline, improvement in several pulmonary function tests occurred after GH treatment. During these study years, caloric intake was similar between groups. Thus, use of GH treatment in children with cystic fibrosis has a substantial beneficial effect, improving growth as well as pulmonary function. This study appears to demonstrate that GH treatment results in less morbidity in children with cystic fibrosis.

J. M. Daly, MD

Gastric vs Small-Bowel Feeding in Critically Ill Children Receiving Mechanical Ventilation: A Randomized Controlled Trial

Meert KL, Daphtary KM, Metheny NA (Wayne State Univ, Detroit; St Louis Univ)

Chest 126:872-878, 2004 8–4

Study Objectives.—To determine the effect of feeding tube position (gastric vs small bowel) on adequacy of nutrient delivery and feeding complications, including microaspiration, in critically ill children.

Design.—Randomized controlled trial.

Setting.—Pediatric ICU in a university teaching hospital.

Patients.—Seventy-four critically ill patients < 18 years of age receiving mechanical ventilation were randomized to receive gastric or small-bowel feeding.

Interventions.—All feeding tubes were inserted at the bedside. Color, pH, and bilirubin concentration of the feeding tube aspirates were used to guide placement. Final tube position was confirmed radiographically. Continuous feedings were advanced to achieve a caloric goal based on age and body weight. Tracheal secretions were collected daily and tested for gastric pepsin by immunoassay.

Measurements and Results.—Thirty-two patients were randomized to the gastric group, and 42 patients were randomized to the small-bowel group. Twelve patients exited the study because a small-bowel tube could not be placed at the bedside, leaving 30 patients in the small-bowel group. Gastric and small-bowel groups were similar at baseline in age, sex, percentage of ideal body weight, serum prealbumin concentration, and pediatric risk of mortality score. The percentage of daily caloric goal achieved was less in the gastric group compared to the small-bowel group (30 ± 23% vs 47 ± 22%, $p < 0.01$). No difference was found in the proportion of tracheal aspirates positive for pepsin between the gastric and small-bowel groups (50 of 146 aspirates vs 50 of 172 aspirates, respectively; $p = 0.3$). No differences were found in the frequency of feeding tube displacement, abdominal distension, vomiting, or diarrhea between groups.

Conclusions.—Small-bowel feeds allow a greater amount of nutrition to be successfully delivered to critically ill children. Small-bowel feeds do not prevent aspiration of gastric contents.

► An almost universally accepted principle is that enteral feeding into the small intestine prevents gastric reflux of enteral nutrients. This prospective, randomized, controlled trial compared gastric feeding with small-bowel feeding using enteral nutrition in critically ill children. The authors noted no difference in the proportion of tracheal aspirates positive for pepsin between the groups. Abdominal complications of enteral feeding were also similar. However, they noted a marked improvement in the amount of calories that could be administered by continuous small-bowel feeding compared with gastric feeding

The important message in this well–carried out study is that the risk of gastric aspiration remains present even when the tip of the feeding tube is beyond the pylorus. Thus, it is important in children to maintain antiaspiration precautions despite the placement of the tip of the feeding tube into the small intestine. Small-bowel feeding does allow for a greater amount of nutritional support and should be utilized as the standard of care.

J. M. Daly, MD

Use of Cholecystokinin-Octapeptide for the Prevention of Parenteral Nutrition-associated Cholestasis

Teitelbaum DH, Tracy TF Jr, Aouthmany MM, et al (Univ of Michigan, Ann Arbor; Brown Med School, Providence, RI; St Vincent's Mercy Children's Hosp, Toledo, Ohio; et al)

Pediatrics 115:1332-1340, 2005 8–5

Objective.—To determine whether cholecystokinin-octapeptide (CCK-OP) would prevent or ameliorate parenteral nutrition-associated cholestasis (PNAC) among high-risk neonates treated with total parenteral nutrition.

Study Design.—This was a multicenter, double-blind, randomized, controlled trial conducted between 1996 and 2001.

Patients.—Neonates at risk for the development of PNAC included very low birth weight neonates and those with major surgical conditions involving the gastrointestinal tract.

Setting.—Tertiary care hospitals.

Intervention.—Patients were randomized to receive CCK-OP (0.04 μg/kg per dose, twice daily) or placebo. Eligible infants were all <30 days of age.

Patients were enrolled within 2 weeks after birth or within 7 days after surgery.

Outcome Measures.—The primary outcome measure was conjugated bilirubin (CB) levels, which were measured weekly. Secondary outcome measures included incidence of sepsis, times to achieve 50% and 100% of energy intake through the enteral route, number of ICU and hospital days, mortality rate, and incidences of biliary sludge and cholelithiasis.

Results.—A total of 243 neonates were enrolled in the study. CCK-OP administration did not significantly affect CB levels (1.76 ± 3.14 and 1.93 ± 3.31 mg/dL for CCK-OP and placebo groups, respectively; mean ± SD). Secondary outcome measures also were not significantly affected by the study drug.

Conclusions.—Use of CCK-OP failed to reduce significantly the incidence of PNAC or levels of CB. CCK-OP had no effect on other secondary measures and should not be recommended for the prevention of PNAC.

► It has been suggested that CCK-OP would prevent or reduce PNAC. This prospective, double-blind, randomized, controlled trial entered 243 neonates receiving total parenteral nutrition. Use of CCK-OP failed to reduce the CB levels or alter secondary outcome measures.

Development of PNAC is a significant complication of parenteral nutrition in neonates. Many methods have been tried to reduce this side effect of parenteral nutrition. Unfortunately, use of CCK-OP is not of benefit in this circumstance.

J. M. Daly, MD

Glutamine Supplement With Parenteral Nutrition Decreases Whole Body Proteolysis in Low Birth Weight Infants

Kalhan SC, Parimi PS, Gruca LL, et al (Case Western Reserve Univ, Cleveland, Ohio)

J Pediatr 146:642-647, 2005 8–6

Objectives.—To examine the effect of supplemental glutamine (0.6 $g{\cdot}kg^{-1}{\cdot}d^{-1}$) on whole body protein/nitrogen and glutamine kinetics in low birth weight (LBW) infants receiving parenteral nutrition in the immediate neonatal period.

Study Design.—Premature infants ≤32 weeks gestation with a birth weight from 694 to 1590 g were randomly assigned to either a glutamine-supplemented group (n = 10) or to a control group (n = 10). Tracer isotope studies were performed when the infants were 6 to 7 days old and had been receiving an amino acid intake of approximately 3.0 $g{\cdot}kg^{-1}{\cdot}d^{-1}$ for at least 3 days. Whole body glutamine and nitrogen kinetics were measured with $[5\text{-}^{15}N]$glutamine, $[^{2}H_5]$phenylalanine, $[1\text{-}^{13}C,^{15}N]$leucine, $[^{15}N_2]$urea, and GC-mass spectrometry.

Results.—Supplemental glutamine was associated with a lower rate of appearance of glutamine (*P* = .003), phenylalanine (*P* = .001), and leucine C

(P = .003). There was no significant difference in leucine N turnover, urea turnover and plasma cortisol, and C-reactive protein levels in the 2 groups.

Conclusion.—Parenteral glutamine supplement in LBW infants was associated with lower whole-body protein breakdown. Because the decrease in whole body proteolysis is associated with protein accretion, parenteral glutamine supplement may be beneficial in selected populations of LBW infants.

► The use of supplemental glutamine in LBW infants may be beneficial in terms of whole-body protein metabolism. This prospective, randomized trial in premature infants evaluated the use of supplemental glutamine. The parenteral glutamine supplement in this study was associated with lower whole-body protein breakdown. This is usually associated with positive nitrogen balance and lean body mass. Thus, parenteral glutamine supplementation may be beneficial in certain LBW infants.

J. M. Daly, MD

Effect of Timing and Method of Enteral Tube Feeding for Dysphagic Stroke Patients (FOOD): A Multicentre Randomised Controlled Trial

Dennis MS, for the FOOD Trial Collaboration (Western Gen Hosp, Edinburgh, England; et al)

Lancet 365:764-772, 2005 8–7

Background.—Undernutrition is common in patients admitted with stroke. We aimed to establish whether the timing and route of enteral tube feeding after stroke affected patients' outcomes at 6 months.

Methods.—The FOOD trials consist of three pragmatic multicentre randomised controlled trials, two of which included dysphagic stroke patients. In one trial, patients enrolled within 7 days of admission were randomly allocated to early enteral tube feeding or no tube feeding for more than 7 days (early versus avoid). In the other, patients were allocated percutaneous endoscopic gastrostomy (PEG) or nasogastric feeding. The primary outcome was death or poor outcome at 6 months. Analysis was by intention to treat.

Findings.—Between Nov 1, 1996, and July 31, 2003, 859 patients were enrolled by 83 hospitals in 15 countries into the early versus avoid trial. Early tube feeding was associated with an absolute reduction in risk of death of 5.8% (95% CI −0.8 to 12.5, p=0.09) and a reduction in death or poor outcome of 1.2% (−4.2 to 6.6, p=0.7). In the PEG versus nasogastric tube trial, 321 patients were enrolled by 47 hospitals in 11 countries. PEG feeding was associated with an absolute increase in risk of death of 1.0% (−10.0 to 11.9, p=0.9) and an increased risk of death or poor outcome of 7.8% (0.0 to 15.5, p=0.05).

Interpretation.—Early tube feeding might reduce case fatality, but at the expense of increasing the proportion surviving with poor outcome. Our data do not support a policy of early initiation of PEG feeding in dysphagic stroke patients.

▶ During approximately a 7-year period, more than 800 patients in 15 countries were enrolled in a trial that evaluated early (<7 days) or no tube feeding (nutrition supplementation with tube feeding) for more than 7 days (early vs avoid) in dysphagic stroke patients. This is the largest randomized, controlled trial to date to investigate this issue of early feeding versus a somewhat delayed feeding in this patient population. A second trial included in this report evaluated PEG feeding versus nasoenteral feeding. While not achieving statistical significance, the results suggested that there was an absolute difference in the risk of death in favor of early feeding. In addition, nasogastric feeding was less of a risk than was the use of PEG tubes.

Studies such as these are enormously difficult to do. This study involved 83 institutions and many countries. Proper quality control is important. The heterogeneity of the dysphagic stroke patients in the degree of injury may also influence results. Nevertheless, it is pointed out that physicians should no longer worry about early intervention with tube feeding in patients who are dysphagic from stroke. If the patient's prognosis is reasonable, nutritional support becomes a method of rehabilitation just as any other that is being used for these patients.

J. M. Daly, MD

Routine Oral Nutritional Supplementation for Stroke Patients in Hospital (FOOD): A Multicentre Randomised Controlled Trial

Dennis MS, for the FOOD Trial Collaboration (Western Gen Hosp, Edinburgh, England; et al)

Lancet 365:755-763, 2005 8–8

Background.—Undernutrition is common in hospital patients with stroke, can develop or worsen in hospital, and is associated with poor outcomes. We aimed to establish whether routine oral nutritional supplements improve outcome after stroke.

Methods.—The FOOD trials are a family of three pragmatic, multicentre, randomised controlled trials. We measured the outcomes of stroke patients who could swallow and who were randomly allocated normal hospital diet or normal hospital diet plus oral nutritional supplements until hospital discharge. The primary outcome was death or poor outcome (modified Rankin scale [MRS] grade 3-5), 6 months after enrollment, measured unaware of treatment allocation. Analysis was by intention to treat.

Findings.—Between Nov 1, 1996, and July 31, 2003, 4023 patients were enrolled by 125 hospitals in 15 countries. Only 314 (8%) patients were judged to be undernourished at baseline. Vital status and MRS at the end of the trial were known for 4012 and 4004 patients, respectively. Supplemented diet was associated with an absolute reduction in risk of death of 0.7%

(95% CI −1.4 to 2.7) and an increased risk of death or poor outcome of 0.7% (−2.3 to 3.8).

Interpretation.—We could not confirm the anticipated 4% absolute benefit for death or poor outcome from routine oral nutritional supplements for mainly well nourished stroke patients in hospital. Our results would be compatible with a 1% or 2% absolute benefit or harm from oral supplements. These results do not support a policy of routine oral supplementation after stroke.

▶ This large study examined over 4000 patients who were given a standard nutrition versus standard nutrition plus food supplements. No statistical benefit was evident to provide routine oral supplementation after stroke. Interestingly, only 8% of the patients were judged to be undernourished at baseline. It has been stated repeatedly in other trials that nutritional supplementation can benefit the undernourished but does not necessarily benefit the well-nourished patient in those undergoing major surgery, major traumatic injury, chemotherapy, or a variety of other situations. One should use nutritional supplementation only in very specific circumstances, including those of an undernourished patient requiring a short-term maximal rehabilitation.

J. M. Daly, MD

Enteral Nutritional Support and Use of Diabetes-Specific Formulas for Patients With Diabetes: A Systematic Review and Meta-Analysis

Elia M, Ceriello A, Laube H, et al (Univ of Southampton, England; Univ of Udine, Italy; Univ of Giessen, Germany; et al)

Diabetes Care 28:2267-2279, 2005 8–9

Objective.—The aim of this systematic review was to determine the benefits of nutritional support in patients with type 1 or type 2 diabetes.

Research Design and Methods.—Studies utilizing an enteral nutritional support intervention (oral supplements or tube feeding) were identified using electronic databases and bibliography searches. Comparisons of interest were nutritional support versus routine care and standard versus diabetes-specific formulas (containing high proportions of monounsaturated fatty acids, fructose, and fiber). Outcomes of interest were measures of glycemia and lipid status, medication requirements, nutritional status, quality of life, complications, and mortality. Meta-analyses were performed where possible.

Results.—A total of 23 studies (comprising 784 patients) of oral supplements (16 studies) and tube feeding (7 studies) were included in the review, and the majority compared diabetes-specific with standard formulas. Compared with standard formulas, diabetes-specific formulas significantly reduced postprandial rise in blood glucose (by 1.03 mmol/l [95% CI 0.58-1.47]; six randomized controlled trials [RCTs]), peak blood glucose concentration (by 1.59 mmol/l [86-2.32]; two RCTs), and glucose area under curve (by 7.96 $mmol \cdot l^{-1} \cdot min^{-1}$) [2.25-13.66]; four RCTs, i.e., by 35%) with no significant effect on HDL, total cholesterol, or triglyceride concentrations. In addition, individual studies reported a reduced requirement for insulin (26-71% lower) and fewer complications with diabetes-specific compared with standard nutritional formulas.

Conclusions.—This systematic review shows that short- and long-term use of diabetes-specific formulas as oral supplements and tube feeds are associated with improved glycemic control compared with standard formulas. If such nutritional support is given long term, this may have implications for reducing chronic complications of diabetes, such as cardiovascular events.

▶ These authors reviewed 23 studies comprising nearly 800 patients who received oral supplements and tube feeding with either standard formulas or diabetes-specific formulas. As expected, diabetes-specific formulas did reduce the food-induced rise in blood glucose, the glucose area under the curve, and other components of glucose metabolism. Thus, if one wishes to achieve better glucose control with enteral feeding, the diabetes-specific type formulas appear to be a benefit. In recent times, it has become much more apparent that critically ill patients should have as near normalization of their blood glucose as possible through the use of either specific feedings or the use of insulin infusions. The latter has been shown in randomized trials to reduce morbidity and mortality rates significantly. It remains to be seen whether use of diabetes-specific formulas, in fact, also reduce the risk of morbidity and mortality in these patients.

J. M. Daly, MD

Clinical and Protein Metabolic Efficacy of Glutamine Granules-supplemented Enteral Nutrition in Severely Burned Patients

Peng X, Yan H, You Z, et al (Third Military Univ, Chongqing, PR China)

Burns 31:342-346, 2005 8–10

Introduction.—As an abundant amino acid in the human body, glutamine has many important metabolic roles that may protect or promote tissue integrity and enhance the immune system. A relative deficiency of glutamine in such patients could compromise recovery and result in prolonged illness and an increase in late mortality. The purpose of this clinical study is to observe the effects of enteral supplement with glutamine granules on protein metabolism in severely burned patients. Forty-eight severe burn patients (total burn surface area 30-75%, full thickness burn area 20-58%) who met the requirements of the protocol joined this double-blind randomized controlled clinical trial. Patients were randomly divided into two groups: burn control group (B group, 23 patients) and glutamine treated group (Gln group, 25 patients). There was isonitrogenous and isocaloric intake in both groups, glutamine and B group patents were supplemented with glutamine granules or placebo (glycine) at 0.5 g/kg per day for 14 days with oral feeding or tube feeding, respectively. The level of plasma glutamine, plasma protein content, urine nitrogen and urine 3-methylhistidine (3-MTH) excretion were determined, wound healing rate of the burned area and hospital stay were recorded. The results showed that there were significant reductions in plasma glutamine level and abnormal protein metabolism. After supplement with glutamine granules for 14 days, the plasma glutamine concentration was significantly higher than that in B group (607.86 ± 147.25 μmol/L versus 447.63 ± 132.38 μmol/L, $P < 0.01$) and the plasma prealbumin and transferrin in Gln group were remarkably higher than those in B group ($P < 0.01$), but the concentration of total protein and albumin were not significantly changed compared with B group ($P > 0.05$). On the other hand, the amount of urine nitrogen and 3-MTH excreted in Gln group were significantly lower than that in B group. In addition, wound healing was faster and hospital stay days were shorter in Gln group than B group (46.59 ± 12.98 days versus 55.68 ± 17.36 days, $P < 0.05$). These indicated that supplement glutamine granules with oral feeding or tube feeding could abate the degree of glutamine depletion, promote protein synthesis, inhibit protein decompose, improve wound healing and reduce hospital stay.

► Glutamine is one of the most abundant amino acids in humans. These authors evaluated the effects of an enteral supplement with glutamine granules on protein metabolism in severely burned patients. This double-blind, randomized, controlled clinical trial divided burn patients into control and glutamine-treated groups. Significant reductions in plasma glutamine levels and abnormal protein metabolism occurred in controls. Supplementation with glutamine granules increased plasma glutamine concentrations, as well as plasma prealbumin and transferrin levels. Wound healing appeared faster and hospital length of stay was shorter in the glutamine group compared with the control group. Thus, these authors demonstrate in severely burned patients that supplementation with glutamine granules along with oral feeding or tube feeding improves protein synthesis and wound healing, and reduces hospital length of stay.

J. M. Daly, MD

Enteral Nutrition as a Primary Therapy for Intestinal Lymphangiectasia: Value of Elemental Diet and Polymeric Diet Compared with Total Parenteral Nutrition

Aoyagi K, Iida M, Matsumoto T, et al (Fukuoka Univ, Japan; Kyushu Univ, Fukuoka, Japan)

Dig Dis Sci 50:1467-1470, 2005 8–11

Introduction.—Intestinal lymphangiectasia (IL) is a rare disease requiring oral fat restriction. The aim of this study was to evaluate the efficacy of enteral nutrition compared to that of total parenteral nutrition (TPN). We retrospectively reviewed nine patients with IL presenting with protein-losing enteropathy. Of these, seven patients not responding to a low-fat diet were treated with elemental diet (ED), polymeric diet (PD) containing medium-chain triglycerides, or TPN. Improvement in serum total protein was observed in two of three on ED and in one of two on PD, compared with three of three on TPN. Enteric protein loss was improved in two of two on ED, one of two on PD, and two of two on TPN. Outpatients who continued to receive enteral nutrition maintained a total protein level. Enteral nutrition appears to be as effective as TPN for patients with IL, and it may provide a valid and safe alternative therapy.

► Aoyagi and others treated 7 patients with IL with either TPN, ED, or PD. It appeared from this prospective study that enteral nutrition was as effective as TPN for patients with IL. In these and other types of patients, long-term TPN may result in IV complications and sepsis. Thus, it is important that these authors have proved that enteral nutrition is a safe alternative therapy providing for maintenance of nutritional attributes, such as total serum protein levels, in this unique group of patients.

J. M. Daly, MD

Early Enteral Feeding by Nasoenteric Tubes in Patients With Perforation Peritonitis

Kaur N, Gupta MK, Minocha VR (Univ of Delhi, India)

World J Surg 29:1023-1028, 2005 8–12

Introduction.—Malnutrition is well recognized as a potential cause of increased morbidity and mortality in surgical patients. Early postoperative enteral nutrition through a feeding jejunostomy has been shown to improve results in patients undergoing major resections for gastrointestinal malignancies, trauma, and perforation peritonitis. We conducted a prospective study to assess the feasibility and short-term efficacy of early enteral feeding through a nasoenteric tube placed intraoperatively in patients with nontraumatic perforation peritonitis with malnutrition. One hundred patients with nontraumatic perforation peritonitis with malnutrition undergoing exploratory laparotomy were randomly divided into a test group (TG) and a control group (CG) of 50 patients each. TG patients had a nasoenteric tube placed at the time of surgery and were started on an enteral feeding regime 24 hours postoperatively. Patients in CG were allowed to eat orally once they passed flatus. The differences between the two groups with respect to nutritional intake in terms of energy and protein, changes in nutritional status as assessed by anthropometric, biochemical, and hematological values, amount of nasogastric aspirate, return of bowel motility, and complication rates were analyzed. The nasoenteric feeding was well tolerated. Total calorie and protein intake in TG was significantly higher than in CG: 981 vs. 505 kcal ($p < 0.01$), protein 24 vs. 0 g on day 3 and 1498 vs. 846 kcal ($p < 0.01$), protein 44 vs. 23 g ($p < 0.01$) on day 7, respectively. There was reduction in the amount of nasogastric aspirate in TG compared with that in CG: 431 vs. 545 ml/24 h on day 2 and 301 vs. 440 ml/24 h on day 3, respectively. There was much faster recovery of bowel motility in TG than in CG at 3.34 vs. 4.4 days ($p < 0.01$). Complications developed in 39 of 50 patients in TG and in 47 of 50 in CG. The major complications occurred in 6 patients in TG and 12 patients in CG ($p < 0.05$). Patients with perforation peritonitis with malnutrition are likely to develop large energy deficits postoperatively, resulting in higher incidence of infective complications. Early enteral feeding through a nasoenteric tube is well tolerated by these patients and helps to improve energy and protein intake, reduces the amount of nasogastric aspirate, reduces the duration of postoperative ileus, and reduces the risk of serious complications.

► Malnutrition occurs commonly in patients with bowel perforation. In the past, these patients were treated routinely with total parenteral nutrition. However, this clinical study reviewed 100 patients with nontraumatic, perforation-induced peritonitis. Fifty patients in the TG had a nasoenteric tube placed for enteral nutrition, and 50 patients served as controls receiving IV fluids. The nasoenteric feeding was well tolerated. The TG patients demonstrated a reduction in nasogastric aspirate and a faster recovery of bowel motility. Complications occurred in 78% of enteral-fed patients and 94% of controls. Thus, even patients with perforation-induced peritonitis are able and should be fed enterally. Early enteral feeding promotes energy and protein intake, reduces the duration of postoperative ileus, and appears to reduce the risk of serious complications.

J. M. Daly, MD

Randomized Clinical Trial of the Anabolic Effect of Hypocaloric Parenteral Nutrition After Abdominal Surgery

Schricker T, Wykes L, Eberhart L, et al (McGill Univ, Montreal; Philipps Univ, Marburg, Germany)

Br J Surg 92:947-953, 2005 8–13

Background.—The observed failure of hypocaloric nutrition to establish an anabolic state after surgery may reflect inadequate control for the type and quality of analgesia in the studies performed. This study was designed to test the hypothesis that hypocaloric nutrition induces anabolism in patients who receive effective segmental pain relief using perioperative epidural analgesia.

Methods.—Sixteen patients who underwent colorectal surgery and received epidural analgesia were randomly assigned to receive intravenous glucose either without (glucose only) or with amino acids (nutrition). Feeding was administered over 48 h from surgical skin incision until the second day after operation. Glucose provided 50 per cent of the patient's resting energy expenditure (REE). Amino acids were infused at rates that provided 20 per cent of REE. Leucine rate of appearance (R_a), leucine oxidation and non-oxidative leucine disposal (NOLD) were assessed by measuring L-[1-^{13}C]leucine kinetics. A positive leucine balance, that is the difference between NOLD and leucine R_a, indicated anabolism.

Results.—After surgery, leucine R_a in the nutrition group was lower than that in the glucose only group (mean(s.d.) 88(25) *versus* 131(22) µmol per kg per h). The leucine balance remained negative in the glucose only group, whereas it became positive in the nutrition group (mean(s.d.) −24(3) *versus* 38(12) μmol per kg per h; $P < 0.001$).

Conclusion.—Patients who receive hypocaloric parenteral nutrition can be rendered anabolic after colorectal surgery in the presence of epidural analgesia.

▶ Previously, it has been described that administration of hypocaloric glucose with amino acids was ineffective as metabolic therapy. However, the ability to reduce the metabolic rate of postoperative patients by administration of epidural analgesia may substantially affect protein metabolism and permit benefit to hypocaloric nutrition. These authors evaluated the use of glucose alone or glucose plus amino acids providing 50% of the patient's REE. In those receiving glucose plus amino acids, leucine balance became positive compared with the controls receiving glucose alone. Use of epidural analgesia is extremely effective as pain control in postoperative patients. This metabolic study suggests that reducing pain decreases energy requirements, allowing a hypocaloric glucose infusion along with amino acids to provide positive amino acid balances. It remains to be seen whether these short-term metabolic effects have any relevance in terms of clinical outcome in patients undergoing major operations.

J. M. Daly, MD

The Economic Impact of Early Enteral Feeding in Gastrointestinal Surgery: A Prospective Survey of 51 Consecutive Patients

Lucha PA Jr, Butler R, Plichta J, et al (Naval Med Ctr, Portsmouth, Va)

Am Surg 71:187-190, 2005 8–14

Introduction.—Early postoperative oral feeding has been demonstrated to be safe and not increase postoperative morbidity. There are conflicting reports about its effect on postoperative length of stay. Some patients will fail attempts at early postoperative feeding and may be relegated to a longer postoperative course. Few studies to date have attempted to identify cost savings associated with early oral support, and those identified address nasoenteric support only. Fifty-one consecutive patients were randomized into either a traditional postoperative feeding group or an early postoperative feeding group after their gastrointestinal surgery. Length of hospital stay, hospital costs (excluding operating room costs), morbidity, and time to tolerance of a diet were compared. There was a tendency toward increased nasogastric tube use in the early feeding arm, but the morbidity rates were similar. Length of hospital stay and costs were similar in both arms. Early postoperative enteral support does not reduce hospital stay, nursing workload, or costs. It may come at a cost of higher nasogastric tube use, however, without an increase in postoperative morbidity.

► Early enteral feeding in patients undergoing gastrointestinal surgery has been suggested in some reports to reduce morbidity and hospital length of stay. These authors evaluated 51 consecutive patients undergoing open, elective gastrointestinal operations who were randomized to early enteral feeding versus control. This study demonstrated no major beneficial economic effect with the use of early enteral feeding. The study was powered at 0.80 to detect a 20% difference in economic cost. One wonders whether it is realistic to demonstrate such a difference in perioperative costs, comparing early enteral feeding to controls, with such a small number of patients and given the major costs of hospitalization. Some studies suggest that major upper gastrointestinal procedures such as esophageal, gastric, or major pancreatic surgery may demonstrate a reduced length of stay and a decreased morbidity with the use of enteral feeding. However, if one takes all patients with intestinal surgery, those with lower bowel surgery do not appear to benefit as much. Thus, one wonders whether this study was large enough, admitting only approximately 25 patients per group, to demonstrate benefit. In elective, open abdominal surgery in patients who are well nourished, there does not seem to be much rationale to intervene with early enteral nutrition.

J. M. Daly, MD

A Prospective Randomized Trial Demonstrating Valved Implantable Ports Have Few Complications and Lower Overall Cost Than Nonvalved Implantable Ports

Carlo JT, Lamont JP, McCarty TM, et al (Baylor Univ, Dallas)
Am J Surg 188:722-727, 2004 8–15

Background.—The purpose of the current study was to evaluate whether a totally implanted valved subcutaneous port system would have fewer complications as compared to a standard nonvalved port.

Methods.—Study subjects requiring port placement were randomized to receive a valved port (PASV; Boston Scientific, Natick, MA) or a nonvalved port (BardPort; Bard Access Systems, Salt Lake City, UT). Each port was placed with standard operative technique. Difficulty with blood return, excess time spent accessing the port, and required interventions were reported over the initial 180 days of port usage.

Results.—Seventy-three patients were randomized to receive either a valved port (n = 37) or a nonvalved port (n = 36). No major complications were identified from port placement, and there were no differences in rates of infection between the 2 ports. A reported inability to withdraw blood was noted in the valved port group on 21 of 364 (5.8%) port accessions and in the nonvalved port group on 37 of 341 (11%) accessions ($P = 0.02$). Significantly more total time was spent ensuring adequate blood draw from nonvalved ports as opposed to valved ports (750 minutes vs. 1545 minutes, respectively) ($P < 0.03$).

Conclusions.—This study revealed that the PASV valved port is associated with significantly fewer instances of poor blood return and less nursing access time, indicating that a port with a PASV valve may be superior to a nonvalved device.

▶ The use of chronic central venous catheterization is beneficial for IV access, not only for drug and parenteral nutrition infusion but also for blood sampling. It is well known that clots develop on the tips of these catheters in many, inhibiting blood sampling once these catheters have been placed for a period of time. These authors studied patients receiving a valved port to see whether blood drawing could be improved over time compared with nonvalved ports. The use of valved ports in this study resulted in a marked improvement in the ability to withdraw blood, with 94.2% of port accessions resulting in successful blood withdrawal compared with 89% of accessions in patients who received the nonvalved port. The rates of infections were similar in both groups. Thus, those patients requiring frequent blood sampling will do better with the use of a valved port for central venous catheterization.

J. M. Daly, MD

Decreasing Use of Percutaneous Endoscopic Gastrostomy Tube Feeding for Veterans With Dementia: Racial Differences Remain

Braun UK, Rabeneck L, McCullough LB, et al (Michael E DeBakey VA Med Ctr, Houston; Baylor College of Medicine, Houston; Univ of Toronto; et al)
J Am Geriatr Soc 53:242-248, 2005 8–16

Objectives.—Percutaneous endoscopic gastrostomy (PEG) tube placement is a widely used method for long-term enteral feeding of demented patients unable to take sufficient food by mouth. National time trends in PEG tube use over the last decade have not been previously reported. The objective of this study was to determine whether use of PEG tubes for patients with dementia has changed over time and by race.

Design.—Retrospective cohort study.

Setting.—All Veterans Affairs hospitals.

Participants.—Using an administrative database of the Veterans Health Administration, all veterans with dementia and all veterans who received a PEG tube were identified between fiscal years 1990-2001.

Measurements.—Proportion of PEG tube placement for dementia patients over time and by race.

Results.—Four hundred thirteen thousand six hundred twenty-seven dementia patients aged 60 and older were identified, of whom 6,464 (1.6%) received a PEG tube. Use of PEG tubes for dementia patients increased during the first half of the decade but subsequently decreased almost to baseline after peaking in 1996 (1990: 1.2%, 1996: 1.8%, 2001: 1.3%). Time trends in the use of PEG tube feeding for dementia patients varied by race. Specifically, the relative risk for PEG tube placement in African-American dementia patients increased from 1.65 (95% confidence interval (CI) = 1.25-2.17, FY 1990) to 1.97 (95% CI = 1.62-2.4, FY 2001).

Conclusion.—Although the overall use of PEG tube feeding for dementia patients decreased over time, rates in use and changes in use over time varied significantly by race. Reasons for the differential use of this procedure should be explored.

► The authors studied the use of PEG tubes in patients in Veterans Affairs hospitals. They identified 413,627 dementia patients aged 60 and older, of whom 1.6% received a PEG tube. An increase in usage occurred in the 1996 period, followed by a decrease in most patients thereafter. However, they noted that the relative risk for PEG tube placement continued to increase in African American patients, from 1.65 in 1990 to 1.97 in 2001. Thus, while there is a decreased use of these tubes overall, racial differences in the use of these tubes may be present.

J. M. Daly, MD

A Nutrition Support Team Led by General Surgeons Decreases Inappropriate Use of Total Parenteral Nutrition on a Surgical Service

Saalwachter AR, Evans HL, Willcutts KF, et al (Univ of Virginia, Charlottesville)
Am Surg 70:1107-1111, 2004 8–17

Introduction.—The purpose of this study was to decrease the number of inappropriate orders for total parenteral nutrition (TPN) in surgical patients. From February 1999 through November 2000 and between July 2001 and June 2002, the surgeon-guided adult nutrition support team (NST) at a university hospital monitored new TPN orders for appropriateness and specific indication. In April 1999, the NST was given authority to discontinue inappropriate TPN orders. Indications, based on the American Society for Parenteral and Enteral Nutrition (ASPEN) standards, included short gut, severe pancreatitis, severe malnutrition/catabolism with inability to enterally feed ≥5 days, inability to enterally feed >50 per cent of nutritional needs ≥9 days, enterocutaneous fistula, intra-abdominal leak, bowel obstruction, chylothorax, ischemic bowel, hemodynamic instability, massive gastrointestinal bleed, and lack of abdominal wall integrity. The number of inappropriate TPN orders declined from 62/194 (32.0%) in the first 11 months of the study to 22/168 (13.1%) in the second 11 months ($P < 0.0001$). This number further declined to 17/215 (7.9%) in the final 12 months of data collection, but compared to the second 11 months, this decrease was not statistically significant ($P = 0.1347$). The involvement of a surgical NST was associated with a reduction in inappropriate TPN orders without a change in overall use.

► Utilizing a NST led by a general surgeon decreased the number of inappropriate TPN interventions from 32% to 13% over 1 year. This further declined to 7.9% in the final 12 months of this study. This report demonstrates what numerous others have shown in the past. The use of a dedicated nutrition team and strict protocols decreases the inappropriate use of TPN support. It is unfortunate that hospital administrators do not recognize this result. Unfortunately, during the past decades, many once strong and vibrant NSTs have been abandoned by hospital administrators wishing to reduce hospital costs. Better evaluation of economics would show that the use of such teams could reduce not only inappropriate use of TPN, but also the incidence of catheter-related infections, the use of antibiotic, and the length of hospital stays.

J. M. Daly, MD

Supplemental Enteral Arginine Is Metabolized to Ornithine in Injured Patients

Tsuei BJ, Bernard AC, Barksdale AR, et al (Univ of Kentucky, Lexington)
J Surg Res 123:17-24, 2005 8–18

Background.—Arginine has been added to immune enhancing diets that may improve patient outcomes, but little is known about the metabolic fate of supplemental arginine. We hypothesize that supplemental enteral arginine in injured patients is metabolized to ornithine by increased activity of the enzyme arginase.

Materials and Methods.—Twenty-five adult patients with injury severity scores ≥20 received up to 14 days of enteral nutrition supplemented with arginine (30 g/day) or placebo in a prospective, randomized, blinded study. Plasma arginine, citrulline, and ornithine concentrations and peripheral blood mononuclear cell (PBMC) arginase activity were measured at baseline and on days 1, 3, 5, 7, 10, and 14. Clinical data collected included demographics, injury patterns, lengths of stay, and infectious complications. Data were analyzed using ANOVA and *t* test.

Results.—PBMC arginase activity was elevated in all patients. In the supplemented group, plasma arginine concentrations increased at days 7, 10, and 14 when compared to baseline ($P < 0.05$) and were higher at day 14 when compared to those of controls ($P < 0.05$). Citrulline concentrations in both groups were unchanged over time. Ornithine concentration increased within 24 h of arginine supplementation and remained elevated when compared to baseline ($P < 0.01$). Ornithine concentration in the supplemented group was higher at days 1, 3, 5, and 7 when compared to that of controls ($P < 0.05$). There were no differences in clinical outcomes.

Conclusions.—Supplemental enteral arginine is absorbed in injured patients and increases arginine levels. Supplemental arginine appears to be metabolized to ornithine. Increased arginase enzyme activity in peripheral blood mononuclear cells may be a contributor.

▶ Twenty-five adult patients were randomly assigned to receive arginine supplementation at 30 g per day or placebo. These authors noted dramatic increases in ornithine concentrations in the arginine-supplemented group. There were no differences in citrulline concentrations in either group. No differences in clinical outcomes were noted. However, this study was not powered to evaluate clinical outcomes. This interesting metabolic study concludes that after injury, supplemental arginine is metabolized to ornithine. Increased arginase activity in PBMCs appears to be at least one contributor to this metabolic outcome.

J. M. Daly, MD

Clinical Outcome of Immunonutrition in a Heterogeneous Intensive Care Population

Kieft H, Roos AN, van Drunen JDE, et al (Isala Clinics, AB Zwolle, The Netherlands; Catharina Hosp Eindhoven, The Netherlands; Numico Research, CA Wageningen, The Netherlands)

Intensive Care Med 31:524-532, 2005 8–19

Objective.—To study the effect of a high-protein enteral formula enriched with arginine, glutamine, and antioxidants and containing ω3 fatty acids and a mixture of fibers, on the clinical outcome of a heterogeneous intensive care (ICU) population.

Design and Setting.—A randomized, prospective, double blind, controlled, two-center clinical trial in two intensive care units in The Netherlands.

Patients and Participants.—A total of 597 adult ICU patients expected to require enteral tube feeding for more than 2 days were randomized to receive immunonutrition or an isocaloric control formula.

Interventions.—Patients received either the immunonutrition or the control feed.

Measurements and Results.—Intention-to-treat and per-protocol analyses showed no statistically significant difference in clinical outcome parameters between the two groups. Results of the intention-to-treat analysis in control vs. immunonutrition were: median ICU length of stay in days, 8.0 (IQR 5.0-16.0) vs. 7.0 (4.0-14.0); median hospital length of stay in days, 20.0 (IQR 10.0-34.0) vs. 20.0 (10.0-35.0); median days of ventilation, 6.0 (IQR 3.0-12.0) vs. 6.0 (IQR 3.0-12.0); ICU mortality, 26.8% vs. 28.2%; in-hospital mortality, 36.4% vs. 38.5%; infectious complications, 41.7% vs. 43.0%.

Conclusions.—The results of this largest randomized, controlled trial found that in the general ICU population immunonutrition has no beneficial effect on clinical outcome parameters. These results are consistent with the literature that is currently available.

► A randomized, prospective, double-blind, controlled clinical trial was carried out in 597 adult ICU patients. These patients received enteral tube feeding with either an immunonutrition or an isocaloric control enteral formula. This is the largest randomized, controlled trial in ICU patients comparing 2 forms of enteral nutrition. The results of this study showed no differences when results were analyzed using intention-to-treat and per-protocol analyses in clinical outcome parameters between the 2 groups.

This excellent study was carried out at 2 major centers in ICU patients. Previous studies in ICU patients have shown immunonutrition to be beneficial in selected subgroups. In those who were septic, one study has suggested there might be harm, and in another trial, cessation of patient entry occurred because of concerns over harm in patients who were septic upon entering the ICU. Studies in elective surgical patients have generally shown benefit in patients receiving immunonutrition. Thus, this large clinical trial in ICU patients is extremely important in providing information for us regarding the appropriate use of enteral immunonutrition.

J. M. Daly, MD

A Review of the True Methodological Quality of Nutritional Support Trials Conducted in the Critically Ill: Time for Improvement

Doig GS, Simpson F, Delaney A (Univ of Sydney, Australia; Royal North Shore Hosp, Sydney, Australia; Foothills Med Centre, Calgary, Alta, Canada)
Anesth Analg 100:527-533, 2005 8–20

Introduction.—In this review we sought to appraise the true methodological quality of nutritional support studies conducted in critically ill patients and to compare these findings to the methodological quality of sepsis trials. An extensive literature search revealed 111 randomized controlled trials conducted in critically ill patients evaluating the impact of nutritional support interventions on clinically meaningful outcomes. Compared with sepsis trials, nutritional support studies were significantly less likely to use blinding (32 of 40 versus 35 of 111, $P < 0.001$) or present an intention-to-treat analysis (37 of 40 versus 64 of 111, $P < 0.001$). There was a trend toward the less frequent use of randomization methods that are known to maintain allocation concealment (12 of 40 versus 19 of 111, $P = 0.10$). Although nutritional support studies demonstrated a significant increase in the use of blinding after the publication of the CONSORT statement in 1996 (9 of 47 versus 26 of 64 post-CONSORT, $P = 0.023$), there were no improvements in other key areas. Previous publications have described the overall methodological quality of sepsis trials as "poor." Nutritional support studies were significantly worse than sepsis trials in all aspects of methodological quality, and there were few improvements noted over time. To detect important differences in clinically meaningful outcomes in critical care, the methodological quality of future studies must be improved.

► These authors evaluated 111 randomized, controlled studies in critically ill patients receiving nutritional support interventions. They noted methodological problems in most of these studies, with poor use of blinding, lack of an intention-to-treat analysis, and less frequent use of randomization methods. The improvement in blinding occurred after 1996. Thus, the authors note that in order to detect important differences in outcomes in critical care patients, the methodological quality of future studies must be improved. In reviewing the bibliography of this article, one is struck by the absence of prospective randomized, blinded trials using an improved methodology conducted *by these authors* in their home institutions. One looks forward to studies by Doig, Simpson, and Delaney demonstrating the improved use of methodologies to allow for evaluation of any clinical outcome benefits in the use of nutritional intervention in critically ill patients. It is relatively easy to critique retrospectively, but far more difficult to lead by example. We eagerly await their example.

J. M. Daly, MD

Time Course of the Hepatic Adaptation to TPN: Interaction With Glycogen Depletion

Chen S-S, Torres-Sanchez CJ, Hosein N, et al (Vanderbilt Univ, Nashville, Tenn)
Am J Physiol Endocrinol Metab 288:E163-E170, 2005 8–21

Introduction.—In response to chronic (5 days) TPN, the liver becomes a major site of glucose disposal, removing ~45% (4.5 mg·kg^{-1}·min^{-1}) of exogenous glucose. Moreover, ~70% of glucose is not stored but released as lactate. We aimed to determine in chronically catheterized conscious dogs the time course of adaptation to TPN and the glycogen depletion impact on early time course. After an 18-h (n = 5) fast, TPN was infused into the inferior vena cava for 8 (n = 5) or 24 h (n = 6). A third group, of 42-h-fasted animals (n = 6), was infused with TPN for 8 h. TPN was infused at a rate designed to match the dog's calculated basal energy and nitrogen requirements. NHGU (−2.3 ± 0.1 to 2.2 ± 0.7 to 3.9 ± 0.6 vs. −1.7 ± 0.3 to 1.1 ± 0.5 to 2.9 ± 0.4 mg·kg^{-1}·min^{-1}, basal to 4 to 8 h, 18 vs. 42 h) and net hepatic lactate release (0.7 ± 0.3 to 0.6 ± 0.1 to 1.4 ± 0.2 vs. −0.6 ± 0.1 to 0.1 ± 0.1 to 0.8 ± 0.1 mg·kg^{-1}·min^{-1}, basal to 4 to 8 h) increased progressively. Net hepatic glycogen repletion and tracer determined that glycogen syntheses were similar. After 24 h of TPN, NHGU (5.4 ± 0.6 mg·kg^{-1}·min^{-1}) and net hepatic lactate release (2.6 ± 0.4 mg·kg^{-1}·min^{-1}) increased further. In summary, *1*) most hepatic adaptation to TPN occurs within 24 h after initiation of TPN, and 2) prior glycogen depletion does not augment hepatic adaptation rate.

► These authors evaluated hepatic adaptation to TPN. It is well known that alterations in glycogen metabolism as well as fatty acids and triglycerides occur in the liver of individuals receiving TPN. They noted in this animal model that hepatic adaptation to TPN occurred within 24 hours of initiation. Prior depletion of glycogen did not appear to improve this hepatic adaptation.

Studies such as these are important to understand better the liver dysfunction that occurs in individuals receiving TPN. At least one method of improvement, that is, depletion of glycogen before initiation, does not appear to have any effect on liver adaptation to TPN.

J. M. Daly, MD

Effects of Total Parenteral Nutrition on Rat Enteric Nervous System, Intestinal Morphology, and Motility

Ekelund M, Ekelund M, Qader SS, et al (Lund Univ, Sweden)
J Surg Res 124:187-193, 2005 8–22

Introduction.—Total parenteral nutrition (TPN) is often crucial for patients not being able to feed enterally or having intestinal absorptive deficits. Enteral nutrition is, however, frequently regarded vital for maintaining functional and structural intestinal integrity. The aim of this study was to investigate possible effects of TPN on rat distal small intestine compared to enterally fed identically housed controls, regarding the enteric nervous system (ENS), motility *in vitro*, and morphology. This study shows that motor responses evoked by electrical stimulation or exposure to vasoactive intestinal peptide (VIP), pituitary adenylate cyclase activating peptide-27 (PACAP-27), and nitric oxide (NO) donor were unchanged. By using immunohistochemistry, the numbers of submucous ($P < 0.05$) and myenteric ($P < 0.05$) nerve cells were found to increase, expressed as numbers per unit length. The percentage of neurons expressing VIP, PACAP-27, NO-synthase, and galanin remained unchanged, however. By *in situ* hybridization the number of submucous neurons expressing neuropeptide Y-mRNA was found to decrease ($P < 0.05$); the other populations were unaltered. Morphometry revealed an increased submucosal thickness ($P < 0.05$), while intestinal circumference markedly decreased ($P < 0.0001$) in TPN-treated rats. In conclusion, TPN treatment resulted in reduced intestinal circumference leading to condensation of enteric neurons. No marked changes in neurotransmitter expression of the enteric neurons or in motor activity were noted.

▶ It has been well known that longer-term use of TPN results in atrophy of the intestinal tract. Studies previously have shown that this relates to a decrease in muscle thickness as well as mucosal atrophy. Thus, patients receiving long-term parenteral nutrition are benefited by administration of enteral nutrition to some extent. Enteral nutrition results in continued stimulation of the intestinal tract, allowing for more normal structure and function. The effects of TPN on ENS and bowel motility are unknown. In this study, rats were given TPN or fed enterally. TPN resulted in reduced intestinal circumference, but there were no major changes in the neurotransmitter expression of enteric neurons or in motor activity.

J. M. Daly, MD

The Nutritional Status Modulates Preservation-Reperfusion Injury in Rat Fatty Liver

Caraceni P, Domenicali M, Pertosa AM, et al (Univ of Bologna, Italy; Univ of Bari, Italy)

J Surg Res 127:190-196, 2005 8–23

Background.—Microcirculation disturbances are essential factors of preservation injury in fatty liver. However, hepatocyte injury is also markedly excessive in fatty liver resulting, at least in part, from energy metabolism impairment and oxidative stress. Thus, this study aimed to determine whether nutritional status influences preservation injury in fatty liver and whether energetic substrate supplementation, alone or with a vasodilator, is protective.

Materials and Methods.—Normal or fatty livers induced by a choline-deficient diet were isolated from fed and fasted rats, preserved in University of Wisconsin solution at 4°C for 18 h, and then reperfused with Krebs-Henseleit solution at 37°C for 120 min. Fasted rats with fatty liver were also treated as follows: (1) *Glucose supplementation*: rats had access to a glucose solution for 18 h prior procurement; (2) *Prostaglandin (PG)*: alprostadil was continuously infused during reperfusion; (3) *Combined treatment*: Glucose supplementation + PG.

Results.—Fasting-induced liver injury was significantly greater in fatty than normal liver. In fatty livers from fasted rats, all treatments reduced the alanine aminotransaminase release. Hepatic oxygen consumption improved in the glucose and glucose + PG groups, while PG infusion had no effect. Glucose supplementation did not affect portal pressure, which, in contrast, was reduced in livers receiving PG. Finally, all treatments lowered oxidative injury.

Conclusions.—Preservation injury in fatty liver is greatly related to nutritional status. Energetic substrate supplementation may represent a clinically feasible protective strategy and a multistep approach adding vasodilators could offer further benefit by acting on different pathogenetic mechanisms.

► The liver responds to injury by becoming fatty due to alterations in choline metabolism and other cellular metabolic events that prevent lipid from leaving hepatocytes. Impaired microcirculation has been proposed as the key event in the pathogenesis of preservation-reperfusion injury in fatty livers. Caraceni et al evaluated this injury in normal and fatty livers in rats induced by a choline-deficient diet. Animals were treated with glucose supplementation, PG infusion, or combined treatment with glucose supplementation and PG infusion. Fasting-induced liver injury was greater in fatty livers compared with normal livers. All treatments reduced alanine aminotransaminase release and lowered oxidative injury. It appears that one could prescribe protective PG and glucose infusions into the donor before transplantation in an effort to reduce the microcirculation impairment after liver transplantation. Given the high incidence of fatty livers in ill patients, this methodology holds great promise in humans.

J. M. Daly, MD

Lack of Enteral Nutrition: Effects on the Intestinal Immune System

Wildhaber BE, Yang H, Spencer AU, et al (Univ of Michigan, Ann Arbor)
J Surg Res 123:8-16, 2005 8–24

Background.—Total parenteral nutrition (TPN) results in a loss of mucosal immune function by alterations in both phenotype and function of intraepithelial lymphocytes (IEL). We hypothesized that the observed changes with TPN administration are caused by the lack of enteral feeding, and not to the TPN solution itself.

Methods.—Mice received oral feeding (Control), TPN alone (TPN), or TPN plus oral feeding (TPN+Food). Mice were killed after 7 days, and bacteriological cultures from spleen, liver, and mesenteric lymph nodes obtained, with bacterial translocation (BT) being defined as a positive culture. IEL phenotype was analyzed by flow cytometry. IEL messenger RNA (mRNA) cytokine expression used reverse transcriptase polymerase chain reaction (RT-PCR). Apoptosis was detected by terminal deoxynucleotidyl transferase biotin-dUTP nick end labeling (TUNEL) staining.

Results.—BT significantly ($P < 0.05$, with analysis of variance [ANOVA]) increased in the TPN group (53%) compared with Control (9%) and TPN+Food (14%) groups. TPN also resulted in a significant ($P < 0.01$) increase in epithelial cell apoptosis: TPN 7.6 ± 1.1% *versus* Control 2.9 ± 1.1% and TPN+Food 2.1 ± 0.3% (mean ± SD). Height of the villus-crypt complex was significantly decreased in TPN mice (315 ± 16 μm) compared with Control (431 ± 27 μm) and TPN+Food (421 ± 26 μm) groups. IEL phenotypes significantly changed with TPN administration: $CD4^+$ $CD8^-$ as well as $CD4^+$ $CD8^+$ subpopulations were reduced compared with Control or TPN+Food mice; as were the $CD8\alpha\beta^+$ thymus-dependent, and $CD8^+$ $CD44^+$ mature IEL. IEL cytokine mRNA expression was also significantly altered with TPN: IL-2 and IL-10 expression declined, and IL-4 IL-6, interferon gamma (IFN-γ), transforming growth factor β_1 (TGF-β_1), and tumor necrosis factor-α (TNF-α) were increased, when compared with Control or TPN+Food mice.

Conclusions.—This study demonstrates that the major factor responsible for TPN-induced BT and IEL-changes is the lack of enteral feeding and not the administration of the TPN solution itself.

▶ The use of TPN is associated with intestinal atrophy, BT, and changes in intestinal immune cell function as well as biliary immunoglobulin levels. In the past, some have suggested that this was due to TPN itself rather than the lack of food in the intestinal tract. Results of this study demonstrate that it is the lack of enteral feeding and not the administration of TPN solution that causes these adverse intestinal events. This study reinforces the dictum that in all patients, when possible, enteral nutrition should be given as part of their nutritional support regimen in an effort to maintain structure, function, and immunologic capabilities of their intestinal tracts.

J. M. Daly, MD

L-Selectin and α4β7 Integrin, But Not ICAM-1, Regulate Lymphocyte Distribution in Gut-Associated Lymphoid Tissue of Mice

Reese SR, Kudsk KA, Genton L, et al (William S Middleton Mem Veterans Hosp, Madison, Wis; Univ of Wisconsin, Madison)

Surgery 137:209-215, 2005 8–25

Background.—Adhesion molecules on lymphocytes (L-selectin and α4β7) and endothelium (MAdCAM-1 and ICAM-1) direct lymphocytes into the gut-associated lymphoid tissue (GALT) of mice. Parenteral nutrition and MAdCAM-1 blockade reduce GALT cell mass. This study examined the effects on GALT cell mass of blockade of L-selectin, α4β7, and ICAM-1 with saturating doses of monoclonal antibodies.

Methods.—In experiment 1, L-selectin and α4β7 expression were measured by flow cytometry in chow-fed mice. In experiment 2, 49 mice randomly received chow, parenteral nutrition, chow + intravenous (IV) anti-CD62L, chow + IV anti-LPAM-1, or chow + IV isotype control antibody. After 4 days, lymphocyte yields in GALT and respiratory and intestinal IgA levels were measured. In experiment 3, 27 mice randomly received chow, parenteral nutrition, chow + IV anti-ICAM-1 monoclonal antibody, or chow + IV isotype control antibody for 5 days. Lymphocyte counts and IgA levels were determined as in experiment 2.

Results.—Some 80% of all circulating lymphocytes were positive for L-selectin and α4β7. Lymphocyte counts in the Peyer's patches, lamina propria, and intraepithelial space were lower in the L-selectin and α4β7 blockade groups (3.1, 1.8, and 0.9 $\times 10^6$ and 2.1, 1.9, and 0.7 $\times 10^6$, respectively) than in the chow group (5.9, 3.0, and 1.7 $\times 10^6$; $P < .02$ vs the L-selectin group and $P < .001$ vs the α4β7 group) and similar to the levels in the parenteral group. Respiratory and intestinal IgA levels are maintained in all groups except the parenteral group ($P < .04$ vs the chow group). ICAM-1 blockade did not influence cell counts or IgA levels.

Conclusion.—Most circulating lymphocytes have GALT homing potential. Their distribution into GALT is hindered by blockade of L-selectin or α4β7, but not by ICAM-1.

► It is well known that mucosal-associated lymphoid tissue contains over 50% of total immunity and produces the majority of the body's immunoglobulin. These authors evaluated lymphocytes and their distribution into GALT in mice. They noted that most circulating lymphocytes have GALT homing potential that was hindered by blockade of L-selectin or α4β7, but not by ICAM-1. Studies such as these are important to understand the homing capability of circulating lymphocytes. GALT is extremely important in immune function, and mechanisms to enhance GALT forming and efficiency are important.

J. M. Daly, MD

9 Wound Healing

Introduction

Efforts continue to evaluate methods of improving the healing of chronic wounds, particularly complex chronic wounds. The biologic basis of wound healing has been studied for hundreds of years. However, new factors continue to be identified that may play a role in wound healing. Opportunities also exist for the discovery of agents that may accelerate wound healing.

Wilgus et al (Abstract 9–1) noted the impact of COX-2 on inflammation in scarless fetal wound healing. They noted that COX-2 is clearly involved in scarless versus scar forming fetal skin wounds. The authors suggested that COX-2 inhibition during the inflammatory phase of wound healing may be of benefit in controlling the wound healing process, resulting in less scar tissue. Care must be taken to be sure that this early inflammatory inhibition does not result in poorer overall wound healing, which may affect the developing strength of the wound.

Many studies evaluated methods to prevent postoperative adhesions. In one such study, Bulbuller et al (Abstract 9–2) evaluated angiotensin-converting enzyme (ACE) inhibitors to prevent postoperative adhesions. These ACE inhibitors appear useful in preventing peritoneal adhesions in an animal model. It will be important for studies to ultimately evaluate the situation in humans, perhaps those undergoing second-look laparotomy such as patients undergoing treatment for ovarian carcinoma. Greene et al (Abstract 9–3) evaluated prevention of intra-abdominal adhesions using COX-2 inhibitors. Again, modulation of the inflammatory phase in animals certainly seems to reduce postoperative peritoneal adhesions. Katada et al (Abstract 9–4) studied COX-2 in a model of mechanical stimulated induced peritoneal adhesions in mice. Again, these results warrant further experimental studies to determine the true therapeutic efficacy of COX-2 inhibitors. Cohen et al (Abstract 9–5) evaluated the use of a novel bioresorbable membrane. Many such studies will be published over the next several years as investigators attempt to design the ideal bioresorbable membrane. It should have strength for a period of time but then dissolve, and clearly should reduce the number of adhesions. This randomized prospective study was carried out in 120 patients who underwent a diverting loop ileostomy. This new bioresorbable membrane created by adding glycerol to the formula appeared to improve handling.

Many studies evaluated methods to accelerate wound repair. Hassanain et al (Abstract 9–6) evaluated human *Rac* 1 in acceleration of cutaneous wound repair. Taly et al (Abstract 9–7) studied the efficacy of multiwavelength light therapy in the treatment of pressure ulcers in subjects with disorders of the spinal cord. In this prospective randomized trial, they found no effect in terms of clinical outcome benefit. Negative studies such as these are extraordinarily important to help us understand what often becomes a fad in various therapeutic settings.

It is clear to many surgeons that incisional hernia repair after a repair of wound dehiscence is often fraught with difficulties. However, in a study from The Netherlands, the incidence of risk factors for recurrent hernia after the initial repair of the incisional hernia was quite high. The cumulative incidence of incisional hernia developing after the initial repair was nearly 70% at 10 years. Thus, we need to work harder in this area to improve the results in patients who have developed a wound dehiscence and undergo initial repair. The number of times the incisional hernia is further repaired seemed to result in a decrease in the likelihood of permanent repair.

Moderate hyperoxia increases antioxidant levels in mouse tissue. These studies suggest a metabolic correlate to clinical data, noting that the administration of oxygen results in higher tissue oxygen levels and improved healing. In a study by DuBay et al (Abstract 9–9), they noted that an animal model of incisional hernia formation accurately recreated the wound pathology expressed in mature incisional hernias. Development of this animal model is extremely important as it lends itself to clinical situations. As shown in the large trial from The Netherlands, incisional hernia repair is often fraught with difficulties and less success than one would like to believe. Thus, creation of this animal model will be helpful in identifying factors that can improve clinical results.

It had been thought that reinforcement of subcuticular continuous suture closure may improve healing. In fact, Yavuzer et al (Abstract 9–12) noted exactly the opposite. The subcuticular continuous suture closure was quite good, whereas the use of gum mastic diminished benefit. The use of steri-adhesive strips with the continuous closure was the best methodology for both cosmesis and healing.

The evaluation of ischemic flaps and ischemic myocutaneous tissues is extremely important. Contaldo et al (Abstract 9–15) evaluated a new generation of hemoglobin-based oxygen carriers in this experimental situation. Clearly, the safety and efficacy of this approach should be tested in other animal models and then proceed to clinical trials when such efficacy is established. These early studies suggest clear benefit. Harder et al (Abstract 9–17) noted the evolution of a falx lunatica in demarcation of critically ischemic myocutaneous tissue. Komori et al (Abstract 9–18) noted that a single local application of recombinant human basic fibroblast growth factor accelerated the initial angiogenesis during wound healing. Again, these studies need to be carried out in a variety of animal models and then move progressively towards the clinical situation if efficacy is borne out. It was noted by Kurten et al (Abstract 9–21) that coordinating epidermal growth factor–induced motility promoted efficient wound closure. Finally, the application of dermatotraction for primary skin closure was determined. This method appeared to be very effective for obtaining primary closure of major wounds without the use of a skin-stretching system. This appeared to have benefit in terms of cost and time.

Thus, studies this year in wound healing were focused more on the scientific evaluation of wound biology and methods to improve healing in a variety of animal models. Continued progression to clinical studies is important to define usefulness in a variety of circumstances.

John M. Daly, MD

The Impact of Cyclooxygenase-2 Mediated Inflammation on Scarless Fetal Wound Healing

Wilgus TA, Bergdall VK, Tober KL, et al (Ohio State Univ, Columbus)

Am J Pathol 165:753-761, 2004 9–1

Introduction.—Cyclooxygenase-2 (COX-2) and the prostaglandin products generated as a result of COX-2 activity mediate a variety of biological and pathological processes. Scarless healing occurs in fetal skin in the first and second trimesters of development. This scarless healing process is known to proceed without a significant inflammatory response, which appears to be important for the lack of scarring. Because the COX-2 pathway is an integral component of inflammation, we investigated its role in the fetal repair process using a mouse model of scarless fetal wound healing. COX-2 expression in scarless and fibrotic fetal wounds was examined. In addition, the ability of exogenous prostaglandin E_2 to alter scarless fetal healing was evaluated. The results suggest that the COX-2 pathway is involved in scar production in fetal skin and that targeting COX-2 may be useful for limiting scar formation in adult skin.

► It is well known that inflammation is a major component in the early phase of wound healing. It has been suggested that the reason for scarless healing in fetal skin is the absence of a major inflammatory component. COX-2 and prostaglandins appear important in the scarless healing of fetal wounds. In this study, COX-2 was clearly involved in scarless versus scar-forming fetal skin wounds. Increasing prostaglandin E_2 (PGE_2) levels in scarless wounds resulted in the conversion to a wound that generates a scar. It is possible that PGE_2 increases acute inflammation, delays the healing process, or disrupts the PGF-β signaling pathways. But the increasing fibroblast proliferation result in a scar. The take-away message is that inhibition of COX-2 may result in less scar formation in cutaneous wounds. Taken together with another article in this series (Abstract 9–4), which demonstrated fewer intraperitoneal adhesions in an animal model, this suggests that COX-2 inhibition may be of benefit in controlling the wound healing process, resulting in less scar.

J. M. Daly, MD

Can Angiotensin Converting Enzyme Inhibitors Prevent Postoperative Adhesions?

Bulbuller N, Ilhan YS, Kirkil C, et al (Firat Univ, Elaziğ, Turkey; SSK Elaziğ Hosp, Turkey)

J Surg Res 125:94-97, 2005 9–2

Background.—Peritoneal adhesions are pathological fibrotic bands developing after mesothelial damage. Transforming growth factor beta-1 (TGF-β1) has mitogenic activities for macrophages and fibroblasts. Overexpression of TGF-β1 has been implicated in the pathogenesis of several fibrotic disorders. Angiotensin II increases the expression of the TGF-β1 in fibroblasts. The aim of the study was to investigate the effect of angiotensin converting enzyme inhibitor (ACE) on intraperitoneal adhesions.

Materials and Methods.—Thirty male Wistar albino rats were divided into two groups. In the first procedure, laparotomy was performed through a 3-cm midline incision. Ileum was divided above 10 cm from ileocecal valve and a single-layer ileoileal anastomosis was performed. Although no treatment was given to rats in group 1, lisinopril (an ACE inhibitor) was given to rats in group 2 for postoperative 7 days in drinking water. Estimated amount of supplied lisinopril was 6.5 mg/kg/day. On postoperative 8th day, relaparotomy was performed and adhesions were evaluated. At the same time, blood samples were taken for TGF-β1 measurements.

Results.—Adhesion severity was significantly less in the ACE inhibitor group ($P < 0.001$). While mean TGF-β1 level was 860.3 ± 108.1 pg/dl (mean ± SD) in control group, it was 335.8 ± 52.4 pg/dl in ACE inhibitor group ($P < 0.001$). There was a significant correlation between serum TGF-β1 levels and grade of adhesions ($r = 0.948$).

Conclusion.—It was concluded that ACE inhibitors might be useful for preventing peritoneal adhesions.

► This study evaluated the effects of ACE inhibitors on TGF-β1 in fibroblasts in an animal model. The authors noted that adhesion severity was significantly less in the ACE inhibitor group compared with controls. Thus, ACE inhibitors may be useful for preventing peritoneal adhesions. The concept of prevention of peritoneal adhesions is extremely important. Patients, both short and long-term, develop peritoneal adhesions. After, they must undergo re-exploration by laparoscopic or open techniques because of bowel obstruction secondary to adhesion formation. Thus, our ability to control the formation of adhesions after surgery is important. Many studies have suggested that laparoscopy reduces the amount of intra-abdominal adhesions. While this has been thought to be due to carbon dioxide instillation, some investigators believe it is simply the reduced manipulation of the intestine that helps to prevent adhesions. The use of other biochemical means to prevent adhesions is less important. Clearly, further studies need to be carried out to determine whether this methodology will be of benefit in a clinical situation.

J. M. Daly, MD

Prevention of Intra-abdominal Adhesions Using the Antiangiogenic COX-2 Inhibitor Celecoxib

Greene AK, Alwayn IPJ, Nose V, et al (Harvard Med School, Boston)

Ann Surg 242:140-146, 2005 9–3

Objective.—To determine the effects of COX-2 specific inhibitors on postoperative adhesion formation.

Summary and Background Data.—Intra-abdominal adhesions are the major cause of intestinal obstruction and secondary infertility after surgical procedures. Because adhesion synthesis requires angiogenesis, and cyclooxygenase-2 enzyme (COX-2) inhibitors have antiendothelial activity, we tested COX-2 inhibitors in a murine model of intra-abdominal adhesion formation.

Methods.—A silicone patch was secured to the lateral abdominal wall of groups of C57BL/6 mice, followed by cecal abrasion to promote adhesion formation. Beginning on the day of surgery, mice were treated with the selective COX-2 agents, celecoxib or rofecoxib, and the nonspecific COX inhibitors, aspirin, naproxen, ibuprofen, or indomethacin. Animals were treated for 10 days and killed. A second group (celecoxib, rofecoxib, aspirin) was treated for 10 days and observed for an additional 25 days. After treatment, intra-abdominal adhesions were scored using a standard method. The patch was subjected to immunohistochemistry with the endothelial-specific marker, CD31.

Results.—Animals treated with selective and nonselective COX-2 inhibitors, except aspirin, had significantly fewer adhesions than control animals. Celecoxib produced a maximal reduction in adhesion formation compared with rofecoxib and the nonselective COX-2 inhibitors at 10 days. After 25 days, celecoxib and rofecoxib, but not aspirin, had fewer adhesions than control mice. Adhesions from mice treated with celecoxib had reduced microvessel density compared with rofecoxib, the nonselective COX inhibitors, and control animals.

Conclusions.—Selective COX-2 inhibitors, in particular celecoxib, provide durable inhibition of intra-abdominal adhesions through an antiangiogenic mechanism.

► Because intra-abdominal adhesions routinely develop after abdominal surgery, studies have looked at a variety of anti-inflammatory agents early after abdominal surgery in an effort to reduce adhesions. In this experimental study in mice, Greene et al treated animals with selective and nonselective COX-2 inhibitors and demonstrated significantly fewer adhesions than in control animals. Thus, selective COX-2 inhibitors may reduce adhesion formation, resulting in less short- and long-term morbidity after abdominal surgery. Studies such as this are difficult to carry out in humans because of the need to quantitatively assess adhesion formation. Thus, these studies need to be further vetted in other animals models, but then utilized in certain subgroups of patients to determine whether short-term use of COX-2 inhibitors can reduce intra-abdominal adhesion formation.

J. M. Daly, MD

Significance of Cyclooxygenase-2 Induced via p38 Mitogen-Activated Protein Kinase in Mechanical Stimulus-Induced Peritoneal Adhesion in Mice

Katada J, Saito H, Ohashi A (Keio Univ, Tokyo)
J Pharmacol Exp Ther 313:286-292, 2005 9–4

Introduction.—Postoperative peritoneal adhesion represents a major complication of surgery, but the molecular mechanism underlying pathogenesis of adhesion is not fully understood. The present study investigated the roles of cyclooxygenase (COX)-1 and COX-2 in peritoneal adhesion induced by scraping the surface of the cecum and abdominal wall in mice. Slight, but macroscopically observable, peritoneal adhesion was induced even on day 1, and the extent of adhesion reached a maximum on day 7 and beyond. COX-1 mRNA was constitutively expressed in the intact cecum, and its expression level was not altered after the mechanical stimulus. In contrast, expression of the COX-2 gene was markedly increased after the stimulus, and maximum expression was observed on days 3 to 7. Mofezolac, a specific COX-1 inhibitor, had no effect on peritoneal adhesion at 30 mg/kg and had only marginal effects on prostaglandin (PG)E_2 levels in the cecum or peritoneal fluid. On the other hand, two highly selective inhibitors for COX-2, NS-398 (*N*-[2-(cyclohexyloxy)-4-nitrophenyl]-methanesulfonamide) and CAY10404 [3-(4-methylsulphonylphenyl)-4-phenyl-5-trifluoromethylisoxazole], dose-dependently inhibited both adhesion formation and the increase in PGE_2 levels (3-30 mg/kg). The effects of NS-398 were eliminated when PGE_2 or (*R*)-butaprost was administered exogenously. A COX-2 antisense oligonucleotide also attenuated adhesion formation. Activation of p38 mitogen-activated protein (MAP) kinase was observed in the traumatized cecum, and an MAP kinase inhibitor, SB202190 [4-(4-fluorophenyl)-2-(4-hydroxyphenyl)-5-(4-pyridyl)-1*H*-imidazole], inhibited adhesion formation (54% inhibition at 15 μM) and also reduced the COX-2 mRNA level and PGE_2 levels. In conclusion, COX-2, but not COX-1, plays a significant role in mechanical stimulus-induced peritoneal formation in the mouse cecum.

► Mechanical stimulus–induced peritoneal adhesions are a major cause of postoperative morbidity in patients undergoing open abdominal operations. The underlying biochemical mechanisms are not clear. These authors studied both COX-1 and COX-2 mRNA after mechanical stimulus to create adhesions. They noted that while COX-1 was slightly elevated, COX-2 was markedly elevated in the peritoneal adhesion group. COX-2 inhibitors markedly decreased both adhesion formation and PGE_2 levels. Thus, COX-2 but not COX-1 plays a major role in this animal model of mechanical stimulus–induced peritoneal formation in the area of the mouse cecum.

COX-2 inhibitors are well recognized as anti-inflammatory agents. The mechanisms of mechanical stimulation of peritoneal adhesion formation are clearly related to the inflammatory response. One wonders whether or not there would be benefit in humans utilizing COX-2 inhibitors not only to decrease postoperative pain, but to reduce mechanical stimulus–induced adhesion formation. The downside of this approach may be some decrease in anastomotic or fascial healing in postoperative patients. Nevertheless, these results warrant further experimental studies to determine the therapeutic role for COX-2 inhibitors.

J. M. Daly, MD

Prevention of Postoperative Abdominal Adhesions by a Novel, Glycerol/Sodium Hyaluronate/Carboxymethylcellulose-Based Bioresorbable Membrane: A Prospective, Randomized, Evaluator-Blinded Multicenter Study

Cohen Z, Senagore AJ, Dayton MT, et al (Univ of Toronto; Cleveland Clinic Found, Ohio; State Univ of New York at Buffalo; et al)

Dis Colon Rectum 48:1130-1139, 2005 9–5

Introduction.—Postoperative abdominal adhesions are associated with significant morbidity and mortality, placing a substantial burden on healthcare systems worldwide. Development of a bioresorbable membrane containing up to 23 percent glycerol and chemically modified sodium hyaluronate/carboxymethylcellulose offers ease of handling and has been shown to provide significant postoperative adhesion prevention in animals. This study was designed to assess the safety of glycerol hyaluronate/carboxymethylcellulose and to evaluate its efficacy in reducing the incidence, extent, and severity of postoperative adhesion development in surgical patients.

Methods.—Twelve centers enrolled 120 patients with ulcerative colitis or familial polyposis who were scheduled for a restorative proctocolectomy and ileal pouch-anal anastomosis with diverting loop ileostomy. Before surgical closure, patients were randomized to no anti-adhesion treatment (control) or treatment with glycerol hyaluronate/carboxymethylcellulose membrane under the midline incision. At ileostomy closure, laparoscopy was used to evaluate the incidence, extent, and severity of adhesion formation to the midline incision.

Results.—Data were analyzed using the intent-to-treat population. Treatment with glycerol hyaluronate/carboxymethylcellulose resulted in 19 of 58 patients (33 percent) with no adhesions compared with 6 of 60 adhesion-free patients (10 percent) in the no treatment control group ($P = 0.002$). The mean extent of postoperative adhesions to the midline incision was significantly lower among patients treated with glycerol hyaluronate/carboxymethylcellulose compared with patients in the control group ($P <$

0.001). The severity of postoperative adhesions to the midline incision was significantly less with glycerol hyaluronate/carboxymethylcellulose than with control ($P < 0.001$). Adverse events were similar between treatment and no treatment control groups with the exception of abscess and incisional wound complications were more frequently observed with glycerol hyaluronate/carboxymethylcellulose.

Conclusions.—Glycerol hyaluronate/carboxymethylcellulose was shown to effectively reduce adhesions to the midline incision and adhesions between the omentum and small bowel after abdominal surgery. Safety profiles for the treatment and no treatment control groups were similar with the exception of more infection complications associated with glycerol hyaluronate/carboxymethylcellulose use. Animal models did not predict these complications.

► This randomized, prospective trial evaluated a bioresorbable membrane in 120 patients with ulcerative colitis or familial polyposis who were undergoing a diverting loop ileostomy. At the time of ileostomy closure, laparoscopy was used to evaluate the incidence, extent, and severity of adhesion formation to the midline incision. Thirty-three percent of the patients receiving the bioresorbable membrane had no adhesions compared with 10% of patients in the control group. Biodegradable membranes have been shown to be of benefit, but are often difficult to manipulate at the time of open abdominal surgery. Thus, this new bioresorbable membrane was created by adding glycerol to improve handling. Results of this study clearly show benefit in terms of reducing midline adhesions, particularly dense adhesions. Studies such as these are important, as subcategories of patients such as those with ovarian carcinoma often undergo repeated abdominal operations. The ability to reduce midline adhesions can result in a safer reoperation when it becomes necessary. Other indications for these membranes may be around the loop ileostomies or temporary diverting colostomies, as it makes the subsequent reversal of the ostomy much easier. One complication was a higher incidence of wound infection and abnormal wound healing identified in the treated patients versus controls. This adverse outcome must be thoroughly investigated to be sure that bioresorbable membranes do not cause harm.

J. M. Daly, MD

Smooth Muscle Cell Expression of a Constitutive Active Form of Human Rac 1 Accelerates Cutaneous Wound Repair

Hassanain HH, Irshaid F, Wisel S, et al (Ohio State Univ, Columbus; Duke Univ, Durham, NC)

Surgery 137:92-101, 2005 9–6

Background.—Hyperoxia has been shown to improve wound healing; however, the mechanism for such therapeutic effects of oxygen remains hypothetical. Rac 1 regulates a wide variety of cellular activities, including cell proliferation and migration, and also is a key regulator for the activity of the nicotinamide dinucleotide phosphate oxidase the enzyme complex responsible for the production of a large fraction of cellular superoxide.

Methods.—We generated transgenic mice that express either the cDNA of a constitutively active mutant of human Rac 1 (V12 mutant or Rac CA) or the dominant negative isoform (V12 and N17 mutant or Rac DN) in the blood vessels using mouse vascular smooth muscle promoter for α-actin. We placed 2 wounds of 6 mm in diameter at the middorsal region of each mouse and allowed about 3 weeks for the wounds to heal.

Results.—The size of the wounds in Rac CA transgenic mice was reduced relative to wild type mice; healing of Rac DN mice was slower than wild type and Rac CA ($P < .05$). Blood vessel formation appeared faster in Rac CA mice, a finding associated with enhanced expression of some angiogenic growth factors.

Conclusion.—The current studies suggest that Rac 1 activation accelerates the wound healing process and is associated with more efficient angiogenesis at the wound site.

▶ These authors evaluated wound healing in transgenic mice with a constitutively active mutant of human Rac 1. They noted that Rac 1 activation accelerated the wound healing process and improved angiogenesis at the wound site. Rac 1 is a member of the small GTPase proteins of the Ras family and regulates a variety of cellular activities, including proliferation. This transgenic animal study suggests that Rac 1 activation in the wound healing process is important.

J. M. Daly, MD

Efficacy of Multiwavelength Light Therapy in the Treatment of Pressure Ulcers in Subjects With Disorders of the Spinal Cord: A Randomized Double-blind Controlled Trial

Taly AB, Nair KPS, Murali T, et al (Natl Inst of Mental Health and Neurosciences, Bangalore, India)

Arch Phys Med Rehabil 85:1657-1661, 2004 9–7

Objective.—To study the efficacy of multiwavelength light therapy in the treatment of pressure ulcers in subjects with spinal cord disorders.

Design.—Randomized controlled trial.

Setting.—Neurologic rehabilitation ward of a referral center in India.

Participants.—Thirty-five subjects with spinal cord injury, with 64 pressure ulcers (stage 2, n=55; stage 3, n=8; stage 4, n=1), were randomized into treatment and control groups. One subject refused consent. Mean duration of ulcers in the treatment group was 34.2±45.5 days and in the control group, 57.1±43.5 days.

Interventions.—Treatment group received 14 sessions of multiwavelength light therapy, with 46 probes of different wavelengths from a gallium-aluminum-arsenide laser source, 3 times a week. Energy used was 4.5 J/cm^2. Ulcers in the control group received sham treatment.

Main Outcome Measures.—Healing of the ulcer, defined as the complete closure of the wound with healthy scar tissue, time taken for the ulcer to heal, and stage of the ulcer and Pressure Sore Status Tool score 14 days after last treatment.

Results.—There was no significant difference in healing between the treatment and control groups. Eighteen ulcers in treatment group and 14 in control group healed completely (P=.802). Mean time taken by the ulcers to heal was 2.45±2.06 weeks in the treatment group and 1.78±2.13 weeks in the control group (P=.330). Time taken for stage 3 and 4 ulcers to reach stage 2 was 2.25±0.5 weeks in treatment group and 4.33±1.53 weeks in control group (P=.047).

Conclusions.—Multiwavelength light therapy from a gallium-aluminum-arsenide laser source did not influence overall healing pressure ulcers. Limited evidence suggested that it improved healing of stage 3 and 4 pressure ulcers.

▶ Previous studies have suggested that multiwavelength light therapy improved the treatment of pressure ulcers in individuals with disorders of the spinal cord. These authors randomized 35 patients with 64 pressure ulcers to treatment and control groups. There was no effect on overall healing of pressure ulcers. Some improvement in healing of stage 3 and 4 pressure ulcers occurred. Studies such as these are critically important because they evaluate in a randomized prospective fashion interventional therapies for pressure ulcers. The fact that multiwavelength therapy was not of benefit is important to note in the literature. Even though lasers promote fibroblast proliferation, collagen production, and epithelialization, in these patients there was little clinical outcome benefit noted.

J. M. Daly, MD

Incisional Hernia After Repair of Wound Dehiscence: Incidence and Risk Factors

van 'T Riet M, de vos van Steenwijk PJ, Bonjer HJ, et al (Erasmus Univ, Rotterdam, The Netherlands)

Am Surg 70:281-286, 2004 9–8

Introduction.—The true incidence of incisional hernia after wound dehiscence repair remains unclear because thorough long-term follow-up studies are not available. Medical records of all patients who had undergone wound dehiscence repair between January 1985 and January 1999 at the Erasmus University Medical Center Rotterdam were reviewed. Long-term follow-up was performed by physical examination of all patients in February 2001. One hundred sixty-eight patients underwent wound dehiscence repair. Of those, 42 patients (25%) died within 60 days after surgery. During a median follow-up of 37 months (range, 3-146 months), 55 of the remaining 126 patients developed an incisional hernia. The cumulative incidence of incisional hernia was 69 per cent at 10 years. Significant independent risk factors were aneurysm of the abdominal aorta (10-year cumulative incidence of 84%, $P = 0.02$) and severe dehiscence with evisceration (10-year cumulative incidence of 78%, $P = 0.01$). Wound dehiscence repair by interrupted sutures had no better outcome than repair by continuous sutures. Suture material did not influence incidence of incisional hernia. Incisional hernia develops in the majority of patients after wound dehiscence repair, regardless of suture material or technique. Aneurysm of the abdominal aorta and severe dehiscence with evisceration predispose to incisional hernia.

► These authors evaluated long-term follow-up in patients who developed wound dehiscence and underwent repair. Twenty-five percent of those with wound dehiscence died within 60 days after operation. Of those who survived, the cumulative incidence of incisional hernia was nearly 70%. Independent risk factors were abdominal aortic aneurysms and severe dehiscence with evisceration. The method of repair did not seem to have any relevance to the later development of ventral hernias. It is important to note the high mortality associated with wound dehiscence in hospitalized patients. Secondly, those who developed severe dehiscence and those who have undergone open abdominal aortic aneurysm repair are at major risk to develop a further ventral hernia. Studies such as these are important as they provide a long-term follow-up (10 years).

J. M. Daly, MD

Progressive Fascial Wound Failure Impairs Subsequent Abdominal Wall Repairs: A New Animal Model of Incisional Hernia Formation

DuBay DA, Wang X, Adamson B, et al (Univ of Michigan, Ann Arbor)

Surgery 137:463-471, 2005 9–9

Background.—Fascial wound failure alters the phenotype of the abdominal wall. This study introduces a novel animal model of progressive failure of the ventral abdominal wall fascia, which generates large incisional hernias.

Material and Methods.—A mechanistic model of incisional hernia was compared with a model of acute myofascial defect hernia repair. Using biological tissue repair markers, tensiometric measurements and recurrent hernia rate, we measured the mechanism by which incisional hernias regenerate abdominal wall structure and function after mesh and suture herniorrhaphy.

Results.—Recurrent incisional hernia formation was significantly increased after repairs of the hernia model, compared with the myofascial defect model (6/16 vs 0/16, $P < .05$). In the hernia model, there were significant decreases in the recovery of wound strength, energy, and extensibility before mechanical disruption, compared with the myofascial defect model. Unexpectedly, excision of fascial hernia wound edges did not significantly improve tissue repair outcomes in the hernia model group.

Conclusions.—Clinically accurate animal modeling can recreate the wound pathology expressed in mature incisional hernias. Progressive fascial wound failure decreases the fidelity of subsequent incisional hernia repair, compared with identically sized acute abdominal wall defect repairs. The mechanism appears to include decreased fascial wound strength and decreased tissue compliance after herniorrhaphy.

► Abdominal ventral hernias occur with some frequency in patients undergoing major complex abdominal surgery. It is well known that a failed primary repair of an abdominal ventral hernia leads to a continued increasing failure rate with subsequent repairs. Mechanisms are not clear. Thus, this animal model of fascial wound failure provides an opportunity to control factors related to repair of these ventral defects. These authors utilized a mechanistic model of incisional hernia and compared it to an acute model of acute myofascial defect. The former showed great similarities to that which occurs in the clinical situation. Thus, examination of changes in fascial wound strength and tissue compliance after herniorrhaphy can be determined in an animal model such as this, providing applications of new therapeutic interventions in the clinical situation.

J. M. Daly, MD

Moderate Hyperoxia (40%) Increases Antioxidant Levels in Mouse Tissue

Lee ES, Smith WE, Quach HT, et al (Univ of California Davis, Sacramento; Univ of Minnesota, Minneapolis)

J Surg Res 127:80-84, 2005 9–10

Background.—Oxygen is routinely administered to patients to improve clinical outcome. Since studies have shown that administering 100% oxygen can cause unwanted side effects, intermediate concentrations of 40% oxygen are used in clinical practice. In this study, we examined whether the breathing of 40% oxygen causes beneficial effects upon tissue levels of antioxidants such as vitamin E, vitamin C, and glutathione.

Methods.—Four-month-old mice were separated into two groups: control ($n = 11$) and experimental ($n = 11$). The treatment group was administered 40% oxygen for 10 days. Brain, heart, lung, liver, testes, and skeletal muscle were harvested and tissue antioxidant levels were determined by HPLC.

Results.—Vitamin E concentrations were higher in brain, heart, lung, liver, and testes of the treatment group ($P < 0.05$). Glutathione concentrations were higher in the lung tissue only ($P < 0.05$). No differences were found in vitamin C levels.

Conclusions.—The data suggest that mice respond to oxidative stress by increasing tissue vitamin E incorporation and cellular synthesis of glutathione in the lung when exposed to moderate levels (40%) of hyperoxia.

► In ill patients, oxygen is routinely administered to improve clinical outcome. However, administering too high concentrations of oxygen can cause side effects, particularly pulmonary side effects. In this study, young mice were separated into groups consisting of animals receiving normal oxygen levels versus animals who received 40% oxygen for 10 days. In the treated mice, vitamin E concentrations were higher in multiple tissues, but glutathione concentrations were higher in lung tissue only. Thus, mice responded to oxidative stress by increasing tissue vitamin E incorporation. These studies suggest a metabolic correlate to clinical data noting that administration of oxygen resulting in higher tissue oxygen levels significantly decreases mortality compared with controls in high-risk surgical patients. Results of this study by Lee et al suggest other mechanisms for this beneficial effect whereby increased oxygen concentrations in tissues improve vitamin E concentrations and antioxidant activity.

J. M. Daly, MD

Peritoneal Regeneration Induced by an Acellular Bovine Pericardial Patch in the Repair of Abdominal Wall Defects

Lai P-H, Chang Y, Liang H-C, et al (Natl Tsing Hua Univ, Hsinchu, Taiwan, ROC; Natl Yang-Ming Univ, Taipei, Taiwan, ROC)

J Surg Res 127:85-92, 2005 9–11

Background.—This study was to evaluate the feasibility of using an acellular bovine pericardium fixed with genipin (AGP) to repair an abdominal wall defect created in a rat model.

Materials and Methods.—The glutaraldehyde-fixed acellular pericardium (AGA), the genipin-fixed cellular pericardium (GP), and a commercially available polypropylene mesh were used as controls.

Results.—Gross examination at 3-month post-operatively revealed that dense adhesions to the visceral organs were observed for the polypropylene mesh and the AGA patch, while a filmy to dense adhesion was seen for the GP patch. In contrast, no adhesion to the visceral organs was observed for the AGP patch. Histologically, inflammatory cells were found mainly surrounding the GP patch. In contrast, host cells (inflammatory cells, fibroblasts, and neo-capillaries) were able to infiltrate into the AGA and AGP patches. Unlike the AGA patch, the AGP patch retrieved at 1-month post-operatively became well integrated with the host tissue near the suture line. Additionally, there were some mesothelial cells, identified by the van Gieson stain, observed on the AGP patch. At 3-month post-operatively, a neo-peritoneum was observed on the AGP patch. The neo-peritoneum consisted of organized vascularized connective tissues covered by an intact layer of mesothelial cells. The calcium contents of the polypropylene mesh and the AGA patch increased significantly at 3-month post-operatively, while those of the GP and AGP patches stayed minimal throughout the entire course of the study.

Conclusions.—The results obtained in the study revealed that the AGP patch effectively repaired abdominal wall defects in rats and successfully prevented the formation of post-surgical abdominal adhesions.

▶ In this study, Lai and colleagues evaluated glutaraldehyde-fixed acellular pericardium in an effort to try to improve the feasibility of such a device to repair abdominal wall defects. In rats, use of this substance effectively repaired abdominal wall defects and prevented the formation of postsurgical abdominal adhesions. Patients undergoing large complex open abdominal surgery with triangular incisions, obese patients undergoing open surgery, patients with pulmonary comorbidities such as chronic bronchitis and chronic obstructive pulmonary disease, those taking immunosuppressants, and many others are at risk for ventral hernia development. Repair often involves artificial materials. The study findings, if reproduced in humans, suggest another methodology for effectively repairing abdominal wall defects. These authors showed that a neoperitoneum had organized, vascularized connective tissues covered by an intact layer of mesothelial cells. These results demonstrate benefit in this animal model with the use of acellular pericardium as a ventral hernia patch.

J. M. Daly, MD

Reinforcement of Subcuticular Continuous Suture Closure With Surgical Adhesive Strips and Gum Mastic: Is There Any Additional Strength Provided?

Yavuzer R, Kelly C, Durrani N, et al (Providence Hosp, Southfield, Mich; Inst for Craniofacial and Reconstructive Surgery, Southfield, Mich)

Am J Surg 189:315-318, 2005 9–12

Background.—This study aimed to compare the burst strength of suture closure versus the use of suture and strip together.

Methods.—On cadavers, 50 skin incisions were closed as follows: group 1—subcuticular continuous suture; group 2—same suturing with placement of strips; group 3—same as group 2 except gum mastic was applied prior to strips; group 4—strips alone; and group 5—strips with gum mastic application. The separation forces were measured using a tensilometer.

Results.—The mean separation forces were as follows: group 1, 14.17 kg; group 2, 14.37 kg; group 3, 15.39 kg; group 4, 1.52 kg; and group 5, 3.85 kg. There were no statistically significant differences between groups 1, 2, and 3. When compared with group 4, group 5 required markedly more force to separate the wound.

Conclusions.—Strip reinforcement with/without gum mastic did not provide any additional strength when sutures were used. Gum mastic increased the adherence of strips and this was important when strips were the only means of wound closure.

► The use of absorbable continuous subcuticular suture is common in the closure of surgical incisions and provides an improved cosmetic result. However, surgeons use many different preferences in addition to the subcuticular closure in an effort to improve cosmetic outcome further and reduce postoperative wound complications. Some use subcuticular closure alone, while others use suturing with placement of Steri-Strips or Steri-Strips with an adhesive bond applied to the skin before placement of the strips. In this study, suture alone, suturing with strips, and suturing plus strips applied after gum mastic had the highest mean wound separation forces. Strips alone and strips with gum mastic application had markedly lower mean wound separation forces. These results suggest that the best method for wound closure is the use of continuous subcuticular suturing with an absorbable material. Placement of Steri-Strips or strips plus adhesive bonding material did not appear to add significantly to mean separation forces in this model.

J. M. Daly, MD

Tissue Factor as a Link Between Wounding and Tissue Repair

Chen J, Kasper M, Heck T, et al (Univ of Heidelberg, Germany; Baylor College of Medicine, Houston; Technical Univ of Dresden, Germany; et al)

Diabetes 54:2143-2154, 2005 9–13

Introduction.—The initial phase of wound repair involves inflammation, induction of tissue factor (TF), formation of a fibrin matrix, and growth of new smooth muscle actin (α-SMA)-positive vessels. In diabetes, TF induction in response to cutaneous wounding, which ordinarily precedes increased expression of vascular endothelial growth factor (VEGF) and α-SMA transcription, is diminished, though not to a degree causing excessive local bleeding. Enhanced TF expression in wounds of diabetic mice caused by somatic TF gene transfer increased VEGF transcription and translation and, subsequently, enhanced formation of new blood vessels and elevated blood flow. Furthermore, increased levels of TF in wounds of diabetic mice enhanced wound healing; the time to achieve 50% wound closure was reduced from 5.5 days in untreated diabetic mice to 4.1 days in animals undergoing TF gene transfer (this was not statistically different from wound closure in nondiabetic mice). Thus, cutaneous wounds in diabetic mice display a relative deficiency of TF compared with nondiabetic controls, and this contributes to delayed wound repair. These data establish TF expression as an important link between the early inflammatory response to cutaneous wounding and reparative processes.

► It is well known that diabetic patients have impaired wound healing. The exact mechanisms for this are unclear since this impairment appears to be multifactorial. It may relate to changes in vascular supply, elevated glucose levels leading to impaired inflammatory cell functions, or other mechanisms. These authors suggest that reduced induction of TF may play a major role. Thus, TF gene transfer in diabetic mice was shown to increase VEGF transcription and translation. Subsequently, increased formation of new blood vessels and elevated blood flow occurred. In these animals, increased levels of TF in wounds of diabetic mice markedly enhanced wound healing. Thus, the use of TF gene transfer may be important in improving VEGF production locally in wounds of diabetics and increasing wound healing.

J. M. Daly, MD

Hypertrophic Scar Cells Fail to Undergo a Form of Apoptosis Specific to Contractile Collagen: The Role of Tissue Transglutaminase

Linge C, Richardson J, Vigor C, et al (RAFT Inst of Plastic Surgery, Middlesex, England; Procyon Biopharma Inc, Dorval, Quebec)

J Invest Dermatol 125:72-82, 2005 9–14

Introduction.—Failure of apoptosis has been postulated to cause the hypercellularity and thus excess scar-tissue formation of hypertrophic scars (HTS). Here, we have examined the susceptibility of fibroblasts derived from normal or HTS to apoptosis induced during collagen-gel contraction, a wound-healing model. Normal scar (NS) fibroblasts underwent significant apoptosis (>40% total) in contractile collagen, whereas apoptosis was not detected in HTS cells. This inability was specific to apoptosis induced by contractile collagen because apoptosis could be induced using diverse modalities. Since chronic fibrotic tissue is known to be excessively cross-linked, we next examined whether collagen matrix that had been conditioned by HTS fibroblasts became refractory to enzymatic breakdown and indeed, found that it is resistant to breakdown by both collagenase D and matrix metalloproteinase-2. Newly formed extracellular matrix is stabilized by the enzyme, tissue transglutaminase, which we demonstrated to be overexpressed by HTS fibroblasts *in vivo* and *in vitro*. Reducing tissue transglutaminase activity in collagen gels containing HTS fibroblasts permitted induction of apoptosis on gel contraction, whereas increasing enzymic activity in NS cell-containing gels completely abrogated collagen-contraction-induced-apoptosis. Together, these observations show that HTS fibroblasts exhibit resistance to a specific form of apoptosis elicited by contraction of collagen gels, and that this phenomenon is dependent on excess activity of cell surface tissue transglutaminase.

► Failure of apoptosis in HTS formation is controversial. These authors cultured fibroblasts derived from normal scars or HTS, evaluating the development of apoptosis induced during collagen-gel contraction. They noted reduced tissue transglutaminase activity in HTS fibroblasts. Thus, resistance to specific forms of apoptosis does appear to be a major cause of HTS formation due to abnormal fibroblast functions. Further experiments will be required for the authors to demonstrate the mechanisms of inducing apoptosis at the appropriate time in HTS tissue fibroblasts to determine a method to benefit patients.

J. M. Daly, MD

New Generation of Hemoglobin-Based Oxygen Carriers Evaluated for Oxygenation of Critically Ischemic Hamster Flap Tissue

Contaldo C, Plock J, Sakai H, et al (Inselspital Univ, Berne, Switzerland; Waseda Univ, Tokyo)

Crit Care Med 33:806-812, 2005 9–15

Objectives.—The aim of this study was to investigate and compare the effects of a traditionally formulated, low-viscosity, right-shifted polymerized bovine hemoglobin solution and a highly viscous, left-shifted hemoglobin vesicle solution (HbV-HES) on the oxygenation of critically ischemic peripheral tissue.

Design.—Randomized, prospective study.

Setting.—University laboratory.

Subject.—A total of 40 male golden Syrian hamsters.

Interventions.—Island flaps were dissected from the back skin of anesthetized hamsters. The flap included a critically ischemic, hypoxic area that was perfused via a collateralized vasculature. One hour after completion of the preparation, the animals received a 33% blood exchange with 6% hydroxyethyl starch 200/0.5 (HES, n = 9), HbV suspended in HES (HbV-HES, n = 8), or polymerized bovine hemoglobin solution (n = 9).

Measurements and Main Results.—Three hours after the blood exchange, microcirculatory blood flow (laser-Doppler flowmetry) was increased to 262% of baseline for HbV-HES ($p < .01$) and 197% for polymerized bovine hemoglobin solution ($p < .05$ vs. baseline and HbV-HES). Partial tissue oxygen tension (bare fiber probes) was only improved after HbV-HES (9.4 torr to 14.2 torr, $p < .01$ vs. baseline and other groups). The tissue lactate/pyruvate ratio (microdialysis) was elevated to 51 in the untreated control animals, and to 34 ± 8 after HbV-HES ($p < .05$ vs. control) and 38 ± 11 after polymerized bovine hemoglobin solution (not significant).

Conclusions.—Our study suggests that in critically ischemic and hypoxic collateralized peripheral tissue, oxygenation may be improved by normovolemic hemodilution with HbV-HES. We attributed this improvement to a better restoration of the microcirculation and oxygen delivery due to the formulation of the solution.

► Tissue skin flaps are susceptible to ischemia and reperfusion injury. These authors studied the use of hemoglobin vesicle solutions on oxygenation in ischemic peripheral tissues of hamster flaps. Their results demonstrated that oxygenation can be improved by normovolemic hemodilution with the hemoglobin vesicle solution. This was specific to this hamster model utilizing critically ischemic and hypoxic collateralized peripheral tissues. Further studies are indicated to evaluate the safety and efficacy of this approach in other animal models, proceeding to clinical trials when this has been established.

J. M. Daly, MD

The Novel Cytokine p43 Stimulates Dermal Fibroblast Proliferation and Wound Repair

Park SG, Shin H, Shin YK, et al (Natl Creative Research Initiatives Ctr for Aminoacyl-tRNA Synthetase (ARS) Network, Seoul, Korea; Imagene Company Biotechnology Incubation Ctr, Seoul, Korea)
Am J Pathol 166:387-398, 2005 9–16

Introduction.—The multifunctional cytokine p43 acts on endothelial and immune cells to control angiogenesis and inflammation. In this report, we describe an additional activity of p43 that specifically promotes fibroblast proliferation and wound repair. In skin wound regions from mice, tumor necrosis factor-α induced p43 expression and secretion from macrophages recruited to the site. p43 also promoted fibroblast proliferation through its 146-amino acid N-terminal domain as revealed by deletion mapping. This p43-induced fibroblast proliferation was mediated by extracellular signal-regulated kinase (Erk). Depletion of endogenous p43 in mice by gene disruption retarded wound repair, whereas exogenous supplementation of recombinant human p43 to the wound area stimulated dermal fibroblast proliferation, collagen production, and wound closure. Thus, we have identified a novel p43 activity involving the stimulation of fibroblast proliferation, which could be applied therapeutically to aid wound repair.

► The authors studied the effects of the multifunctional cytokine p43 on endothelial and immune cells as well as on fibroblast proliferation. p43 induces fibroblast proliferation in a mouse model. Depletion of endogenous p43 in mice decreased wound repair, while exogenous supplementation using recombinant human p43 in the wound area stimulated fibroblast proliferation, collagen, and wound closure. The ability to control wound healing is truly the "holy grail" of surgical science. Continued studies such as these demonstrating mechanisms for novel genes and novel cytokines may one day allow us to improve wound healing in those in whom it is impaired, as well as control wound healing in normal individuals.

J. M. Daly, MD

Evolution of a "Falx Lunatica" in Demarcation of Critically Ischemic Myocutaneous Tissue

Harder Y, Amon M, Georgi M, et al (Univ of Saarland, Homburg/Saar, Germany; Univ of Berne, Switzerland)
Am J Physiol Heart Circ Physiol 288:H1224-H1232, 2005 9–17

Introduction.—Using intravital microscopy in a chronic in vivo mouse model, we studied the demarcation of myocutaneous flaps and evaluated microvascular determinants for tissue survival and necrosis. Chronic ischemia resulted in a transition zone, characterized by a red fringe and a distally adjacent white falx, which defined the demarcation by dividing the proximally normal from the distally necrotic tissue. Tissue survival in the red zone was determined by hyperemia, as indicated by recovery of the transiently reduced functional capillary density, and capillary remodeling, including dilation, hyperperfusion, and increased tortuosity. Angiogenesis and neovascularization were not observed over the 10-day observation period. The white rim distal to the red zone, appearing as "falx lunatica," showed a progressive decrease of functional capillary density similar to that of the necrotic distal area but without desiccation, and thus transparency, of the tissue. Development of the distinct zones of the critically ischemic tissue could be predicted by partial tissue oxygen tension (PtO_2) analysis by the time of flap elevation. The falx lunatica evolved at a PtO_2) between 6.2 ± 1.3 and 3.8 ± 0.7 mmHg, whereas tissue necrosis developed at <3.8 ± 0.7 mmHg. Histological analysis within the falx lunatica revealed interstitial edema formation and muscle fiber nuclear rarefaction but an absence of necrosis. We have thus demonstrated that ischemia-induced necrosis does not demarcate sharply from normal tissue but develops beside a fringe of tissue with capillary remodeling an adjacent falx lunatica that survives despite nutritive capillary perfusion failure, probably by direct oxygen diffusion.

▶ Harder et al evaluated demarcation in critically ischemic myocutaneous tissue. They noted a white rim distal to the red zone appearing as a falx lunatica. PtO_2 was between 3.8 and 6.2 mm Hg on average, whereas tissue necrosis developed at less than 3.8 mm Hg. Thus, ischemia-induced necrosis does not demarcate sharply from normal tissue but does develop near a fringe of tissue with capillary remodeling. It appears that diffusion may be responsible for this more distal site. This implicates therapies that may be beneficial in trying to improve flap survival in critically ischemic tissues.

J. M. Daly, MD

A Single Local Application of Recombinant Human Basic Fibroblast Growth Factor Accelerates Initial Angiogenesis During Wound Healing In Rabbit Ear Chamber

Komori M, Tomizawa Y, Takada K, et al (Tokyo Women's Med Univ)
Anesth Analg 100':830-834, 2005 9–18

Introduction.—Local angiogenic therapy with recombinant human basic fibroblast growth factor (rhbFGF) has been used to promote wound healing. To obtain useful information for the development of optimal angiogenic therapy, we chronologically evaluated the effects of a single local application of rhbFGF on angiogenesis in a rabbit ear chamber model of wound healing by observing the subcutaneous vessel bed intravitally. New vessel formation during wound healing was macroscopically and microscopically evaluated for 5 wk. Each rabbit ear chamber received a single dose of 6 μg rhbFGF (treatment B1: $n = 13$), 18 μg rhbFGF (treatment B2: $n = 16$), or physiological saline as control ($n = 13$). At 1 wk the newly vascularized area was significantly larger in groups B1 and B2 than in control. At 2 wk, the vascularized areas in groups B1, B2, and control were similar. At 5 wk, the percentage of rabbits with complete vascularization was significantly larger in group B1 than in control. Capillary density at 5 wk was similar among the three groups. These results suggest that locally applied rhbFGF accelerated angiogenesis during early wound healing in rabbits; however, this effect was transient and no increase in capillary density occurred at the completion of vascularization.

► Kamori et al studied the local application of rhbFGF. These authors noted an increase in early angiogenesis compared with controls using a rabbit ear chamber model. However, capillary density at 5 weeks was similar among all groups, including controls. Thus, while angiogenesis was accelerated during early wound healing in rabbits, this effect was transient. The importance of this study is that it evaluated not only the early phase of wound healing, but looked sequentially over time to demonstrate whether the early effects were long lasting. Unfortunately, the early acceleration was not perpetuated.

J. M. Daly, MD

Enhancement of Dorsal Random-Pattern Skin Flap Survival in Rats With Topical Lidocaine and Prilocaine (EMLA): Enhancement of Flap Survival by EMLA

Karaçal N, Ambarcioğlu Ö, Topal U, et al (Karadeniz Technical Univ, Trabzon, Turkey)

J Surg Res 124:134-138, 2005 9–19

Background.—Various topical pharmacologic agents have been investigated for their efficacy in preventing or reversing skin flap ischemia. Most of these studies have focused on agents that act on the vascular smooth muscles to cause vasodilatation and improve circulation in the flap. Most of local anesthetics relax vascular smooth muscle and produce peripheral vasodilatation. Topical lidocaine administration was shown that it was an effective and prompt resolution of mechanically induced vasospasm. The topical analgesia cream, EMLA is a mixture of the substances lidocaine and prilocaine. EMLA causes a biphasic vascular response comprising initial blanching and vasoconstriction (maximal after 1.5 h of application) and late erythema and vasodilatation at application times longer than 3 h.

Materials and Methods.—To investigate the effect of EMLA on random flap survival, 40 rats were divided in 2 groups of 20 animals. Caudally based random pattern skin flaps were elevated on dorsa of the rats in 10 × 3 cm dimensions. In group 1 which was the treatment group, topical EMLA was applied and covered with Opsite™ for 1 week whereas in group 2 which was the control group, carrier for EMLA was applied to the flaps. At the end of treatment period, the areas of flap necrosis were measured and percentages of flap survivals were calculated.

Results.—The mean percentages of flap survivals in group 1 and 2 were 81.2 ± 1.2 percent and 58.7 ± 2.3 percent, respectively.

Conclusion.—Topically administered EMLA might lead to a significant improvement in flap survival. In addition, it is safe, cost-effective, easily applied, and clinically available.

► These authors evaluated the use of topical lidocaine and prilocaine to improve flap survival. The use of these substances did lead to an improved flap survival of 81% in treated rats compared with 59% in controls. These drugs appear to cause an early vasoconstriction but a later erythema and vasodilation. These studies are among a number that have applied local medications to flaps in an effort to improve their outcome. Local application of these drugs along with oxygen supplementation may be of value in ischemic flaps.

J. M. Daly, MD

Improvement of Nutritive Perfusion After Free Tissue Transfer by Local Heat Shock-Priming-Induced Preservaton of Capillary Flowmotion

Rücker M, Kadirogullari B, Vollmar B, et al (Univ of Saarland, Homburg/Saar, Germany; Univ of Rostock, Germany)

J Surg Res 123:102-108, 2005 9–20

Background.—Capillary flowmotion protects pedicled flaps during critical perfusion conditions. However, free tissue transfer, causing ischemia-reperfusion and surgical trauma, have been shown to blunt these protective blood flow fluctuations. Because heat shock priming protects tissue after transfer, we herein studied whether heat shock protein expression is capable to preserve critical perfusion-induced capillary flowmotion in transferred composite flaps.

Methods.—In Sprague Dawley rats (n = 16), osteomyocutaneous flaps were subjected to critical perfusion after harvest and 1 h and 4 h after free transfer. In eight animals additional heat shock priming was induced 24 h before flap harvest. Microcirculation including capillary flowmotion was analyzed using intravital fluorescence microscopy.

Results.—After harvest, critical perfusion induced capillary flowmotion in skeletal muscle tissue of all flaps. By this, functional capillary density (FCD), an indicator of nutritive perfusion, was maintained not only in muscle but also in periosteum, subcutis, and skin. In contrast, 1 h after flap transfer muscle capillary flowmotion was completely abrogated, resulting in a significant decrease of FCD in all tissues. Heat shock-priming completely restored capillary flowmotion, and, by this, maintained tissue FCD.

Conclusions.—The loss of muscle capillary flowmotion after free tissue transfer-associated ischemia-reperfusion can be prevented by heat shock-priming. This may represent the mechanism of protection by local heat application.

► It is known that heat shock priming protects tissue that is subject to critical ischemia and reperfusion injury. These authors evaluated in Sprague-Dawley rats osteomyocutaneous flaps. They noted that heat shock priming completely restored capillary flow motion and maintained tissue FCD. The authors note that this may be one mechanism whereby local heat application may improve ischemia-reperfusion injury. Studies such as these are important to continue to identify biologic mechanisms for ischemic injury in flaps and methods to quantify efforts to reduce such injury.

J. M. Daly, MD

Coordinating Epidermal Growth Factor-Induced Motility Promotes Efficient Wound Closure

Kurten RC, Chowdhury P, Sanders RC Jr, et al (Univ of Arkansas, Little Rock; Univ of Florida, Gainesville)
Am J Physiol Lung Cell Mol Physiol 288:C109-C121, 2005 9–21

Introduction.—Wound healing is a response to injury that is initiated to reconstruct damaged tissue. In skin, reepithelialization involves both epithelial cells and fibroblasts and contributes to the reformation of a barrier between the external environment and internal milieu. Growth factors including epidermal growth factor (EGF) play important roles in promoting this process. In the present studies we employed CV-1 fibroblasts in a tissue culture model of reepithelialization to develop strategies for optimizing wound closure stimulated by EGF. We found that EGF enhanced cell motility within 6-8 h of EGF treatment in serum-free medium but wounds failed to close within 24 h. However, if medium on these cultures was exchanged for medium containing serum, cells pretreated with EGF closed new scrape wounds more rapidly than did cells that were not pretreated. These results indicate that serum factors work in concert with EGF to coordinate cell motility for efficient wound closure. Indeed, EGF enhanced the rate of wound closure in the presence of serum, and this effect also persisted for at least 24 h after EGF was removed. This coordination of EGF-induced cell motility was accompanied by an increase in the transient phosphorylation of ERK1 and ERK2. The persistent effects of EGF were blocked by transient exposure to reversible inhibitors of transcription and translation, indicating that the expression of new proteins mediated this response. We propose that EGF-stimulated CV-1 fibroblast motility is coordinated by a serum component that induces cell-cell adhesive properties consistent with an epithelial phenotype, thereby enhancing the reepithelialization process.

► These authors evaluated growth factors improving reepithelialization in an in vitro cell culture model. They noted that serum factors are important along with EGF to induce motility and promote epithelialization in this in vitro model. EGF-induced cell motility was accompanied by an increase in phosphorylation of ERK1 and ERK2. Closure of wounds required reepithelialization and contraction. Motility of endothelial cells is important in this process. Thus, this in vitro study provides important information that may help in in vivo circumstances of reepithelialization.

J. M. Daly, MD

The Application of Dermatotraction for Primary Skin Closure

Marek DJ, Copeland GE, Zlowodzki M, et al (Univ of Minnesota, St Paul; Univ of Arkansas, Little Rock)

Am J Surg 190:123-126, 2005 9–22

Background.—Management of an open wound is frequently necessary in the treatment of fractures. The traditional methods other than primary closure—skin grafting, rotational flaps, free flaps, and healing by secondary intention—all add significant cost, time, and risk of morbidity to the patient. Thus, it is important to obtain primary closure of open wounds whenever possible. This may be assisted with the use of the viscoelastic properties of the skin. A technique is described that uses the natural stretching ability of the skin to enable primary closure of wounds.

Methods.—The equipment needed for this technique includes two 18-gauge spinal needles and 2 towel clips. The spinal needles are inserted subdermally at approximately 5 mm from the wound margins. The tongs of the clamps are then placed with the tips around the spinal needles. The clamps are then used to slowly advance the skin edges. After 10 to 15 minutes of stress–relaxation, the tension will have decreased, and the towel clips may be gradually advanced. Once the skin edges are approximated, the wound can be closed using either sutures or staples.

> *Case Report.*—Man, 23, was seen at the emergency department after a gunshot wound to the left forearm at close range. Radiographs revealed an isolated midshaft ulna fracture. The patient underwent open reduction and internal fixation of the ulna through a dorsal incision. The dermatotraction technique described in this report was used to slowly advance the skin edges over a 20-minute period, after which time the skin edges were brought together. The subcutaneous tissues were loosely approximated with 4-0 vicryl sutures, and the skin was closed with 3-0 nylon sutures.

Conclusions.—The dermatostretching technique described in this report is an effective method for obtaining primary closure of substantial wounds without the use of the Sure-Closure skin-stretching system, at significant cost and time savings.

▶ This study demonstrates the remarkable ability of skin and subcutaneous tissues to stretch, which allows for closure of primary wounds, particularly encountered in the treatment of open fractures. Dermatotraction is able to stretch the skin to achieve primary closure of large wounds in this simplified approach. Thus, this method may prove useful in trauma patients with compound fractures who benefit by primary skin closure.

J. M. Daly, MD

10 Gastrointestinal

Introduction

Surgical gastroenterology continues to dominate this volume of scientific contributions to the surgical literature, as is evident in selected articles for the 2006 YEAR BOOK OF SURGERY that remain of seminal interest to our readership. For the 2006 edition, the editors have again attempted to select principle contributions that depict representative basic and applied scientific contributions of importance in the clinical aspects of patient care. As in the past, the editors of the YEAR BOOK are highly selective in their choices of contributions to the field to recognize the inclusion of anatomic, pathophysiologic, and technical measures that are essential in the general surgeon's management of the patient with various abnormalities of gastrointestinal origin. Further, as in previous editions of the YEAR BOOK, we again include contemporary contributions from basic science that provide surgeons the important tools for the future practice of surgical science. The editor and contributing editors have therefore provided selections that continue to highlight benchmark clinical trials and translational research that is directed to the surgical management of diseases of importance to scientific progress of gastrointestinal tract research and clinical care.

The laypress has increasingly recognized the importance of morbid obesity in our Western societies. With the emergence of laparoscopic technical approaches for abdominal surgery approximately 15 years earlier, laparoscopic gastric banding currently represents one of the most commonly performed procedures for weight control. Bariatric surgery using laparoscopic approaches is minimally invasive and is associated with low operative morbidity and low mortality. Moreover, the outcomes and patient satisfaction are exceptional, as it provides rapidly achievable satisfactory weight loss that is superior to any oral or systemic pharmacologic or drug preparation. However, as indicated in the paper by Suter et al,[1] a significant number of patients develop reflux symptoms requiring proton-pump inhibitors and/or band deflation. Some patients progress to esophageal dilation and "pseudo-achalasia."

Suter and associates confirm that esophageal dysmotility and gastroesophageal reflux are not uncommon in the postoperative era after gastric banding. Thus, in these morbidly obese patients, preoperative testing should be considered on a routine basis. The authors have emphasized that distal esophageal low-amplitude contractions with evidence of increased esophageal acid exposure should be considered a contraindication to the gastric banding procedure. Rather than offer such patients the banding approach, their morbid obesity control is best managed with *Roux-en-Y* gastric bypass.

Surgeons at St Mark's Hospital, United Kingdom, provide an 11-year experience in a major tertiary referral center to evaluate current practice and outcomes in the management of enterocutaneous fistulas. This feared complication of abdominal surgery results soon after surgery, although inflammatory bowel disease, ischemic bowel disease, malignancy, trauma, radiotherapy, and diverticulitis are co-contributors. Before the advent of proper nutritional support via the central venous route and attention to sepsis, malnutrition, and fluid/electrolyte/metabolic balance, enterocutaneous fistulas were regarded as an entity with high morbidity and mortality. Recent reports by West et al,[2] Makhdoom et al,[3] and Halversen et al[4] suggest a significant reduction in mortality rate from 65% to approximately 20%; McIntyre et al[5] and Conter et al[6] note that mortality rates more than 10% are infrequent.

West was specifically interested in evaluating current strategies and outcomes for management of this surgical malady. This study emphasizes the importance of the enteral rather than the parenteral measure for nutritional support, as enteral feeding promotes rapid bowel and tissue repair, enhances immune function, and has diminution in the frequency of sepsis. As many have emphasized, a second critical point is the early recognition and control of sepsis and proper nutritional and blood management to reduce mortality. Specifically, surgical management is delayed, often longer than 6 months, to allow maturation of tissue and quieting of the inflammatory response after fistula maturation. Specific bowel management includes resection of involved skin, irrespective of the volume of bowel sacrificed in the procedure. Such strategies have enhanced the favorable results and are detailed in this review.

The past decade has witnessed an evolution in surgical strategies commonly employing minimally invasive techniques. Such is the circumstance of managing the most common intra-abdominal malady—appendicitis—with or without peritonitis. Minimally invasive approaches have decreased hospital stay, and in many cases, have made management outcome principally an outpatient procedure. As various studies have drawn upon the importance of consideration of laparoscopy to diagnose acute, complex, and perforated appendicitis, Mancini et al[7] of the University of Tennessee, Knoxville, evaluated a retrospective, nonrandomized cohort of 92 patients undergoing laparoscopic appendectomy (LA) for acute appendicitis with peritonitis, perforation, or abscess.

It is evident that laparoscopy remains a valuable and evolving tool in the management of acute, complex, and simple presentations of inflammation of this organ. It would appear that no clinical data are especially helpful to the surgeon to predict the severity of disease that will be encountered in the operating room or the likely necessity for open conversion. Of interest, Mancini and associates note a 61% success rate in cases of complex appendicitis; the open conversion rate was 39% for all cases. We agree that there is little risk of the probability for adverse outcomes with attempted LA and copresentations of peritonitis, perforation, or abscess formation. Further, the severity of the presentation of appendicitis accounts for a higher complication rate in the group converted to an open procedure. It would appear that the conversion to an open procedure represents an "indicator" of the severity of the organ disease.

Semm[8] first described LA in 1983; subsequently, various randomized studies have compared LA with open appendectomy. Various meta-analyses confirm that LA is safe and provides a more rapid return to normal activity with fewer complications; LA does have a longer operating time. As several papers in the current series utilized in the 2006 YEAR BOOK OF SURGERY describe, the importance of preoperative ultrasound and CT for diagnosis of appendicitis, the expectant findings at surgery of disease of the organ is possible in greater than 80%. Diagnostic laparoscopy represents a safe, accurate, and low-complication procedure (0%-1.4%),[9-12] and when the appendix is normal it can be safely left *in situ.* The paper by Moberg et al,[13] represents a randomized, blinded study to compare time to full recovery after LA and OA for laparoscopically confirmed appendicitis. These authors confirm no differences in time to full recovery for either procedure after laparoscopic confirmation of disease. A trend toward better and faster physical activity (and thus return to work) was evident and trended toward the laparoscopic approach. These data would suggest that the laparoscopic approach is less traumatic; despite these findings, the clinical relevance can remain disputed, as the hospital stay and time to full recovery are similar.

It has been emphasized that diverticulitis management is often formulated on single-institutional case series and has biased outcomes based upon selection and publication prejudice. The paper by Salem and associates[14] from the University of Washington, Seattle, emphasizes the management strategy changes over the past 2 decades for known diverticulitis and include CT scanning, effective oral antimicrobials, percutaneous imaging drainage, and pain management. Despite the evolution of usage of modern diagnostic, imaging, and therapeutic strategies, the extent these applications have on outcomes is unclear. The authors were therefore interested in studying temporal trends in the use of surgical and percutaneous interventions in the management of the disease to enhance outcomes. Of great interest, there was minimal enhancement in the frequency of diverticulitis admissions over time in this large database that exceeded 25,000 patients. Expectantly, an increase in the use of percutaneous imaging and drainage procedures was associated with a decrease in emergency operative procedures (eg, perforation, peritonitis, abscess). Further, the proportion of patients who underwent colostomy remained stable (range, 49%-61%) as did the proportion of patients undergoing prophylactic colectomy after initial nonsurgical management (approximately 10%). Thus, there did not appear to be a significant usage of the one-stage procedure after colectomy in the management of diverticulitis. While diverticulitis still accounts for nearly one third of all colectomies and colostomies, the frequency of the emergent procedure for this disease has decreased over time as the frequency of percutaneous drainage with radiographic imaging has increased. Further, despite the increasing evidence-based medicine regarding the safety of the primary anastomosis in diverticular peritonitis, *colostomy has not decreased* over time. These temporal trends and observations suggest the need for rigorous clinical trials to define the role of the colostomy-sparing surgery in the treatment of diverticulitis. In addition, the frequency of colostomy concurrent to colectomy in elective procedures did not vary significantly by year, and averaged 16%, ranging from 13% to 20%.

The important paper provided by the Surgical Site Infection Prevention Guideline Writers' Work Group is summarized in the advisory statement by Bratzler and Houck.[15] This study concludes that surgical site infections (SSIs) represent the second most common cause of nosocomial infections.[16,17] Moreover, 2% to 5% of patients having *clean* extra-abdominal operations, and as great as 20% undergoing intra-abdominal operations, develop an SSI.[18] The Centers for Disease Control and Prevention currently estimates that approximately 500,000 SSIs occur in the United States annually.[19] The consequences of an SSI have great upside risk for morbidity and mortality, as documented by Kirkland et al,[20] as these patients are five times as likely to be readmitted, 60% more likely to spend time in an ICU, and have twice the mortality rate compared with patients without SSI. These are events that occur, notwithstanding those of the significant healthcare costs related to the SSI.

This advisory statement by the Surgical Site Infection Prevention Group also emphasizes to surgeons that "infusion of the first antimicrobial drug should begin within 60 minutes *before* surgical incision." Moreover, these authors suggest that "prophylactic antimicrobial agents should be discontinued within 24 hours of the end of surgery." In addition to these specific guidelines, the authors have provided an advisory statement that provides an overview for other issues that relate to antimicrobial prophylaxis. This statement also includes specific suggestions regarding the *selection of the antibacterial agent* recommended based on the type of procedure; this recommendation also includes caveats regarding dosage, infusion time, and redosing intervals. Thus, the readership of the 2006 YEAR BOOK OF SURGERY is strongly advised to consider review of this important mandate.

Surgeons in the United Kingdom have recently completed a randomized clinical trial to assess the impact of light- versus heavy-weight mesh on chronic pain after inguinal hernia repair. O'Dwyer and associates[21] acknowledge the severe chronic pain syndrome associated as a serious long-term problem after inguinal hernia repair. In this analysis of more than 320 patients, a comparison was utilized in this randomized prospective trial comparing pain severity at 12 months after inguinal hernia repair with a partially-absorbable light-weight mesh (LW group) versus a non-absorbable heavy-weight mesh (HW group). LW mesh was associated with less chronic pain, but patients experienced an increase in recurrence of hernia with long-term follow-up. This observation is perhaps related to technical factors associated with fixation of the mesh rather than an inherent defect in the construct of this biomaterial. The authors conclude that a reduction in total volume of the mesh left *in situ* after repair will reduce chronic pain; it would appear that the higher recurrence rates may be therefore relate to the *size of the suture purchase* within the mesh rather than to inherent defects.

The routine application of the temporary loop ileostomy for diversion after restorative proctocolectomy remains controversial as a result of the reported morbidity that is associated with not only the creation, but closure, of the ileostomy. A study by Wong and associates[22] of the Cleveland Clinic Foundation, Ohio, reviews their extensive experience in more than 1500 patients with loop ileostomy closure after restorative proctocolectomy. The authors were interested in overall complication rates, as well as rates related to the hand-sewn versus staple closure methods. Of interest, no significant differences in complication rates and length of hospital stay were evident between the types of closure. However, odds ratio for developing wound infection of ileostomy closure at or after 3.2 months produced substantial differences. Infection rates were 2.2% with closures at less than 3.2 months (early closure) versus 0.7% for closures at or after 3.2 months (late closure), $p = 0.015$. Such objective evidence should be strongly considered by the general surgeon in practice who inquires regarding the timing of closure of loop ileostomy after restoration of the colonic segment.

A review of Diagnostic-Related Group (DRG) assignment for laparoscopic versus open colectomy provides insight into the financial implications for both the payer and the health provider. Senagore and associates[23] provide the first study to demonstrate that DRG assignment can change solely based upon *differential rates of operative complications* for the 2 competing approaches (laparoscopic vs open). It is not surprising that open colectomy results in a significant increase in cost for the insurer under a prospective payment program (PPP). Of interest, savings to the institution coupled with shortened length of stay offsets the potential loss of revenue to the institution. These data provide substantive outcomes for the effects of the laparoscopically assisted colectomy for cost of the PPP and provider reimbursement costs, and emphasize the importance of assessing new technology in light of improvement in both cost and quality for patient outcomes. This paper emphasizes that academic and community medical centers should critically assess *net reimbursement effects* that utilize evolving technology based upon similar quality and outcome measurements for total reimbursement.

The randomized prospective analysis by the Swedish Obese Subject Study provided extensive data on obese subjects undergoing gastric bypass matched contemporaneously with conventionally treated obese control patients. This study identified risks for diabetes, lifestyle, and cardiovascular morbidity-mortality for 10 years after weight reduction bariatric surgery. This landmark study concludes that compared with conventional approaches, bariatric surgical therapy of the obese represents an important option for therapy and results in durable weight loss, enhancement of lifestyle, and with few exceptions (hypercholesterolemia) will reduce the risk factor for cardiovascular disease evident with baseline presentation of weight gain. While evidence confirms that bariatric surgery represents a major contributor to quality-of-life reinstatement of the severely obese, all obesity-associated risk factors were not improved by sustained weight loss. This benchmark analysis further recommends the necessity for obtaining long-term data on the effect of weight reduction on overall mortality and the progressive incidence of cardiovascular and neoplastic transformation.

The importance of prospective analyses evaluating the demographics of cost and efficacy are born out by many of the abstracts included in this 2006 edition of the YEAR BOOK OF SURGERY. The importance of these and other analyses included in the YEAR BOOK further indicate that in our changing healthcare environment, cost and regulations continue to require that we be prudent and examine clinical and fiscal data, all of which comprise critical measures that influence therapeutic strategy and the decision process. The editor again emphasizes that many superb abstracts and full-content papers are not included due to the limitations of page-volume restrictions. This policy of adherence to publication of quality abstracts from highly regarded papers will continue in prospective editions of the YEAR BOOK OF SURGERY.

Kirby I. Bland, MD

References

1. Suter M, Dorfa G, Giusti V, et al: Gastric banding interfered with esophageal motility and gastroesophageal reflux. *Arch Surg* 140:639-643, 2005.
2. West MA: Conservative and operative management of gastrointestinal fistulae in the critically ill patient. *Curr Opin Crit Care* 6:143-147, 2000.
3. Makhdoom ZA, Komar MJ, Still CD: Nutrition and enterocutaneous fistulas. *J Clin Gastroenterol* 31:195-204, 2000.
4. Halversen RC, Hogle HH, Richards RC: Gastric and small bowel fistulas. *Am J Surg* 118:968-972, 1969.
5. McIntyre PB, Ritchie JK, Hawley PR, et al: Management of enterocutaneous fistulas: A review of 132 cases. *Br J Surg* 71:293-296, 1984.
6. Conter RL, Roof L, Roslyn JJ: Delayed reconstructive surgery for complex enterocutaneous fistulae. *Am Surg* 54:589-593, 1988.
7. Mancini GJ, Mancini ML, Nelson HS: Efficacy of laparoscopic appendectomy in appendicitis with peritonitis. *Am Surgeon* 71:1-5, 2005.
8. Semm K: Endoscopic appendectomy. *Endoscopy* 15:59-64, 1983.
9. Moberg AC, Ahlberg G, Leijonmarck CE, et al: Diagnostic laparoscopy in 1043 patients with suspected acute appendicitis. *Eur J Surg* 164:833-840, 1998.
10. Teh SH, O'Ceallaigh S, McKeon JGK, et al: Should an appendix that looks 'normal' be removed at diagnostic laparoscopy for acute iliac fossa pain? *Eur J Surg* 166:388-389, 2000.
11. van den Brock WT, Bijnen AB, de Ruiter P, et al: A normal appendix found during diagnostic laparoscopy should not be removed. *Br J Surg* 88:251-254, 2001.
12. Thorell A, Gröndal S, Schedvins K, et al: Value of diagnostic laparoscopy in fertile women with suspected appendicitis. *Eur J Surg* 165:751-754, 1999.
13. Moberg AC, Berndsen F, Palmquist I, et al: Randomized clinical trial of laparoscopic versus open appendicectomy for confirmed appendicitis. *Br J Surg* 92:298-304, 2005.
14. Salem L, Anaya DA, Flum DR: Temporal changes in the management of diverticulitis. *J Surg Res* 124:318-323, 2005.
15. Bratzler DW, Houck PM: Antimicrobial prophylaxis for surgery: an advisory statement from the National Surgical Infection Prevention Project. *Am J Surg* 189:395-404, 2005.
16. Burke JP: Infection control—a problem for patient safety. *N Engl J Med* 348:651-656, 2003.

17. National Nosocomial Infections Surveillance: Data summary from October 1986-April 1996, issued May 1996: A report from the National Nosocomial Infections Surveillance (NNIS) System. *Am J Infect Control* 24:380-388, 1996.
18. Auerbach AD: Prevention of surgical site infections. In: Shojania KG, Duncan BW, McDonald KM, et al, editors. *Making Health Care Safer: A Critical Analysis of Patient Safety Practices.* Evidence Report/Technology Assessment No. 43. AHRQ Publication No. 01-E058, Rockville, MD: Agency for Healthcare Research and Quality 2001;221-244.
19. Wong ES: Surgical site infection. In: Mayhall DG, editor. *Hospital Epidemiology and Infection Control.* 2nd ed. Philadelphia, PA: Lippincott;1999:189-210.
20. Kirkland KB, Briggs JP, Trivette SL, et al: The impact of surgical site infections in the 1990s: Attributable mortality, excess length of hospitalization and extra costs. *Infect Control Hosp Epidemiol* 20:725-730, 1999.
21. O'Dwyer PJ, Kingsnorth AN, Molloy RG, et al: Randomized clinical trial assessing impact of a lightweight or heavyweight mesh on chronic pain after inguinal hernia repair. *Br J Surg* 92:166-170, 2005.
22. Wong K-S, Remzi FH, Gorgun E, et al: Lopp ileostomy closure after restorative proctocolectomy: Outcome in 1,504 patients. *Dis Colon Rectum* 48:243-250, 2005.
23. Senagore AJ, Brannigan A, Kiran RP, et al: Diagnosis-related group (DRG) assignment in laparoscopic and open colectomy: Financial implications for payer and provider. *Dis Colon Rectum* 48:1016-1020, 2005.

Antimicrobial Prophylaxis for Surgery: An Advisory Statement From the National Surgical Infection Prevention Project

Bratzler DW, for the Surgical Infection Prevention Guideline Writers Workgroup (Oklahoma Found for Medical Quality, Oklahoma City)

Am J Surg 189:395-404, 2005 10–1

Introduction.—In January 2003, leadership of the Medicare National Surgical Infection Prevention Project hosted the Surgical Infection Prevention Guideline Writers Workgroup meeting. The objectives were to review areas of agreement among the published guidelines for surgical antimicrobial prophylaxis, to address inconsistencies, and to discuss issues not currently addressed. The participants included authors from most of the published North American guidelines for antimicrobial prophylaxis and several specialty colleges. The workgroup reviewed currently published guidelines for antimicrobial prophylaxis. Nominal group process was used to draft a consensus paper that was widely circulated for comment. The consensus positions of the workgroup include that infusion of the first antimicrobial dose should begin within 60 minutes before surgical incision and that prophylactic antimicrobial agents should be discontinued within 24 hours of the end of surgery. This advisory statement provides an overview of other issues related to antimicrobial prophylaxis including specific suggestions regarding antimicrobial selection.

► The National Surgical Infection Prevention Project posted the Surgical Infection Prevention Guideline Writers Working Group in January of 2003. This advisory statement provided in the April, 2005 issue of the *American Journal of Surgery* provides an overview of issues related to antimicrobial prophylaxis, including specific suggestions regarding antimicrobial selection. The objectives of this working group were to review areas of agreement among published guidelines for antimicrobial prophylaxis and to address the inconsistencies of these previously published recommendations. In addition, the authors wanted to elaborate on issues that were not previously addressed, but which the working group thought were important. This review article provides a consensus paper that has been widely circulated for comment and agreed upon by the working group members.

Bratzler and Houck provide a consensus position of the Prevention Guideline Committee that includes infusion of the first antimicrobial dose of chemotherapeutics within 60 minutes before the surgical incision; the consensus group further elaborates on the issue that prophylactic antimicrobial agents should be discontinued within 24 hours of the surgical procedure.

K. I. Bland, MD

The Advancing Art and Science of Endoscopy

Vitale GC, Davis BR, Tran TC (Univ of Louisville, Ky)

Am J Surg 190:228-233, 2005 10–2

Introduction.—Flexible endoscopy continues to advance encompassing treatment of a variety of diseases traditionally managed surgically. This review describes and evaluates many of these new endoscopic approaches with an eye toward the future. Gastroesophageal reflux disease is now treated with several endoscopic, non-operative techniques. A procedure using radiofrequency energy delivered by a peroral catheter with small needles inserted into the wall of the esophagus causes collagen deposition and ablates transient lower esophageal sphincter relaxation, both of which reduce reflux. With this treatment, >80% of patients will reduce or stop their medication for reflux. Trials involving new injectable materials show promise with a 75-80% improvement in heartburn-related quality-of-life scores and reduced medication use. Endoscopic suture and stapling devices restore the antireflux barrier with sutures that create a pleat or plication at the gastroesophageal junction. Early results indicated that 62-74% of patients had significant improvement. Long-term results are not available for any of these new techniques and there seems to be a drop off in effectiveness over time. Gastrointestinal bleeding has been more effectively managed with the recent introduction of small clips and detachable snares to control bleeding vessels. Banding and sclerotherapy for variceal bleeding has all but eliminated urgent operation for that diagnosis. In the biliary-pancreas realm, endoscopic management of pancreatic pseudocysts, stenting of pancreatic or biliary strictures and fistulae have reduced operative indications in those disease processes. Pseudocyst drainage involves creation of a transenteric communication between the pseudocyst and the stomach or duodenum. Complete cyst resolution without recurrence can be expected in 85% of patients. While endoscopic palliation of malignant biliary strictures has been accepted for years, experience with endoscopic management of iatrogenic strictures indicates that it may serve as an alternative option without surgery in many patients. Enteric stenting using metallic self-expanding stents in the esophagus, duodenum, and colon allows alleviation of obstruction without surgery for palliantation and in the colon may relieve obstruction to avoid colostomy prior to an elective resection. On the horizon stands the flexible endoscopic route to the abdominal cavity via the transgastric route and the promise of combined endoscopic-laparoscopic approaches to complex abdominal problems. General surgeons should rekindle their interest in flexible endoscopy or risk losing entire categories of disease to other specialties or to a small specialized group of endoscopic surgeons.

► The authors emphasize the importance of flexible endoscopy to advance the therapy of a variety of diseases traditionally managed only by open surgery. This review article provides an encompassing perspective that describes and evaluates evolving endoscopic approaches for a potpourri of surgical options used in the management of gastrointestinal diseases. This article will generate keen interest because of its importance to the practicing general surgeon who must enhance their interest in flexible endoscopy. It is highly probable that many of these various categories of diseases will be relegated to other specialties or to smaller specialized groups of endoscopic surgeons unless there is a rekindling of interest in these endoscopic approaches. It is also incumbent upon the Association of Program Directors in Surgery (APDS) and the Residency Review Committee in Surgery (RRC-S) to vigorously support and enlarge the expectations of endoscopic approaches by residents in their surgical training.

K. I. Bland, MD

Are Young Surgeons Competent to Perform Alimentary Tract Surgery?

Prystowsky JB (Northwestern Univ, Chicago)

Arch Surg 140:495-502, 2005 10–3

Background.—Assessment of competency during residency training has received increased attention recently. There has been less attention given to the competency of residents after training.

Hypothesis.—Patient outcomes for alimentary tract surgery (ATS) should be similar for surgeons who recently completed their residency training compared with more experienced surgeons, indicating that the younger surgeons had achieved clinical competency on completion of their residency training.

Design.—Retrospective analysis of Illinois inpatient discharge data (January 1, 1996-December 31, 1999).

Setting.—All 205 nonfederal acute care hospitals in Illinois.

Patients.—The patients were 120,160 adult Illinois residents who underwent ATS in Illinois.

Main Outcome Measures.—Mortality rate, morbidity rate, and hospital length of stay.

Results.—Regression analyses demonstrated that surgeon experience was a significant determinant of mortality and morbidity rates, with worse outcomes observed for patients of young surgeons undergoing high-complexity ATS (ie, procedures other than appendectomy and cholecystectomy).

Conclusions.—For high-complexity ATS, there was a significant disparity in outcomes between young and more experienced surgeons, whereas for low-complexity ATS, there was no disparity. Attention to competency during residency training is warranted, especially as it relates to high-complexity ATS. Furthermore, patient outcomes provide an opportunity to assess competency after training that can complement assessments during training and together identify educational strengths and weaknesses of residency training.

► In 1999, the Accreditation Council for Graduate Medical Education (ACGME) defined attributes considered important and required to properly train competent physicians for them to discharge their duties as physicians (and surgeons).[1] The ACGME defined 6 general competencies that represent skill sets that all physicians should know and include: patient care, medical knowledge, practice-based learning, interpersonal and communications skills, professionalism, and systems-based practice. Such competencies have subsequently been embraced and required by the American Board of Surgery (ABS).

In this article by Prystowsky, the author assumes that outcomes of patient care of ATS should be similar for surgeons recently completing their residency training when compared with more experienced surgeons. Such an assumption suggests that the younger surgeon achieves clinical competency after completion of their residency training. However, there is a significant disparity in the outcomes evaluated in this regression analysis by the author. This indicates that surgical experience represents a significant determinant of morbidity and mortality; worse outcomes were observed in the young surgeon undergoing high complexity ATS.

Although such outcomes are not unexpected, the best learning devices are repetition and prolongation of experience in patient management. The ABS certificate awarded the postresident practicing surgeon cannot ensure competency across all spectrums of the alimentary tract as is evident in this analysis. Clinical outcomes according to surgical experience identify no variance in low complexity procedures. Analysis demonstrates a significant relationship, however, for less experienced surgeons to increase morbidity and mortality but no significant relationship to length of stay. Such empiric data suggest that surgical investigators must continue the pursuit of evidence-based guidelines that can be developed for achieving technical proficiency in specific operations. However, the quote "there is no substitute for experience" remains an adage to be beholden by surgeons completing residency within the past 5 years. Their goal should be to aim and strive for an increasing knowledge base in a specific disease and its management, and rely on the experience of their colleagues to assist in proper outcomes.

K. I. Bland, MD

Reference

1. Accreditation Council for Graduate Medical Education: *General Competencies*, version 1.3. Chicago, Accreditation Council for Graduate Medical Education, 2000.

Laparoscopic Heller Myotomy for Achalasia

Cacchione RN, Tran DN, Rhoden DH (Univ of Louisville, Ky; Univ of Oklahoma, Tulsa)

Am J Surg 190:191-195, 2005 10–4

Background.—Achalasia is an uncommon illness affecting 1 per 100,000 patients yearly. There is evidence to suggest viral, autoimmune, and hereditary etiologies. There are many treatment options available including medications, botulinum toxin injection, pneumatic dilation, and surgical myotomy.

Methods.—We present a retrospective review of patients undergoing laparoscopic-modified Heller myotomy at a large referral and surgical training center.

Results.—There were 36 patients identified. Thirty patients had undergone prior treatment with botulinum toxin injection, pneumatic dilation, previous Heller myotomy, or esophageal stenting. Immediate complications included mucosal perforation (2), spleen injury (1), and trocar-site infection (1). There were no postoperative esophageal leaks. Three patients suffered reflux requiring the daily use of a proton pump inhibitor 9 months after surgery. Three patients suffered recurrent dysphagia.

Conclusions.—Presently, there are little data to suggest an ideal management strategy in patients with achalasia. Our patient population consists predominantly of failures of other treatment methods submitted for laparoscopic myotomy. Our data suggest that laparoscopic Heller myotomy can be safely undertaken in this population, without a higher than expected rate of recurrent symptoms or reflux.

▶ The frequency of achalasia (1:100,000 patients per year) suggests that this primary disorder of the esophagus is an uncommon but nonrare presentation. Achalasia is recognized in all age groups but peaks between the third and fifth decades of life. With the enhanced understanding of the pathophysiology of degeneration of the myenteric plexus as a common pathway, and understanding of its treatment options both medical and surgical, effective therapies have evolved. Its cause includes: viral,[1] hereditary,[2] and autoimmune mechanisms.[3] De Oliveira et al[4] note the sparing of postganglionic cholinergic excitatory fibers with evident selective excitation of inhibitory nerves to suggest loss of the vasoactive intestinal peptide and nitric oxide synthatase as etiologic. Thereafter, there is functional impairment of the gastroesophageal (GE) junction to initiate achalasia symptoms, which are explained by these findings of unopposed excitatory input levels with impairment of LES (lower esophageal sphincter) relaxation.

Cacchione et al provide a retrospective evaluation of patients undergoing laparoscopic-modified Heller myotomy at a large referral center. Of 36 intensively studied patients, 30 had undergone prior therapy with botulinum-toxin injection, pneumatic dilation, Heller myotomy, or esophageal stenting. The authors identify that multiple prior reviews have provided minimal data of value suggesting that an ideal management strategy in these patients with achalasia is unavailable. It would appear that the Heller myotomy performed laparoscopically for this disorder is a safe and highly regarded measure that can be completed in referral centers with excellent outcomes, inclusive of excellent control of recurrent symptoms and reflux.

K. I. Bland, MD

References

1. Ruiz-de-Leon A, Mendoza J, Sevilla-Mantilla C, et al: Myenteric antiplexus antibodies and class II HLA in achalasia. *Dig Dis Sci* 47:15-19, 2002.
2. Castagliuolo I, Brun P, Costantini M, et al: Esophageal achalasia: Is the herpes simplex virus really innocent? *J Gastrointest Surg* 8:24-30, 2004.
3. Clark SB, Rice TW, Tubbs RR, et al: The nature of the myenteric infiltrate in achalasia: An immunohistochemical analysis. *Am J Surg Pathol* 24:1153-1158, 2000.
4. de Oliveira JM, Birgisson S, Doinoff C, et al: Timed barium swallow: A simple technique for evaluating esophageal emptying in patients with achalasia. *AJR Am J Roentgenol* 169:473-479, 1997.

EUS Followed by EMR for Staging of High-Grade Dysplasia and Early Cancer in Barrett's Esophagus

Larghi A, Lightdale CJ, Memeo L, et al (Columbia Univ, New York)
Gastrointest Endosc 62:16-23, 2005 10–5

Background.—Accurate staging of high-grade dysplasia and of early cancer in Barrett's esophagus is important in the selection of patients for endoscopic therapy.

Methods.—Patients with Barrett's esophagus and biopsy specimen proven high-grade dysplasia and adenocarcinoma in focal nodular lesions or in endoscopically unapparent flat lesions in short-segment Barrett's esophagus were initially staged with EUS. In patients with disease limited to the mucosa on EUS, cap-assisted EMR was performed. The depth of tumor invasion on EMR specimens was classified in a similar manner to squamous-cell cancer of the esophagus: m1 (epithelial layer, dysplasia), m2 (lamina propria invasion), m3 (muscularis mucosae invasion), sm (submucosal invasion).

Results.—EUS was performed in 48 consecutive patients (27 with focal nodular lesions and 21 with microscopic lesions), and submucosal invasion was diagnosed in 8 (confirmed in 7/8 at surgery). EMR was carried out in the remaining 40 patients without significant complications. In the 25 patients with high-grade dysplasia on prior biopsy specimens, EMR confirmed m1 disease in 19; whereas in 6 (24%), invasive adenocarcinoma was detected (to m2 in 4; to m3 in 2). In the 15 patients with invasive cancer on prior biopsy specimens and staged as intramucosal cancer on EUS, intramucosal carcinoma was confirmed in 9 (m2 in 3; m3 in 6); whereas, in 6 patients (40%), submucosal invasion was found. Overall, EUS provided accurate staging in 41/48 patients (85%) with one patient overstaged and 6 patients understaged compared with pathologic staging obtained by surgery or EMR. Of the 34 patients with m1 to m3 staging after EMR, 29 were treated endoscopically and had no evidence of cancer after a mean follow-up of 22.9 months(standard deviation 9.2 months).

Conclusions.—EMR provides pathologic staging information that, in addition, may be helpful after EUS if a stage-determined approach is used in the management of high-grade dysplasia and of early cancer in Barrett's esophagus. EMR may be particularly useful for staging of focal nodules or in short-segment Barrett's esophagus with microscopic lesions when endoscopic therapy is an option.

► The accompanying article by Vitale et al in this issue of the 2006 YEAR BOOK OF SURGERY (Abstract 10–2) reiterates the importance of comprehensive surgical training to treat a variety of diseases with flexible endoscopy. This review by Larghi et al of Columbia University emphasizes the importance of accurate staging of high-grade dysplasia (HGD) and early cancer (EC) in Barrett's esophagus for the selection of patients for endoscopic therapy. These patients who were initially staged with endoscopic ultrasonography (EUS) had cap-assisted endoscopic mucosal resection (EMR) when disease was limited to the mucosa on EUS. The abstract above depicts the depth of tumor invasion on EMR for epithelium, lamina propria, muscularis mucosal, and submucosal invasion.

The authors conclude that EMR in this prospective, single-center study of HGD and EC with Barrett's can be accurately performed using initial EUS, followed by EMR. It is essential that the readership understand that this is of importance and applicable only for lesions that are confined to the mucosa. Long-term follow-up will be essential to activate such approaches. However, it is evident that EMR provides pathologic staging of mucosal and submucosal invasion, and indicates that a staging classification similar to that used for squamous-cell neoplasia of the esophagus can be applied in short-segment Barrett's esophagitis and for focal nodules of the mucosa.

K. I. Bland, MD

The Frequency of Barrett's Esophagus in High-Risk Patients With Chronic GERD

Westhoff B, Brotze S, Weston A, et al (Univ of Kansas, Kansas City, Mo)
Gastrointest Endosc 61:226-231, 2005 10–6

Background.—The reported frequency of Barrett's esophagus (BE) in patients with reflux symptoms varies from 5% to 15%. The exact frequency of long-segment BE (LSBE) (>3 cm) and short-segment BE (SSBE) (<3 cm) in patients with chronic symptoms of GERD is uncertain. The aim of this study was to determine the frequency of LSBE and SSBE in consecutive patients presenting for a first endoscopic evaluation with GERD as the indication.

Methods.—Consecutive patients presenting to the endoscopy unit of a Veterans Affairs Medical Center for a first upper endoscopy with the indication of GERD were prospectively evaluated. Demographic information (gender, race, age), data on tobacco use and family history of esophageal disease, and body mass index (BMI) were recorded for all patients. Before endoscopy, all patients completed a validated GERD questionnaire. The diagnosis of BE was based on the presence of columnar-appearing mucosa in the distal esophagus, with confirmation by demonstration of intestinal metaplasia in biopsy specimens. All patients with erosive esophagitis on the initial endoscopy underwent a second endoscopy to document healing and to rule-out underlying BE. Patients with a history of BE, alarm symptoms (dysphagia, weight loss, anemia, evidence of GI bleeding), or prior endoscopy were excluded.

Results.—A total of 378 consecutive patients with GERD (94% men, 86% white; median age 56 years, range 27-93 years) were evaluated. A diagnosis of BE was made in 50 patients (13.2%). The median length of Barrett's esophagus (BE) was 1.0 cm (range 0.5-15.0 cm). Of the patients with BE, 64% had short-segment BE (SSBE) (overall SSBE frequency 8.5%). The overall frequency of long-segment BE (LSBE) was 4.8%. A hiatal hernia was detected in 62% of the patients with BE. Of the 50 patients with BE (median age 62 years, range 29-81 years), 47 (94%) were men and 98% were white. Eighteen patients (36%) were using tobacco at the time of endoscopy; 23 (46%) were former users. The median body mass index (BMI) of patients with BE was 27.3 (overweight). There were no significant differences between patients with LSBE and SSBE with respect to age, gender, ethnicity, BMI, and GERD symptom duration (Table 1).

Conclusions.—The frequency of BE in a high-risk patient group (chronic GERD, majority white men, age > 50 years) who sought medical attention is

TABLE 1.—Comparison of Patients With LSBE Vs. SSBE

	LSBE	SSBE	*p*Value
N	18	32	
Male gender	100%	91%	0.5445
White	94%	100%	0.3600
Median age, y	62 (range 37-76)	61.5 (range 29-81)	0.6130
Median heartburn duration (y)	5.5 (range 1-7)	5 (range 1-7)	0.7219
Median regurgitation duration (y)	5 (range 1-7)	5 (range 1-7)	0.3911
Tobacco use (current and past)	83% (33% and 50%)	81% (37% and 44%)	0.9274
Family history of GERD	17%	28%	0.4973
Family history of BE or esophageal cancer	0%	6%	0.5298
Hiatal hernia	67%	59%	0.7637
Median hiatal hernia length (cm)	3.5 (range 2-6)	3 (range 2-6)	0.0490
Median body mass index	28.7 (range 16.1-36.7)	27.2 (range 14.9-39.6)	0.2322
Median Barrett's mucosa length (cm)	4.5 (range 3-15)	1 (range 0.5-2)	<0.0001

Abbreviationa: LSBE, Long-segment Barrett's esophagus; *SSBE,* short-segment Barrett's esophagus.

(Courtesy of Westhoff B, Brotze S, Weston A, et al: The frequency of Barrett's esophagus in high-risk patients with chronic GERD. *Gastrointest Endosc* 61:226-231, 2005.)

13.2%, with the majority (64%) having SSBE. These data suggest that the frequency of BE in patients with GERD has not changed. The true prevalence of BE in the general population, including those who do not seek care, is undoubtedly lower, currently and historically. The majority of patients with BE are overweight and have a hiatal hernia. Demographic data for patients with LSBE and SSBE are similar, indicating that these are a continuum of the same process.

▶ These authors determine the frequency of LSBE and SSBE (<3 cm) in patients with chronic symptoms of GERD. As indicated in the article, the prevalence of Barrett's is primarily found in the white male older than 50 years with sustained reflux. This frequency of 13% seeking medical attention is significant, and the majority of patients (64%) had SSBE. Further, the risk factors are those of this male population who are overweight and have a documented hiatal hernia.

Table 1 confirms the demographic features of the 2 variants of Barrett's; it confirms only a difference in the length of the mucosa that differentiates the 2, and the fact that there is a longer hiatal hernia length (cm). The authors have confirmed the true prevalence of BE in the general population, including individuals who did not seek medical attention is undoubtedly lower, at present and historically. LSBE and SSBE remain consistently similar pathophysiologic events related to obesity and reflux. Thus, the data suggest that the frequency of Barrett's in those with GERD has not changed substantially.

K. I. Bland, MD

Quality of Life After Transhiatal Compared With Extended Transthoracic Resection for Adenocarcinoma of the Esophagus

de Boer AGEM, van Lanschot JJB, van Sandick JW, et al (Academic Med Ctr, Amsterdam; Erasmus Med Ctr, Rotterdam, the Netherlands)

J Clin Oncol 22:4202-4208, 2004 10–7

Purpose.—To assess 3 years of quality of life in patients with esophageal cancer in a randomized trial comparing limited transhiatal resection with extended transthoracic resection.

Patients and Methods.—Quality-of-life questionnaires were sent at baseline and at 5 weeks; 3, 6, 9, and 12 months; and 1.5, 2, 2.5, and 3 years after surgery. Physical and psychological symptoms, activity level, and global quality of life were assessed with the disease-specific Rotterdam Symptom Checklist. Generic quality of life was measured with the Medical Outcomes Study Short Form-20.

Results.—A total of 199 patients participated. Physical symptoms and activity level declined after the operation and gradually returned toward baseline within the first year ($P < .01$) (Fig 1). Psychological well-being consistently improved after baseline ($P < .01$), whereas global quality of life showed a small initial decline followed by continuous gradual improvement ($P < .01$). Quality of life stabilized in the second and third year. Three months

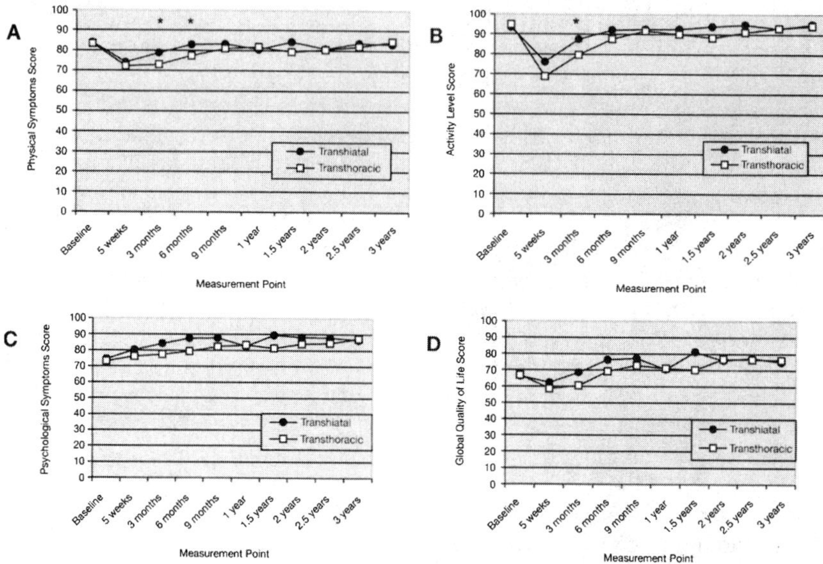

FIGURE 1.—Physical symptoms, activity level, psychological symptoms, and global quality of life measured with the Rotterdam symptom Checklist during 3 years for patients randomly assigned to transhiatal esophagectomy or transthoracic esophagectomy with extended en bloc lymphadenectomy. (*), statistically significant; $P, \leq .01$. (Courtesy of de boer AGEM, van Lanschot JJB, van Sandick JW, et al: Quality of life after transhiatal compared with extended transthoracic resection for adenocarcinoma of the esophagus. *J Clin Oncol* 22:4202-4208, 2004. Reprinted with permission from the American Society of Clinical Oncology.)

after the operation, patients in the transhiatal esophagectomy group (n = 96) reported fewer physical symptoms ($P = .01$) and better activity levels ($P < .01$) than patients in the transthoracic group (n = 103), but no differences were found at any other measurement point. For psychological symptoms and global quality of life, no differences were found at any follow-up measurement. A similar pattern was found for generic quality of life.

Conclusion.—No lasting differences in quality of life of patients who underwent either transhiatal or transthoracic resection were found. Compared with baseline, quality of life declined after the operation but was restored within a year in both groups.

▶ De Boer et al from the Departments of Medical Psychology and Surgery, Amsterdam, and the Department of Surgery, Rotterdam, Netherlands, provide a 3-year quality of life (QOL) assessment for patients with esophageal carcinoma randomly assigned to a trial comparison of the limited transhiatal resection with that of the extended resection variant. With participation of nearly 200 patients, physical symptoms and activity level declined after operation but gradually returned to baseline within the first year ($P < .01$). Of importance, the authors confirm no lasting differences in the QOL for patients undergoing either transhiatal or extended resections. While QOL compared with baseline declined after operation, same was restored within a year of surgery for both groups.

In the article, the authors compare 96 transhiatal versus 103 transthoracic esophagectomies regarding physical symptoms, activity levels, psychologic symptoms, and global QOL measured with the Rotterdam Symptom Checklist (RSCL). As is evident, only physical symptoms scores were statistically significant at 3 and 6 months with improvement that was superior in the transhiatal approach versus the total resection variant. For activity level, the transhiatal patients performed better and with greater activity at 3 months when compared with the transthoracic resection esophagectomy. In addition, psychologic symptoms show a consistent improvement after baseline in the first year after esophagectomy, but stabilized, whereas there is only a small initial decline in global QOL. It would appear from this important study that no lasting differences were evident in QOL among patients with esophageal carcinoma undergoing either operation. Baseline scores declined following operation, as it would be expected, but were restored within a year of either therapy.

K. I. Bland, MD

Neoadjuvant Chemoradiotherapy for Esophageal Carcinoma: A Meta-analysis

Greer SE, Goodney PP, Sutton JE, et al (Dartmouth-Hitchcock Med Ctr, Lebanon, NH; Dept of Veterans Affairs Med Ctr, White River Junction, Vt)

Surgery 137:172-177, 2005 10–8

Background.—The effectiveness in improving survival of neoadjuvant chemoradiotherapy (NCRT) in patients undergoing surgery for esophageal carcinoma remains unclear.

Methods.—MEDLINE, the Cochrane Database of Systematic Reviews, BIOSIS Previews, and other resources were searched from January 1966 through January 2003. Randomized trials were selected on the basis of study design (NCRT followed by surgery vs surgery alone). Of 21 potential studies identified by abstract review, 6 (29%) met the inclusion criteria.

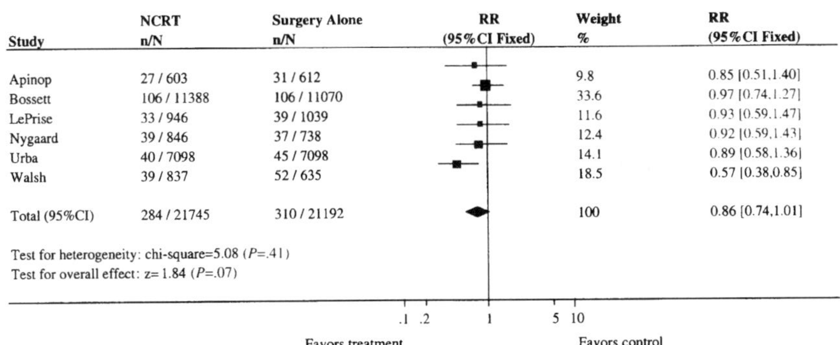

Study	NCRT n/N	Surgery Alone n/N	RR (95%CI Fixed)	Weight %	RR (95%CI Fixed)
Apinop	27 / 603	31 / 612		9.8	0.85 [0.51,1.40]
Bossett	106 / 11388	106 / 11070		33.6	0.97 [0.74,1.27]
LePrise	33 / 946	39 / 1039		11.6	0.93 [0.59,1.47]
Nygaard	39 / 846	37 / 738		12.4	0.92 [0.59,1.43]
Urba	40 / 7098	45 / 7098		14.1	0.89 [0.58,1.36]
Walsh	39 / 837	52 / 635		18.5	0.57 [0.38,0.85]
Total (95%CI)	284 / 21745	310 / 21192		100	0.86 [0.74,1.01]

Test for heterogeneity: chi-square=5.08 (*P*=.41)
Test for overall effect: z= 1.84 (*P*=.07)

FIGURE 2.—Relative risk (RR) of death for NCRT followed by surgery compared with surgery alone, measured by number of deaths (n)/patient-months of follow-up (N). (Courtesy of Greer SE, Goodney PP, Sutton JE, et al: Neoadjuvant chemoradiotherapy for esophageal carcinoma: A meta-analysis. *Surgery* 137:172-177, 2005. Copyright 2005 by Elsevier.

Results.—Across 6 studies, a total of 374 patients underwent NCRT followed by surgery and 364 underwent surgery alone. In 5 of the 6 studies in our meta-analysis, there was a small, non-statistically significant trend toward improved survival with NCRT. Only 1 study demonstrated a statistically significant benefit to NCRT. In our summary measure for all 6 studies, we found a small, non-statistically significant trend toward improved long-term survival in the NCRT followed by surgery group (relative risk of death in the NCRT group [RR], 0.86; 95% confidence interval [CI], 0.74 to 1.01; $P = .07$) (Fig 2).

Conclusions.—NCRT followed by surgery is associated with a small, non-statistically significant improvement in overall survival. Whether this benefit is sufficient to warrant the considerable expense and risks associated with NCRT should be the subject of future larger randomized trials.

▶ As is indicated by the authors, effectiveness to improve survival with use of NCRT for patients undergoing surgery for esophageal carcinoma is indeterminate. Thus, the authors have applied a commonly used database methodology to statistically validate, among 6 studies, a total of 374 patients having NCRT after surgery and 364 patients undergoing surgery alone. As is evident in the article, a statistical trend that is nonstatistically significant is evident among the groups receiving NCRT. However, only 1 study has confirmed statistical benefit with this approach. Thus, this benefit may not be sufficient to warrant the considerable expense, morbidity, and risk for use of NCRT with surgery for esophageal carcinoma. We fully concur that the frequency of use of this technique, as well the expense, portends the necessity of a future clinical trial that focuses on outcomes, survival, morbidity, and cost.

K. I. Bland, MD

Prospective Evaluation of Positron Emission Tomography in the Preoperative Staging of Esophageal Carcinoma

Kneist W, Schreckenberger M, Bartenstein P, et al (Johannes Gutenberg-Univ, Mainz, Germany; Johann Wolfgang Goethe Univ, Frankfurt am Main, Germany)

Arch Surg 139:1043-1049, 2004 10–9

Hypothesis.—Positron emission tomography (PET) is a useful tool in the selection of patients with esophageal cancer who may not benefit from esophageal resection.

Design.—Case series.

Setting.—Tertiary care hospital.

Patients.—Eighty-one patients with newly diagnosed esophageal cancer who underwent PET and computer tomography (CT) of the chest and abdomen (and of the neck in 45 patients) within 45 days were included.

Main Outcome Measures.—We calculated the sensitivity and specificity in detecting metastatic sites on the basis of 31 histologically verified lesions.

In addition to results obtained on CT, the information provided by PET was evaluated with a view to the choice of management strategies.

Results.—The PET findings had a higher specificity (89% vs 11%) but a lower sensitivity (38% vs 63%) than CT findings in the detection of metastatic sites. The CT results showed greater agreement with histopathological findings than did PET results. In 8 patients (10%), PET detected distant metastases that were not identified with CT. In 4 patients (5%), PET detected bone metastases only, but in all of these patients metastases in other locations were detected by CT. Although PET led to upstaging (M1) in 2 patients (2%), it did not enable the exclusion of esophageal resection.

Conclusions.—Preoperative PET was not characterized by greater accuracy in the detection of metastatic sites previously identified by CT. Therefore, PET did not lead to a change in the indication for esophagectomy. An increase in the sensitivity and the combined use of CT and PET may lead to new indications for this staging procedure.

▶ The authors provide international data that suggest that PET has higher specificity, but lower sensitivity, than CT in the detection of metastatic sites from esophageal carcinoma. Moreover, the CT results confirm greater agreement with histopathologic findings than did PET results. However, these studies suggest that preoperative PET does not provide greater accuracy in the detection of metastatic sites previously identified by CT. Thus, use of PET does not enhance change in the indications for esophagectomy.[1] The accuracy in adenocarcinoma of the esophagus for either modality was 47%; for squamous cell carcinoma, PET accuracy was 56% (vs 43% for CT). It would appear that the data suggest that PET is able to identify distant metastases that are missed on CT and did not provide the surgeon a valuable aid in the demonstration of secondary tumors (1.6%) for preoperative staging of esophageal carcinoma. The demonstration exclusively by PET for distant metastasis was quite low (1/81).[2]

K. I. Bland, MD

Reference

1. Kneist W, Schreckenberger M, Bartenstein P, et al: Prospective evaluation of positron emission tomography in the preoperative staging of esophageal carcinoma. *Arch Surg* 139:1043-1049, 2004.
2. Landis JR, Koch GG: The measurement of observer agreement for categorical data. *Biometrics* 33:159-174, 1977.

Intrathoracic Leaks Following Esophagectomy Are No Longer Associated With Increased Mortality

Martin LW, Swisher SG, Hofstetter W, et al (Univ of Texas, Houston)

Ann Surg 242:392-402, 2005 10–10

Objectives.—Assess outcomes following intrathoracic leaks after esophagectomy from 1970 to 2004 to evaluate the impact of evolving surgical and perioperative techniques on leak-associated mortality (LAM).

Summary Background Data.—An intrathoracic leak following esophagectomy has historically been considered a catastrophic event, with mortality as high as 71%. Concerns about this complication often affect choice of surgical approach for esophagectomy.

Methods.—A retrospective review of all esophagectomies for cancer from 1970 to 2004 (n = 1223) was performed. Outcomes following intrathoracic anastomoses (n = 621) were analyzed by era: historical 1970-1986 (n = 145) and modern 1987-2004 (n = 476).

Results.—There was no difference in the frequency of leak between the time intervals (4.8% versus 6.3%, $P = 0.5$). Despite a significant increase in the use of preoperative chemoradiation (1% versus 42%, $P < 0.001$) in the historical versus modern era, the overall mortality decreased from 11% to 2.5% ($P < 0.001$). The LAM was markedly reduced from 43% to 3.3% ($P = 0.016$). Factors associated with LAM included failure to use enteral nutrition (HR 13.22, CI 1.8-96.8) and era in which the surgery was performed (HR 18.3, 1.9-180). Other differences included an increased proportion of successful reoperations for leak control (11/30 versus 0/7, $P = 0.08$) and use of reinforcing muscle flaps (7/11). In the modern era, perioperative mortality is not significantly different for patients with or without intrathoracic leaks (3.3% versus 2.5%, $P = 0.55$), nor is long-term survival ($P = 0.16$).

Conclusions.—Modern surgical management of intrathoracic leaks results in no increased mortality and has no impact on long-term survival. Clinical decisions regarding the use of intrathoracic anastomoses should not be affected by concerns of increased mortality from leak.

► Surgical resection is currently the accepted and most successful approach for treatment of esophageal cancer and provides the only chance for a cure. However, the approach to this resection remains controversial. The 2 best and most common approaches are transhiatal esophagectomy and transthoracic, or Ivor Lewis, esophagectomy. Each approach has its proponents. Multiple prospective randomized trials have been unable to demonstrate a significant survival benefit for one approach over the other. However, the proponents of each technique make compelling arguments for their approach. Significant in these arguments are the risks of interthoracic anastomosis and intrathoracic leaks. Historically, the LAM from intrathoracic anastomosis has been listed as high as 50% versus less than 20% from cervical leaks.

The authors of this study retrospectively evaluated the true risks of endothoracic leaks in terms of mortality, comparing historical and modern era treatment. The study included 621 patients who had intrathoracic anastomoses for resection of esophageal cancer. Two eras were evaluated: from 1970 to 1986 and from 1987 to 2004. The first era included only 145 patients; the second era included 476. The results were quite striking. No significant difference was found in the frequency of leaks in the 2 periods; however, a significant decrease was seen in the overall mortality rate in the 2 periods, from 11% to 2.5%. This occurred despite a 40% increase in preoperative chemoradiation. Of note, the LAM was significantly reduced in the 2 periods, from 43% to 3.3%. This study demonstrates that, in the modern era, the LAM is not significantly different from the overall perioperative mortality rate: 3.3% versus 2.5%. The study also demonstrates that some important improvements occurring in the modern surgical era have significantly reduced the LAM related to Ivor Lewis esophagectomies. First, enteral nutrition has been routinely administered to patients because their esophageal cancer has significantly decreased oral intake and they are usually nutritionally compromised. Thus, in this series, patients who underwent an Ivor Lewis esophagectomy routinely had feeding jejunostomies placed. Second, uncontrolled thoracic anastomotic leaks have been aggressively treated. In this series, the patients were routinely reoperated on and had muscle flaps placed as a routine part of closing the anastomotic leak and rebuttressing the anastomosis. In addition, patients who had controlled intrathoracic leaks received aggressive, conservative (ie, antibiotic and nutritional) management. This study elucidates the improvement in the overall intrathoracic LAM related to Ivor Lewis esophagectomies and proves that this procedure should continue to be used as adequate and appropriate treatment for patients with esophageal cancer.

S. M. Vickers, MD

A Study of 11,003 Patients With Hypertrophic Pyloric Stenosis and the Association Between Surgeon and Hospital Volume and Outcomes

Safford SD, Pietrobon R, Safford KM, et al (Duke Univ, Durham, NC)

J Pediatr Surg 40:967-973, 2005 10–11

Aim.—The availability of large clinical databases allows for careful evaluation of surgical practices, indicators of quality improvement, and cost. We used a large clinical database to compare the effect of surgeon and hospital volume for the care of children with hypertrophic pyloric stenosis (HPS).

Methods.—Patients with International Classification of Diseases-9 codes for HPS and pyloromyotomy were selected from the 1994 to 2000 National Inpatient Samples database. Multiple and logistic regression models were used to evaluate the risk-adjusted association between provider volume and outcomes.

Results.—Postoperative complications occurred in 2.71% of patients. Patients operated on by low- and intermediate-volume surgeons were more likely to have complications compared with those operated on by high-volume surgeons (95% confidence interval [CI], 1.25-3.78 and 95% CI, 1.25-2.69, respectively). Patients operated at low-volume hospitals were 1.6 times more likely to have complications compared with those operated at intermediate- or high-volume hospitals (95% CI, 1.19-2.20). Procedures performed at high-volume hospitals were less expensive than those at intermediate-volume hospitals by a margin of $910 (95% CI, $443-$1377).

Conclusions.—These data represent the largest study to date on the epidemiology, complication rate, and cost for care for HPS. Patients treated by both high-volume surgeons and at high-volume hospitals have improved outcomes at less cost.

▶ This article documents the fact that patients undergoing pyloromyotomy for HPS have better outcomes in hospitals that are high volume for this disease and are managed by surgeons who have a large experience in treating HPS. Complications and hospital costs for pyloromyotomy were higher in those hospitals that had a low-volume experience with pyloric stenosis. Also, low-volume surgeons had a higher complication rate and costs per patient were higher after pyloromyotomy in the hands of low-volume surgeons.

Although general surgeons have traditionally performed pyloromyotomy in infants for HPS, it now appears that these patients are better served if operated on by experienced pediatric surgeons in high-volume centers. With the general availability of pediatric surgeons within a 200 mile radius of almost every area of the United States, it would seem best if most patients with pyloric stenosis were operated on in high-volume centers by pediatric surgeons.

K. E. Georgeson, MD

Pyloromyotomy: A Comparison of Laparoscopic, Circumumbilical, and Right Upper Quadrant Operative Techniques

Kim SS, Lau ST, Lee SL, et al (Univ of Washington, Seattle)

J Am Coll Surg 201:66-70, 2005 10–12

Background.—Ramstedt pyloromyotomy through a right upper quadrant (RUQ) transverse incision has been the traditional treatment for hypertrophic pyloric stenosis. Recently, laparoscopic (LAP) and circumumbilical (UMB) approaches have been introduced as alternative methods to improve cosmesis, but concerns about greater operative times, costs, and complications remain. This study compares the three operative techniques and examines their advantages and complication rates.

Study Design.—We performed a retrospective review of patients undergoing pyloromyotomy at a children's hospital between January 1997 and June 2003.

Results.—Two hundred ninety patients underwent pyloromyotomy by LAP (n = 51), RUQ (n = 190), or UMB (n = 49). Complication rate, time to ad libitum feeding, incidence of emesis, and postoperative length of stay did not differ considerably among groups (Table 2). Two LAP patients were converted to RUQ. Mucosal perforation occurred in three patients each in the RUQ and UMB groups, but none in the LAP group. Operative times were considerably less for LAP (25 ± 9 minutes) than for RUQ (32 ± 9 minutes) and UMB (42 ± 12 minutes) ($p < 0.05$, ANOVA, Bonferroni). Charges re-

TABLE 2.—Intraoperative and Postoperative Data Comparison

Characteristic	LAP ($n = 51$)	RUQ ($n = 190$)	UMB ($n = 49$)	p Value
Operating room time (min)	71 ± 13*	74 ± 14†	83 ± 15‡	<0.0001
Operative time (min)	25 ± 9*‡	32 ± 9†	42 ± 11‡	<0.0001
Postoperative length of stay (d)	1.8 ± 1	1.6 ± 1	1.8 ± 1	0.26
Time to ad lib feedings (h)	26 ± 22	22 ± 14	26 ± 19	0.07
Postoperative emesis (%)	51	56	59	0.53
Conversion rate (%)	2/51 (4)			
Complication rate (%)	4	10	14	0.23
Mucosal perforation	0	3	3	
Wound infection	0	11	3	
Wound dehiscence	1	1	1	
Incisional hernia	0	2	0	
Persistent emesis	1	2	0	
Charges ($)				
Surgery	1,299 ± 331*	1,238 ± 411†	1,574 ± 433‡	<0.0001
Anesthesia	586 ± 137*	578 ± 167†	731 ± 190‡	<0.0001
Recovery room	318 ± 72	301 ± 74	321 ± 46	0.2

Items flagged with the following symbolsindicate that the specified pairwise comparisons were statistically significant at the Bonferroni-adjusted $p < 0.05$.

Data presented at mean ± SD or (%). P value listed for the overall ANOVA, chi-square, or Fisher's exact analysis of all three groups.

*LAP versus UMB.

†RUQ versus UMB.

‡LAP versus RUQ.

Abbreviations: LAP, laparoscopic; *RUQ,* right upper quadrant; *UMB,* circumumbilical.

(Courtesy of Kim SS, Lau ST, Lee SL, et al: Pyloromyotomy: A comparison of laparoscopic, circumumbilical, and right upper quadrant operative techniques. *J Am Coll Surg* 201:66-70, 2005. By permission of the Journal of the American College of Surgeons.)

lated to operations and anesthesia were considerably greater for UMB (operation: $1,574 ± $433; anesthesia: $731 ± $190) compared with the other two groups ($p < 0.05$, ANOVA, Bonferroni), but did not differ between LAP (operation: $1,299 ± $311; anesthesia: $586 ± $137) and RUQ (operation: $1,237 ± $411; anesthesia: $578 ± $167). Data are presented as mean ± SD.

Conclusions.—Advantages of LAP include a shorter mean operative time without higher complications or costs. UMB is associated with the greatest mean operative time and costs. Laparoscopic pyloromyotomy is a safe and effective approach to the treatment of hypertrophic pyloric stenosis.

▶ This interesting study heralds the significance of LAP pyloromyotomy as the gold standard for the treatment of pyloric stenosis in infants when compared with open techniques. The LAP procedure proved to be the fastest and was associated with the least complications. Laparoscopy improved operative times, cost, and intraoperative and postoperative complications. In addition, the LAP approach appeared to be associated with the best cosmetic outcome. For all of these reasons, it seems appropriate that the LAP approach should be adopted by all pediatric surgeons. A comparative study performed 5 or 10 years from now should make LAP pyloromyotomy look even better as the surgical instruments become smaller and better designed. The umbilical approach has significant drawbacks including the difficulty in delivering the pyloric mass through the periumbilical incision without tension. Other problems with the umbilical approach include the increased potential for a wound infection and the sometimes distorted appearance of the umbilicus after the periumbilical incision is healed. As resistance to laparoscopy in infants diminishes among pediatric surgeons, LAP pyloromyotomy should become the gold standard.

K. E. Georgeson, MD

The Efficacy of Fibrin Sealant in Prevention of Anastomotic Leak After Laparoscopic Gastric Bypass

Nguyen NT, Nguyen CT, Stevens CM, et al (Univ of California, Orange)

J Surg Res 122:218-224, 2004 10–13

Background.—Anastomotic leak after laparoscopic gastric bypass (GBP) can result in significant morbidity, mortality, and consumption of healthcare resources. Fibrin sealant has been used clinically in the prevention of leak; however, its efficacy has not been clearly demonstrated. The aims of this study were to (1) develop an iatrogenic leak model in swine, (2) examine the efficacy of fibrin sealant in sealing iatrogenic anastomotic leak, and (3) review our experience with the use of fibrin sealant in 66 patients who underwent laparoscopic GBP.

Methods.—This study was performed in three phases. In phase 1, laparoscopic gastrojejunostomy was performed in adult swine with iatrogenic disruption of the anastomotic staple line. The size of disruption was sequentially increased (6- to 12-F opening) until a leak model was developed. In phase 2, 16 animals underwent laparoscopic gastrojejunostomy with a 12-F disruption of the anastomosis; 10 animals (study group) had fibrin sealant (Tisseel VH) applied on the disrupted anastomosis and 6 animals (control group) did not receive fibrin sealant. Animals were sacrificed on postoperative day 5 or earlier if peritonitis developed and were examined for sealing of the anastomotic disruption and the presence of intraabdominal abscess. In phase 3, the outcome of 66 consecutive patients who underwent laparoscopic GBP with fibrin sealant applied at the gastrojejunostomy was reviewed.

Results.—In phase 1, an anastomotic leak model was developed with a 12-F disruption of the staple line. In phase 2, two control animals required early sacrifice for bile peritonitis; three control animals had intraabdominal abscess discovered at sacrifice and one animal did not have any evidence of intraabdominal abscess or leak. Of the 10 animals in the study group, all survived until sacrifice and none of these animals had evidence of intraabdominal abscess or persistent leak. Therefore, 83% of animals in the control group developed either leak or abscess compared to 0% in the study group ($P < 0.01$, Fisher's exact test). Clinically, no leak or intraabdominal abscess developed in 66 patients who underwent laparoscopic GBP with the use of fibrin sealant.

Conclusions.—An anastomotic leak model was developed in swine with disruption of the stapled gastrojejunostomy to a 12-F opening. The use of fibrin sealant significantly reduces leak and abscess complication. Our re-

TABLE 2.—The Mechanism of Fibrin Sealant in Formation of Fibrin Clots

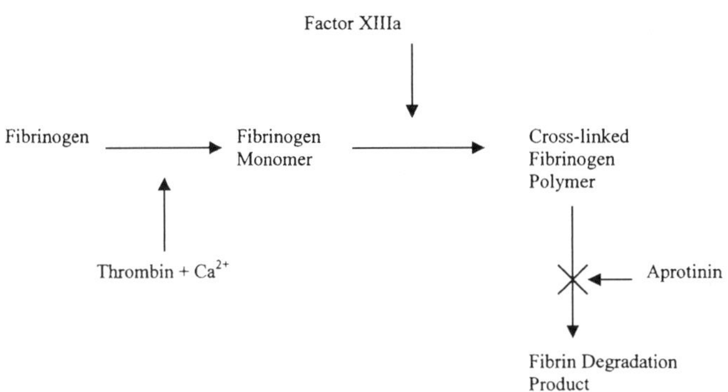

(Courtesy of Nguyen NT, Nguyen CT, Stevens CM, et al: The efficacy of fibrin sealant in prevention of anastomotic leak after laparoscopic gastric bypass. *J Surg Res* 122:218-224, 2004. With permission from Elsevier Science.)

sults support the tissue sealing property of fibrin sealant and its use on high-risk gastrointestinal anastomosis (Table 2).

▶ This interesting study used an animal model to document the efficacy of fibrin sealant application for the prevention of a suture line leak. This study has importance for all internal anastomoses, but specifically for laparoscopic anastomoses that may be more vulnerable to leaks. This article is encouraging in that leak models showed no leak or abscess formation in all 10 animals who were left with a size 12-F defect in the anastomosis. The control animals that did not have the application of the fibrin sealant showed significant leakage with drastic morbidity associated with this leakage. Further studies should follow to verify the positive results of this technique. The costs and the effort to apply the fibrin sealant should be outweighed by the decrease in morbidity and costs from intestinal leaks.

K. E. Georgeson, MD

Lifestyle, Diabetes, and Cardiovascular Risk Factors 10 Years After Bariatric Surgery

Sjöström L, for the Swedish Obese Subjects Study Scientific Group (Sahlgrenska Univ, Göteborg, Sweden; et al)

N Engl J Med 351:2683-2693, 2004 10–14

Background.—Obesity is associated with increased morbidity and mortality. It is assumed that the morbidity is mediated mainly by insulin resistance, diabetes, hypertension, and lipid disturbances, which affect 25% of persons in North America. Studies have shown that in the short term, lifestyle changes that result in weight loss can provide improvements in insulin resistance, diabetes, hypertension, and lipid disturbances and may prevent these conditions. However, several observational epidemiologic studies have suggested that weight loss is associated with increased overall mortality and mortality from cardiovascular disease among thin, normal weight, and obese persons. The goals of the Swedish Obese Subjects (SOS) Study were to address this apparent discrepancy and to determine whether the short-term amelioration and prevention of metabolic and cardiovascular risk associated with weight loss are persistent over time.

Methods.—The SOS Study was a prospective, controlled study involving obese persons who underwent gastric surgery (fixed or variable banding, vertical banded gastroplasty, or gastric bypass) and contemporaneously matched, conventionally treated obese control subjects. Follow-up data were reported for subjects with a mean age of 48 years and a mean body mass index of 41 who had been enrolled for at least 2 years (4047 subjects) or 10 years (1703 subjects) before the analysis. The follow-up rate was 86.6% at 2 years and 74.5% at 10 years.

Results.—At 2 years, weight had increased by 0.1% in the control group and had decreased by 23.4% in the surgery group. At 10 years, weight had increased by 1.6% in the control group and had decreased by 16.1% in the surgery group. Subjects in the surgery group had lower energy intake than the control subjects throughout the study, and the proportion of physically active subjects was higher in the surgery group than in the control group (Fig 2). Recovery rates at 2 and 10 years from diabetes, hypertriglyceridemia, low levels of high-density lipoprotein cholesterol, hypertension, and hyperuricemia were better in the surgery group than in the control group, but recovery from hypercholesterolemia did not differ between the two groups. The surgery group had lower incidence rates for diabetes, hypertriglyceridemia, and hyperuricemia at both 2 and 10 years compared with the control group. However, there were not detectable differences between the groups in the incidence of hypercholesterolemia or hypertension.

Conclusion.—In comparison with conventional therapy, bariatric surgery appears to be a viable option for the treatment of severe obesity, providing long-term weight loss, improved lifestyle, and (with the exception of hypercholesterolemia) a reduction in risk factors for patients with elevated risk factors at baseline.

▶ This prospective, randomized study by the SOS Study Scientific Group identified obese subjects undergoing gastric bypass who were matched con-

---

FIGURE 2.—Lifestyle Changes Among the Subjects in the Swedish Obese Subjects Study Over a 10-Year Period. Mean energy intake (in kilocalories per day) (**Panel A**) and the percentage of subjects who were physically active during leisure time and at work (**Panels B and C, respectively**) are shown. Energy intake and the proportion of active subjects at baseline (year 0) are unadjusted values, whereas the values during the follow-up have been adjusted for sex, age, body-mass index, and energy intake or physical activity at baseline. All data are from subjects who completed 10 years of the study. *Asterisks* denote *P* <0.01 and daggers *P* <0.05 for the comparison between the groups (by tests for equality). *I bars* represent the 95 percent confidence intervals. (Reprinted by permission of *The New England Journal of Medicine* from Sjöström L, for the Swedish Obese Subjects Study Scientific Group: Lifestyle, diabetes, and cardiovascular risk factors 10 years after bariatric surgery. *N Engl J Med* 351:2683-2693, 2004.)

FIGURE 2

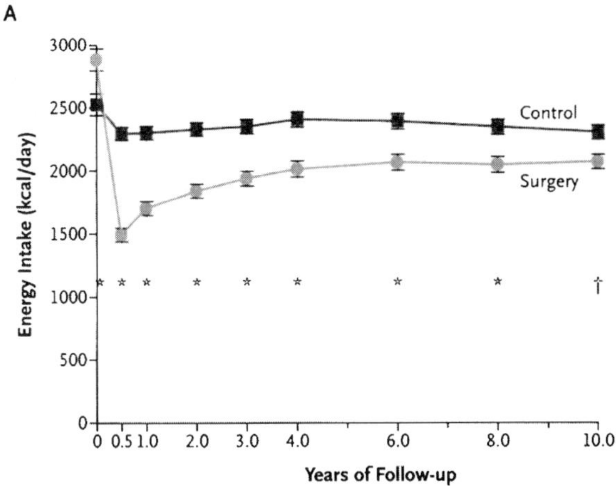
A
Energy Intake (kcal/day)
3000
2500
2000
1500
1000
500
0
Control
Surgery
* * * * * * * * †
0 0.5 1.0 2.0 3.0 4.0 6.0 8.0 10.0
Years of Follow-up

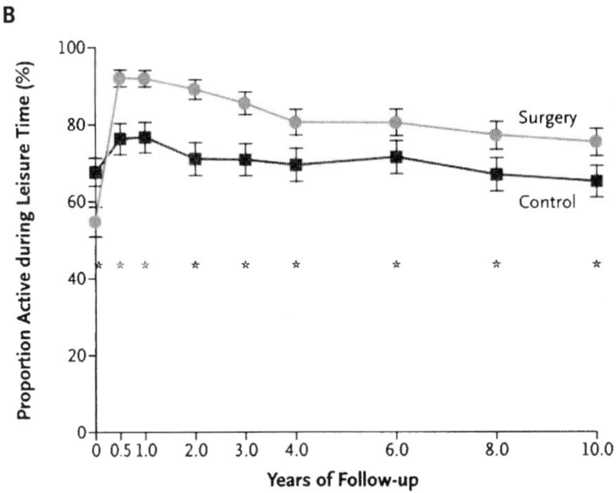
B
Proportion Active during Leisure Time (%)
100
80
60
40
20
0
Surgery
Control
* * * * * * * * *
0 0.5 1.0 2.0 3.0 4.0 6.0 8.0 10.0
Years of Follow-up

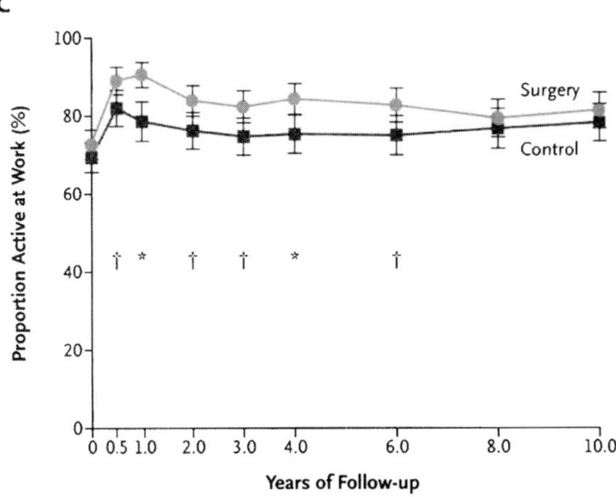
C
Proportion Active at Work (%)
100
80
60
40
20
0
Surgery
Control
† * † † * †
0 0.5 1.0 2.0 3.0 4.0 6.0 8.0 10.0
Years of Follow-up

temporaneously with conventionally treated obese control subjects. This important article identifies risks for lifestyle, diabetes, and cardiovascular morbidity/mortality some 10 years following weight loss following bariatric surgery. The study concludes that, compared with conventional approaches, bariatric surgical therapy of the obese is an important option of therapy and will result in durable weight loss, enhancement of lifestyle, and—with the exception of hypercholesterolemia—will reduce the risk factor for cardiovascular disease evident with the baseline presentation of obesity.

With regard to lifestyle changes, data from subjects completing the 10-year study had a reduction of caloric intake (Fig 2, Panel A), proportional increase in activity during leisure time (Fig 2, Panel B), and an enhancement of proportional activity at work (Fig 2, Panel C). Of additional interest, the mean changes in weight and risk factors were more favorable among patients surgically treated by gastric bypass than among those randomized to banding or vertical-banded gastroplasty.

This landmark study suggests that bariatric surgery is a major contribution to the therapy of severe obesity. However, all of the obesity-associated risk factors were not improved by sustained weight loss, suggesting the need for obtaining long-term data for the effect of weight reduction on overall mortality and the progressive incidence of cardiovascular and neoplastic transformation.

K. I. Bland, MD

Effect of Diabetes and Hypertension on Obesity-Related Mortality

Livingston EH, Ko CY (Univ of Texas, Dallas; VA Greater Los Angeles Health Care System)

Surgery 137:16-25, 2005 10–15

Background.—Obesity is increasing and, along with it, greater mortality resulting from the overweight condition. Weight-reduction surgery is recommended for many obese patients based on a perceived risk of greater obesity-related mortality. However, many of the studies cited to justify this have aggregated patient groups together, making it difficult to apply their findings to individual patients.

Methods.—The combined National Health Interview Survey database from the years 1986-1994 that has been linked to the National Death Index was analyzed. Patients were stratified for their body mass index (BMI) category, the presence or absence of diabetes and hypertension, gender, and race. The contribution of hypertension and diabetes to mortality was determined by Cox proportional hazards modeling. The absolute magnitude that the effect gender, race, BMI, hypertension, and diabetes had on mortality was determined by examination of stratified age-adjusted death rates.

Results.—We analyzed 662,443 records from individuals interviewed between 1986 and 1994. Of these, 49,391 had died in the follow-up period (mean follow-up, 7.2 years; range, 1-14 years). Cox proportional hazards modeling-adjusting for age, race, and gender-revealed that hypertension (hazard ratio = 1.35 [95% CI 1.34-1.35], $P < .0001$) and diabetes (hazard ratio = 2.29 [95% CI 2.28-2.29], $P < .0001$) increased mortality independent of body weight. Serious obesity was associated with an increased mortality by Cox modeling (hazard ratio = 1.72 [95% CI 1.71-1.73], $P < .0001$); however, when assessed by stratified age-adjusted mortality rates, this increase was numerically small because of the relatively low mortality rate for those without hypertension or diabetes. The presence of hypertension or diabetes substantially increased age-adjusted mortality rates. Much of the increased mortality observed in diabetic patients was attributable to complications of diabetes and not necessarily from atherosclerosis.

Conclusion.—Because weight-loss surgery successfully cures hypertension or diabetes in most obese patients, it should be considered for obese patients having these diseases. Based on the greatly elevated mortality associated with diabetes, surgery may be justified for obese diabetic patients with BMIs lower than the currently accepted criteria. In contrast, for the morbidly obese without diabetes or hypertension, mortality is only slightly increased from obesity alone. In terms of mortality, the benefits of weight reduction resulting from weight-loss surgery are less clear if there is no coexistent diabetes or hypertension.

▶ Drs Livingston and Ko of the University of Texas-Southwestern, Dallas, and the VA Greater Los Angeles Health Care System, California, use the National Health Interview Survey Database (1986-1994) and the National Death Index to analyze 662,443 records to evaluate the implications of diabetes and hypertension on obesity-related mortality. The concern of the authors was that the NIH Consensus Conference of 1991 suggested that patient BMI greater than 40 may be considered a surgical candidate for weight reduction. The authors identified comorbidities as an important constituent of the increased mortality experienced in this obese population. Clearly, the examination of this large health information database and their death records allowed introspection into the effect that obesity, exclusive of the presence of diabetes or hypertension, had on mortality.

The authors conclude that based on the greatly elevated mortality associated with diabetes, surgery may be justified for obese diabetic patients with BMIs lower than the currently accepted criteria. This is based on the objective fact that weight-loss surgery has successfully cured hypertension and/or diabetes in most obese patients. In contradistinction, for the morbidly obese without diabetes or hypertension, mortality is only slightly increased from obesity alone. Thus, this important article suggests that the benefits of the reduction from weight loss are less significant in the absence of coexistence diabetes or hypertension. The authors intimate that perhaps this BMI criterion should be lowered to 30, but will require a prospective trial. We agree that BMIs that exceed 35 with obesity-related comorbidities should be strongly considered for a gastric bypass procedure—despite the demand for this surgical procedure. The importance of this article is to emphasize that the obese patient, with absence of diabetes or hypertension, almost certainly will not gain the longevity expectations as do those who have these morbidities coexisting with obesity. We concur that prospective randomized trials that include substantially these risk parameters must be assessed.

K. I. Bland, MD

Gastric Banding Interferes With Esophageal Motility and Gastroesophageal Reflux

Suter M, Dorta G, Giusti V, et al (Centre Hospitalier Universitaire Vaudois, Lausanne, Switzerland)

Arch Surg 140:639-643, 2005 10–16

Background.—Gastroesophageal reflux and progressive esophageal dilatation can develop after gastric banding (GB).

Hypothesis.—Gastric banding may interfere with esophageal motility, enhance reflux, or promote esophageal dilatation.

Design.—Before–after trial in patients undergoing GB.

Setting.—University teaching hospital.

Patients and Methods.—Between January 1999 and August 2002, 43 patients undergoing laparoscopic GB for morbid obesity underwent upper gastrointestinal endoscopy, 24-hour pH monitoring, and stationary esophageal manometry before GB and between 6 and 18 months postoperatively.

Main Outcome Measures.—Reflux symptoms, endoscopic esophagitis, pressures measured at manometry, esophageal acid exposure.

Results.—There was no difference in the prevalence of reflux symptoms or esophagitis before and after GB. The lower esophageal sphincter was unaffected by surgery, but contractions in the lower esophagus weakened after GB, in correlation with preoperative values. There was a trend toward more postoperative nonspecific motility disorders. Esophageal acid exposure tended to decrease after GB, with fewer reflux episodes. A few patients developed massive postoperative reflux. There was no clear correlation between preoperative testing and postoperative esophageal acid exposure, although patients with abnormal preoperative acid exposure tended to maintain high values after GB.

Conclusions.—Postoperative esophageal dysmotility and gastroesophageal reflux are not uncommon after GB. Preoperative testing should be done routinely. Low amplitude of contraction in the lower esophagus and increased esophageal acid exposure should be regarded as contraindications to GB. Patients with such findings should be offered an alternative procedure, such as Roux-en-Y gastric bypass.

► GB is the latest operation promoted by bariatric surgeons to bring about significant weight loss using the least deranging surgical procedure and a laparoscopic approach. This article is another in a growing series of studies that warn that esophageal reflux and dysmotility can develop after placement of a constricting band around the top portion of the stomach. What is not abnormal early may develop at 6 to 18 months afterward by weakening the esophageal musculature.

The authors searched for predictions of postoperative acid reflux or esophagitis in their 43 patients and found none. They excluded patients with large hiatal hernias but found that some patients with preoperative reflux symptoms were asymptomatic after operation. However, those with abnormal preoperative esophageal pH values or poor motility were more likely to have postoperative problems; each time, these problems could be avoided and treated with an alternative Roux-en-Y gastric bypass. The enthusiasm for GB, which is currently high, should be tempered by recognition of these postoperative difficulties and by the variability in weight loss results, which suggests that gastric bypass is more efficacious.

J. J. Gleysteen, MD

Open Repair of Paraesophageal Hernia: Reassessment of Subjective and Objective Outcomes

Low DE, Unger T (Virginia Mason Med Ctr, Seattle)

Ann Thorac Surg 80:287-294, 2005 10–17

Background.—Surgical repair of paraesophageal hernias (PEH) remains a challenging operation. Increasing numbers of patients are undergoing laparoscopic repair. This series provides an up-to-date benchmark of the results of open repair of PEH to compare with current laparoscopic series.

Methods.—All patients undergoing surgical repair of PEH by a single surgeon between April 1996 and November 2001 were included. Follow-up included postoperative SF-36 survey and objective reassessment (barium swallow or endoscopy) at a mean of 29.8 months.

Results.—Seventy-two consecutive patients (mean age, 68.7 years) presented with large PEH. Presenting symptoms included heartburn (60%), dysphagia (43%), chest pain (42%), anemia (39%), and dyspnea (32%). Surgical treatment involved transabdominal open repair including sac excision, crural closure (primary closure 98.6%), and antireflux procedure (Hill procedure, 96%; Nissen fundoplication, 4%). No patient required a Collis procedure. Postoperative assessment (subjective, 97%; objective, 88%) was prospective. Median operative length was 155 minutes. Median length of

TABLE 10.—Comparative Outcomes of Laparoscopic Series* and Current Virginia Mason Medical Center Series of Open Paraesophageal Hernia Repairs

Outcome	Laparoscopic Reports (1997-2003)	Open Repairs Current Report (1996-2001)
Operation length (min)	169-240	155
Hospital length of stay (days)	2.0-4.2	4.5
Visceral injuries (%)	1-12	0
Mortality (%)	0-3	0
Hernia recurrence (%)	14-33	5-18

*See Table 9 in original article.

(Courtesy of Low DE, Unger T: Open repair of paraesophageal hernia: Reassessment of subjective and objective outcomes. *Ann Thorac Surg* 80:287-294, 2005. Reprinted with permission from the Society of Thoracic Surgeons.)

stay was 4.5 days (range, 3 to 12 days). Postoperative complications occurred in 17 of 72 patients (23.6%), but no patient sustained intraoperative or postoperative visceral injuries. In-hospital and 30-day mortality was zero. Heartburn and dysphagia symptom scores demonstrated significant improvement ($p < 0.001$). Postoperative SF-36 scores demonstrated levels better than the general population (six of eight categories) and better than the age-matched population (eight of eight categories). Objective follow-up demonstrated recurrent hernias in 11 patients (18%). Most of these recurrences (73%) were less than 2-cm sliding hernias, and no patients required revisional surgery.

Conclusions.—The results of open repair of PEH have continued to evolve in the same time that has seen the introduction of laparoscopic PEH repairs. Results with the open approach in the modern era can provide excellent outcomes, which are comparable to and in some measures exceed those obtained with the laparoscopic approach (Table 10).

▶ The authors have a sizeable and favorable experience with open PEH repair in patients who have been followed up, on average, for 30 months. The transabdominal operations all involved hernia sac excision with diaphragmatic closure and an antireflux procedure; none involved application of polypropylene mesh. The authors emphasize that the technique and results of open repairs have evolved in recent years, and they compare recent open results to laparoscopic results. They claim that mobilization of the esophagus is extensive and sufficient with both techniques, that the length of stay favors the laparoscopic approach, and that some cases of recurrence are small (<2-cm) sliding hernias, which are not likely to be clinically relevant. The results of recent studies in which laparoscopy was used are compared with those of the current series (Table 10).

J. J. Gleysteen, MD

Mesh in the Hiatus: A Controversial Issue

Targarona EM, Bendahan G, Balague C, et al (Autonomous Univ of Barcelona)
Arch Surg 139:1286-1296, 2004 10–18

Objective.—To analyze the experience acquired to date on the use of prosthetic mesh to prevent recurrence after laparoscopic repair of paraesophageal hernia.

Data Sources.—Current English-language literature review.

Study Selection.—Case reports, series, and opinion articles on the use of mesh for paraesophageal hernia repair.

Data Extraction and Synthesis.—Study type and results were analyzed. Most articles were short case series. Few comparative or randomized trials assessing the procedure have been published to date. The information available showed that the use of a mesh for hiatal repair was safe and prevented recurrence. However, data on the long-term results were lacking, and infrequent but severe complications may arise.

Conclusions.—The mesh should be used selectively, and the decision to proceed should be based on clinical experience. In light of the evidence available, however, it appears to be safe, and the fears expressed in the past have not been confirmed.

▶ This is a review article in which the authors are comprehensive in their collection of articles and provide helpful illustrations of the variety of mesh repairs used for paraesophageal hernia repair. Different configurations of hernias occur in this area, and it is understandable that recurrence rates might be variable (up to 42% and 50% in laparoscopic and open series, respectively).

The real issue in managing this problem has been the potential deleterious effect of the mesh over the long-term. The mesh needs to be nonabsorbable, and polytef has been favored over polypropylene for this use as softer and less desmoplastic. The frequency of complications in articles has been less that 2%, although some serious erosion problems have occurred. Usually, the mesh is placed around the hiatus in a tension-free manner. The mesh needs to stay in place to work, but as seen later on with mesh placed in other places, once ingrowth to the mesh has occurred, the mesh can become incorporated with native tissue and will become stable.

The authors suggest that final answers on effectiveness will come after longer term follow-up but that randomized trials may be required to settle technical issues such as the type of mesh, the location of the mesh, selective versus routine use, Collis esophageal lengthening, and other variables.

J. J. Gleysteen, MD

Surgical Strategies for Necrotising Enterocolitis: A Survey of Practice in the United Kingdom

Rees CM, Hall NJ, Eaton S, et al (Inst of Child Health, London)
Arch Dis Child Fetal Neonatal Ed 90:F152-F155, 2005 10–19

Background.—Strategies for the surgical management of necrotising enterocolitis are various and controversial.

Objective.—To characterise variation in surgical management of this disease across the United Kingdom.

Methods.—Postal survey of 104 consultant paediatric surgeons with a 77% response rate.

Results.—Duration of antibiotic treatment (median 10 days, range 6-14), time until the start of enteral feeding (median 10 days, range 4-21), and absolute indications for surgery all vary between surgeons (Table 1). Peritoneal drainage is used by 95% of surgeons. Forty two percent use it in neonates of all weights, whereas 36% restrict its use to those <1000 g (Table 2). Peritoneal drainage is used for stabilisation by 95% and as definitive treatment by 58%. At laparotomy, operative procedures include diverting jejunostomy, resection and stoma, resection with primary anastomosis, and "clip and drop". All procedures are used in infants of all weights except resection and primary anastomosis, which is used predominantly in larger infants (55%

TABLE 1.—Absolute Indications for Surgical Intervention

Absolute Indication	Percentage of Surgeons Using Indication Laparotomy	Peritoneal Drain
Clinical findings		
Failure of medical therapy	71	14
Abdominal mass	36	1
Thrombocytopenia	3	4
Raised inflammatory markers	3	1
Radiological findings		
Pneumoperitoneum	75	53
Fixed intestinal loop	39	6
Portal venous gas	8	4
Pneumatosis intestinalis	3	0

(Courtesy of Rees CM, Hall NJ, Eaton S, et al: Surgical strategies for necrotising enterocolitis: A survey of practice in the United Kingdom. *Arch Dis Child Fetal Neonatal Ed* 90:F152-F155, 2005. With permission from the BMJ Publishing Group.)

in <1000 g; 77% in >1000g; $p=0.005$). Infants may be considered too unwell for peritoneal drainage by 11% of surgeons compared with 90% for laparotomy ($p<0.0001$).

Conclusions.—There is considerable variation in surgical strategies for necrotising enterocolitis. Peritoneal drainage is used by most surgeons, with controversial indications and expectations. The use of resection and primary anastomosis is influenced by the weight of the neonate.

► Rees et al of the Department of Surgery, Institute of Child Health, London, emphasize the various strategies that have evolved in the surgical management of necrotising enterocolitis and the controversy encountered therein. The authors were intent upon characterizing the variations in management of this entity throughout the United Kingdom; the authors completed a survey of 104 consultant pediatric surgeons, receiving a 77% response rate to the survey questionnaires.

In the most common gastrointestinal emergency encountered in the neonatal population necrotising enterocolitis has a consistent mortality of 20% to 40%, despite exceptional advances in neonatal intensive care. As many as half of all confirmed cases of necrotising enterocolitis may require surgical inter-

TABLE 2.—Use of Peritoneal Drainage and Weight of Patient

Weight Category	Number of Surgeons (n = 74)	%
All weights	31	42
<1000 g	27	36
<1500 g	14	19
<2000 g	2	3

Question asked: In which of these weight categories of infants would you use peritoneal drainage? (pick one only): All; <2000g; <1500 g; <1000 g.

(Courtesy of Rees CM, Hall NJ, Eaton S, et al: Surgical strategies for necrotising enterocolitis: A survey of practice in the United Kingdom. *Arch Dis Child Fetal Neonatal Ed* 90:F152-F155, 2005. With permission from the BMJ Publishing Group.)

vention; of great controversy is the surgical management of the premature neonate less than 1000 g in weight.

Of interest, peritoneal drainage was used by 95% of all pediatric surgeons surveyed in the United Kingdom who managed necrotising enterocolitis; 36% of these surgeons restricted its use to neonates less than 1000 g. Eleven percent of the surgeons do not use peritoneal drainage in infants they consider too ill for its usage.

What became evident in this report by the surveyors is that the use of surgical resection and primary anastomosis is principally influenced by the weight of the neonate.

K. I. Bland, MD

Gastroschisis in the Rat Model Is Associated With a Delayed Maturation of Intestinal Pacemaker Cells and Smooth Muscle Cells

Midrio P, Faussone-Pellegrini MS, Vannucchi MG, et al (Children's Inst for Surgical Sciences, Philadelphia; Univ of Florence, Italy)

J Pediatr Surg 39:1541-1547, 2004 10–20

Background.—A pacemaker system is required for peristalsis generation. The interstitial cells of Cajal (ICC) are considered the intestinal pacemaker, and are identified by expression of the c-*kit* gene—encoded protein. Gastroschisis is characterized by a severe gastrointestinal dysmotility in newborns. In spite of this clinical picture, few studies have focused on smooth muscle cells (SMC) morphology and none on ICC. Therefore, their morphology has been studied in fetuses at term in the rat model of gastroschisis.

Methods.—At 18.5 day's gestation (E18.5), 10 rat fetuses were killed, 10 underwent surgical creation of gastroschisis, and 10 underwent manipulation only. The small intestine of the latter 2 groups was harvested at E21.5. Specimens were processed for H&E, c-*kit* and actin (α smooth muscle antibody [α-SMA]) immunohistochemistry, and transmission electron microscopy (TEM).

Results.—In the controls, SMC were c-*kit*+ and α-SMA+, with labeling intensity increasing by age. At E21.5, some cells around the Auerbach's plexus were more intensely c-*kit*+, and differentiating ICC were seen under TEM at this level. Gastroschisis fetuses had no c-*kit*+ cells referable to ICC. In the more damaged loops, SMC were very faintly c-*kit*+ and α-SMA+. Under TEM, there were few differentiated SMC and no presumptive ICC. In the less-damaged loops, SMC were faintly c-*kit*+ and α-SMA+ and had ultrastructural features intermediate between those of E18.5 and E21.5 controls; ICC were very immature.

Conclusions.—ICC and SMC differentiation is delayed in gastroschisis with the most damaged loops showing the most incomplete picture. These findings might help in understanding the delayed onset of peristalsis and the variable time-course of the recover seen in babies affected by gastroschisis.

► This study identifies delayed differentiation of the intestinal pacemaker cells, the ICC, in a fetus with gastroschisis. The article shows that the environment of the developing intestine influences the rate of maturation of the ICC and also the SMCs. This delayed maturation of the ICC and SMCs is responsible for the dysmotility in infants with gastroschisis. These findings tend to diminish the role of the neonatal management of these patients in determining the rapidity of the return of intestinal function after gastroschisis repair. It might also help to explain the deranged motility and secondary nature of this derangement in other gastrointestinal diseases such as Hirschsprung's disease or proximal intestinal atresia. Rather than providing a solution to a complex problem, this investigation offers an avenue of research that may, over the long haul, help us better understand and manage infants with gastroschisis.

K. E. Georgeson, MD

An 11-Year Experience of Enterocutaneous Fistula

Hollington P, Mawdsley J, Lim W, et al (St Mark's Hosp, Harrow, England)

Br J Surg 91:1646-1651, 2004 10–21

Background.—Enterocutaneous fistula has traditionally been associated with substantial morbidity and mortality, related to fluid, electrolyte and metabolic disturbance, sepsis and malnutrition.

Methods.—A retrospective review of enterocutaneous fistula in 277 consecutive patients treated over an 11-year period in a major tertiary referral centre was undertaken to evaluate current management practice and outcome.

Results.—Most fistulas occurred secondary to abdominal surgery, and a high proportion (52.7 per cent) occurred in association with inflammatory bowel disease. A low rate of spontaneous healing was observed (19.9 per cent). The healing rate after definitive fistula surgery was 82.0 per cent, although more than one attempt was required to achieve surgical closure in some patients. Definitive fistula resection resulted in a mortality rate of 3.0 per cent. In addition, one patient died after laparotomy for intra-abdominal sepsis and an additional 24 patients died from complications of fistulation, giving an overall fistula-related mortality rate of 10.8 per cent.

Conclusion.—Early recognition and control of sepsis, management of fluid and electrolyte imbalances, meticulous wound care and nutritional support appear to reduce the mortality rate, and allow spontaneous fistula closure in some patients. Definitive surgical management is performed only after restitution of normal physiology, usually after at least 6 months.

► This long-term study from a hospital renowned for its collection of gastrointestinal surgical disease information provides a great deal of data on enterocutaneous fistulas (other bowel fistulas excluded). In doing so, the authors emphasize 2 strategic points. The first is that the early goal was to achieve an enteral rather than a parenteral means of nutritional support. Despite initiation with total parenteral nutrition, the effort was made to decrease output to less than 500 mL/d as rapidly as possible with several antimotility drugs (octreotide, if a positive response was shown), proton pump inhibitors, and encouraged oral consumption of Gatorade-like solutions. The reason for this is the conviction that the enteral route promotes more rapid healing and improved immune functioning and helps to avoid sepsis.

The second strategic point is that surgery was delayed, often longer than 6 months, to allow time for fistula maturation, resolution of the inflammatory reaction in the peritoneal cavity, and optimization of the patients' nutritional state. At that time, all diseased bowel tissue, including overlying skin, was resected, irrespective of the amount of bowel lost. These strategies produced the favorable results detailed above.

J. J. Gleysteen, MD

Free Peritoneal Graft for Repair of Severe Seromuscular Defect of Bowel: From Experiment to Clinical Practice

Yin W-Y (Tzu Chi Univ, Chia Yi, Taiwan)

J Surg Res 125:3-8, 2005 10–22

Background.—Severe seromuscular tear of the bowel with impending perforation following enterolysis or trauma is not uncommon in gastrointestinal surgery. It is sometimes complicated with enterocutaneous fistula, intra-abdominal abscess or free perforation, especially of the ileus. In addition, direct serosal repair is often impossible, or complicated by lumen compromise. Serosal patch repair also reportedly is also associated with complications such as dislodgement of the sutured bowel loop, fistula formation, adhesion ileus, or volvulus. Free peritoneal graft (FPG), as in split-thickness skin graft (STSG), can be taken by underlying healthy tissue within 24 to 48 h and used for repair of such defect.

Patients and Methods.—In this study, FPG was used as an alternative to serosal patch repair or resection to cover severe defects of the colon, rectum, duodenum, or small bowel in 30 consecutive patients. All defects were over 8 × 4 cm in size and involved 30 to 80% of the circumference of the bowel wall. Each defect was deep enough to expose the thin mucosal layer, with the intestinal content visible through it. These defects could have been successfully treated by resection or repair using a serosal or mucosal patch instead of FPG. After making sure that the mucosa associated with the defect was alive and not perforated, a patch of intact peritoneum with pre-peritoneal tissue from the lateral abdominal wall (slightly smaller than the defect) was superimposed, with the edges simply sewn to the margin of the defect.

Results.—All patients recovered uneventfully, with no untoward effects determined, even after long-term follow-up.

Conclusion.—We believe that FPG provides a feasible, simple, effective, economic, and safe alternative for repair of severe seromuscular defects; potentially making it widely applicable in clinical practice.

► This article suggests a simple resolution to a problem that has vexed abdominal surgeons: the problem of a severe seromuscular tear of the bowel during release of intestinal adhesions. Seromuscular injury to the bowel often leads to unintended bowel resection when the tear is long and greater than 50% of the circumference of the bowel wall. The author reports the use of a FPG to repair the seromuscular defect. This solution seems almost too easy. It makes one wonder why it has not been used in the past. Perhaps the fear of a dysmotile segment of bowel that does not have adequate motility has been the main deterrent to the use of this technique. The author suggests that this technique is especially beneficial for portions of the bowel that are difficult to resect such as the duodenum and rectum. Although this technique is alluring, additional reports will be necessary before it can fully establish itself in general surgery. Methods to detect the viability of the underlying mucosa are also important to the successful use of this technique. Hopefully this report will stimulate further investigations into this difficult problem.

K. E. Georgeson, MD

Serial Transverse Enteroplasty Is Associated With Successful Short-Term Outcomes in Infants With Short Bowel Syndrome

Javid PJ, Kim HB, Duggan CP, et al (Harvard Med School, Boston)

J Pediatr Surg 40:1019-1024, 2005 10–23

Background.—The serial transverse enteroplasty (STEP) has been shown to improve nutritional indices in an animal model of short bowel syndrome. The aim of this study was to review short-term surgical and nutritional outcomes in the first cohort of infants to undergo the STEP procedure at our institution.

Methods.—All patients who underwent the STEP procedure during a 26-month period from February 2002 to March 2004 were reviewed. Paired *t* tests were used for comparisons between values pre-STEP and post-STEP ($P < .05$ deemed significant). Data are expressed as mean and range.

Results.—The STEP was performed on 5 patients, including 1 newborn. The STEP was used as a primary lengthening operation in 4 patients. Intestinal length was significantly increased in all patients with 18 (10-26) stapler applications (Fig 1). There were no perioperative complications and no evidence of intestinal leak or obstruction on routine postoperative contrast study. Nutritional follow-up was available on 3 subjects at 17 (11-26) months post-STEP (Fig 2). Percentage of enteral nutrition was significantly increased in these subjects ($P < .05$). One subject was fully weaned from total parenteral nutrition 6 weeks after the STEP, and bilirubin in another patient with profound cholestasis who had been listed for liver-small bowel transplant normalized after the STEP. An additional patient, with established cir-

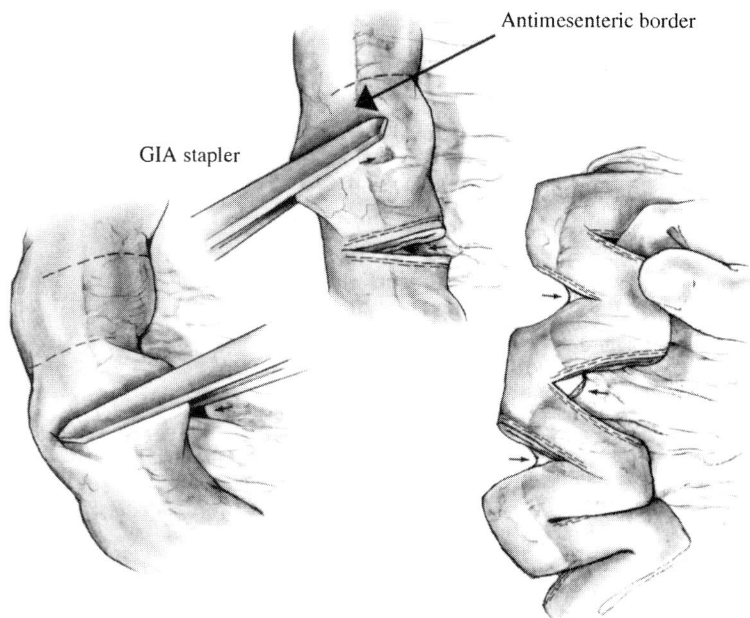

FIGURE 1.—The basic concepts of the STEP procedure. Serial applications of the linear stapler are used to create a zigzag-shaped channel of lengthened small bowel. The stapler is placed perpendicular to the long axis of the bowel, so that all stapler applications are parallel to the mesenteric blood supply. (Courtesy of Javid PJ, Kim HB, Duggan CP, et al: Serial transverse enteroplasty is associated with successful short-term outcomes in infants with short bowel syndrome. *J Pediatr Surg* 40:1019-1024, 2005.)

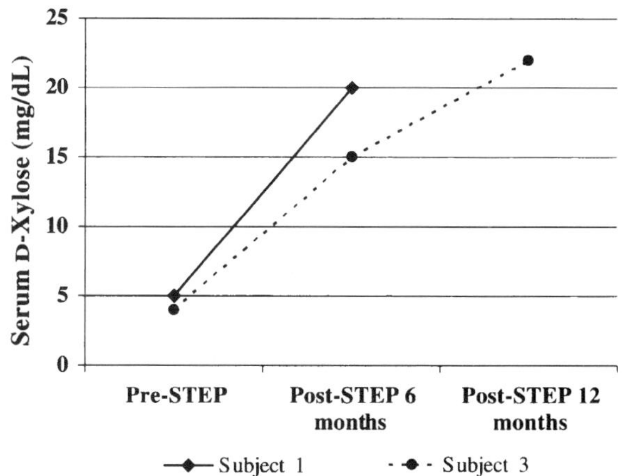

FIGURE 2.—Levels of serum D-xylose pre-STEP and post-STEP. In 2 of the 3 subjects with postoperative short-term nutritional data, levels of D-xylose were abnormally low before STEP procedure. After STEP, both subjects demonstrated a substantial increase to normal levels of D-xylose. D-Xylose is a validated marker for small intestinal mucosal surface area and carbohydrate absorptive capacity. (Courtesy of Javid PJ, Kim HB, Duggan CP, et al: Serial transverse enteroplasty is associated with successful short-term outcomes in infants with short bowel syndrome. *J Pediatr Surg* 40:1019-1024, 2005.)

rhosis before operation, underwent successful liver-small bowel transplantation 8 months after intestinal lengthening.

Conclusion.—The STEP procedure is a simple bowel-lengthening procedure with promising early surgical and nutritional outcomes. Further data from a multicenter registry are needed to demonstrate its long-term efficacy.

▶ STEP is an exciting new operation that has been developed for lengthening the small intestine in patients with short bowel syndrome. This operation takes short, dilated dysmotile bowel and both decreases lumen size for more efficient peristalsis and lengthens the bowel for greater fluid and nutrient absorption. For practitioners familiar with the older Bianchi gut-lengthening technique, the STEP procedure seems simple but elegant. Certainly the potential for complications after the STEP operation and the simplicity of the operation itself advocate for the use of the STEP in preference to the Bianchi technique. However, as with any procedure, the appropriate indications for the operation are important in determining how successful the outcomes will be. This certainly is true for the STEP operation. The authors in this article report excellent short-term success with the STEP operation. It seems that patient selection is important in the successful outcome of this procedure. For example, it is important that the patient have a potential for adequate postoperative motility.

It is possible that with time, continued dilatation of the bowel can diminish peristaltic effectiveness and lead to recurrent dysfunctional motility in these patients. Perhaps a second STEP procedure can be performed in these patients or as patients become older and larger they may be a more suitable candidate for small bowel transplantation. In summary, the STEP operation appears to be a superior procedure when compared with the Bianchi gut-lengthening technique.

K. E. Georgeson, MD

A Pilot Study of the Use of Epidermal Growth Factor in Pediatric Short Bowel Syndrome

Sigalet DL, Martin GR, Butzner JD, et al (Univ of Calgary, Alta, Canada)
J Pediatr Surg 40:763-768, 2005 10–24

Background.—This study examined the effects of enterally administered epidermal growth factor (EGF) on nutrient absorption and tolerance of enteral feeds in pediatric patients with short bowel syndrome (SBS).

Methods.—Patients identified with severe SBS (<25% bowel length predicted for age) were prospectively enrolled in treatment using human recombinant EGF (1-53); 100 μg/kg per day given mixed with enteral feeds and patients were treated for 6 weeks. End points followed were patient weight, tolerance of enteral feeds, nutrient absorption, and intestinal permeability as determined using carbohydrate probes and hematologic values for liver function parameters.

Results.—Five patients were treated with EGF; all showed a significant improvement in carbohydrate absorption (3-0 methylglucose): absorption

24.7% ± 9.7% pretreatment vs 34.1% ± 13.8% posttreatment and improved tolerance of enteral feeds (enteral energy as % of total energy, 25% ± 28% pretreatment vs 36% ± 24% posttreatment; mean ± SD; $P < .05$ by Wilcoxon's signed rank test). Epidermal growth factor treatment was not associated with significant changes in intestinal permeability, the rate of weight gain, or liver function tests. During the treatment phase, no patients developed episodes of sepsis; however, within 2 weeks of discontinuation of EGF treatment, 3 patients developed septic episodes. No adverse effects of EGF administration were noted.

Conclusions.—These results suggest that enteral treatment with EGF in pediatric SBS improves nutrient absorption, increases tolerance with enteral feeds, and may improve the infection rate. Further studies exploring treatment strategies including the timing and duration of EGF administration are indicated.

► Pediatric SBS is an uncommon, but morbid and economically disastrous condition. Although there have been major improvements in outcome after small bowel transplantation, this therapy is expensive and morbid. The use of EGF as a therapeutic aid for increasing absorptive intestinal surface area has been widely documented in animal models, but not in humans. This report of the successful use of EGF in improving patient tolerance for enteral feeds is important. The authors indicated that it may be necessary to continue therapy to retain the benefits obtained from the primary use of EGF in SBS patients. Obviously, this study needs to be broadened and carried out over a much longer period. The early positive results may beckon a new era in the management of SBS, especially for pediatric patients.

K. E. Georgeson, MD

Surgical Management of Bile Duct Injuries Sustained During Laparoscopic Cholecystectomy: Perioperative Results in 200 Patients

Sicklick JK, Camp MS, Lillemoe KD, et al (Johns Hopkins Med Insts, Baltimore, Md; Indiana Univ, Indianapolis)

Ann Surg 241:786-795, 2005 10–25

Objective.—A single institution retrospective analysis of 200 patients with major bile duct injuries was completed. Three patients died without surgery due to uncontrolled sepsis. One hundred seventy-five patients underwent surgical repair, with a 1.7% postoperative mortality and a complication rate of 42.9%.

Summary Background Data.—The widespread application of laparoscopic cholecystectomy (LC) has led to a rise in the incidence of major bile duct injuries (BDI). Despite the frequency of these injuries and their complex management, the published literature contains few substantial reports regarding the perioperative management of BDI.

Methods.—From January 1990 to April 2003, a prospective database of all patients with a BDI following LC was maintained. Patients' charts were retrospectively reviewed to analyze perioperative surgical management.

Results.—Over 13 years, 200 patients were treated for a major BDI following LC. Patient demographics were notable for 150 women (75%) with a mean age of 45.5 years (median 44 years). One hundred eighty-eight sustained their BDI at an outside hospital. The mean interval from the time of BDI to referral was 29.1 weeks (median 3 weeks). One hundred nine patients (58%) were referred within 1 month of their injury for acute complications including bile leak, biloma, or jaundice. Twenty-five patients did not undergo a surgical repair at our institution. Three patients (1.5%) died after delayed referral before an attempt at repair due to uncontrolled sepsis. Twenty-two patients, having intact biliary-enteric continuity, underwent successful balloon dilatation of an anastomotic stricture. A total of 175 patients underwent definitive biliary reconstruction, including 172 hepaticojejunostomies (98%) and 3 end-to-end repairs. There were 3 deaths in the postoperative period (1.7%). Seventy-five patients (42.9%) sustained at least 1 postoperative complication. The most common complications were wound infection (8%), cholangitis (5.7%), and intraabdominal abscess/biloma (2.9%). Minor biliary stent complications occurred in 5.7% of patients. Early postoperative cholangiography revealed an anastomotic leak in 4.6% of patients and extravasation at the liver dome-stent exit site in 10.3% of patients. Postoperative interventions included percutaneous abscess drainage in 9 patients (5.1%) and new percutaneous transhepatic cholangiography and stent placement in 4 patients (2.3%). No patient required reoperation in the postoperative period. The mean postoperative length of stay was 9.5 days (median 9 days). The timing of operation (early, intermediate, delayed), presenting symptoms, and history of prior repair did not affect the incidence of the most common perioperative complications or length of postoperative hospital stay.

Conclusions.—This series represents the largest single institution experience reporting the perioperative management of BDI following LC. Although perioperative complications are frequent, nearly all can be managed nonoperatively. Early referral to a tertiary care center with experienced hepatobiliary surgeons and skilled interventional radiologists would appear to be necessary to assure optimal results.

► These authors from the Johns Hopkins Medical Institution report the largest single institutional series for perioperative management of BDIs after LC. In the highly litigious society in which we live, the general surgeon in practice will commonly have a low threshold to refer these advanced injuries to a tertiary care center allowing the experienced, interventional radiologist and hepatobiliary surgeons to provide optimal outcomes. The authors emphasize that although perioperative complications are frequent in the management of these BDIs, most are managed nonoperatively. The emphasis in this study is the provision for the growing influence supporting the importance of proper early biliary reconstruction at a hepatobiliary center for these life-threatening complications.

K. I. Bland, MD

Effect of Estrogen Therapy on Gallbladder Disease

Cirillo DJ, Wallace RB, Rodabough RJ (Univ of Iowa, Iowa City; Fred Hutchinson Cancer Research Ctr, Seattle; Northwestern Univ, Chicago; et al)
JAMA 293:330-339, 2005 10–26

Context.—Estrogen therapy is thought to promote gallstone formation and cholecystitis but most data derive from observational studies rather than randomized trials.

Objective.—To determine the effect of estrogen therapy in healthy postmenopausal women on gallbladder disease outcomes.

Design, Setting, and Participants.—Two randomized, double-blind, placebo-controlled trials conducted at 40 US clinical centers. The volunteer sample was 22,579 community-dwelling women aged 50 to 79 years without prior cholecystectomy.

Intervention.—Women with hysterectomy were randomized to 0.625 mg/d of conjugated equine estrogens (CEE) or placebo (n = 8376). Women without hysterectomy were randomized to estrogen plus progestin (E + P), given as CEE plus 2.5 mg/d of medroxyprogesterone acetate (n = 14,203).

Main Outcome Measures.—Participants reported hospitalizations for gallbladder diseases and gallbladder-related procedures, with events ascertained through medical record review. Cox proportional hazards regression was used to assess hazard ratios (HRs) and 95% confidence intervals (CIs) using intention-to-treat and time-to-event methods.

Results.—The CEE and the E + P groups were similar to their respective placebo groups at baseline. The mean follow-up times were 7.1 years and 5.6 years for the CEE and the E + P trials, respectively. The annual incidence rate for any gallbladder event was 78 events per 10,000 person-years for the CEE group (vs 47/10,000 person-years for placebo) and 55 per 10,000 person-years for E + P (vs 35/10,000 person-years for placebo). Both trials showed greater risk of any gallbladder disease or surgery with estrogen (CEE: HR, 1.67; 95% CI, 1.35-2.06; E + P: HR, 1.59; 95% CI, 1.28-1.97). Both trials indicated a higher risk for cholecystitis (CEE: HR, 1.80; 95% CI, 1.42-2.28; E + P: HR, 1.54; 95% CI 1.22-1.94); and for cholelithiasis (CEE: HR, 1.86; 95% CI, 1.48-2.35; E + P: HR, 1.68; 95% CI, 1.34-2.11) for estrogen users. Also, women undergoing estrogen therapy were more likely to receive cholecystectomy (CEE: HR, 1.93; 95% CI, 1.52-2.44; E + P: HR, 1.67; 95% CI, 1.32-2.11), but not other biliary tract surgery (CEE: HR, 1.18; 95% CI, 0.68-2.04; E + P: HR, 1.49; 95% CI, 0.78-2.84).

Conclusions.—These data suggest an increase in risk of biliary tract disease among postmenopausal women using estrogen therapy. The morbidity and cost associated with these outcomes may need to be considered in decisions regarding the use of estrogen therapy.

▶ Cirillo et al determined the effect of estrogen therapy in healthy, postmenopausal women on gallbladder disease outcomes. This is the largest such trial to date, as this information is based on portions of the Women Health Initiative Clinical Trials, inclusive of a volunteer sample of 22,579 community-dwelling women, age 50 to 79 years, without prior cholecystectomy. These findings demonstrate for the first time in a randomized, double-blind study that these otherwise healthy postmenopausal women have a substantial increase in the risk of adverse biliary tract outcomes using either estrogen alone or a combination of estrogen plus progesterone (progestin).

Of importance to the general surgeon is the fact that this large randomized trial shows an important increase in the necessity of surgical procedures among women randomly assigned for either oral single agent equine estrogen or the combination of estrogen and progesterone. The estimate of cumulative risk for any gallbladder outcome in estrogen-alone or the combination estrogen trial was confirmed. Both the frequency of disease and necessary gallbladder procedure are enhanced statistically as a consequence of these additive estrogens versus placebo. Thus, the general surgeon must be aware of this frequency when considering causes of biliary tract disease and abdominal pain in the emergency evaluation of patients who use those drugs for hormonal replacement therapy.

K. I. Bland, MD

Hepatic Resection-Related Hypophosphatemia Is of Renal Origin as Manifested by Isolated Hyperphosphaturia

Salem RR, Tray K (Yale Univ, New Haven, Conn; Hartford Hosp, Conn)

Ann Surg 241:343-348, 2005 10–27

Objective.—The objective of this study was to elucidate and define the pathophysiological mechanism(s) responsible for the clinically relevant phenomenon of posthepatic resection hypophosphatemia.

Summary Background Data.—Although biochemically significant hypophosphatemia has been described after major hepatic resection, no mechanism or validated scientific explanation exists. The phenomenon is of considerable clinical relevance because numerous patients, after hepatic resection, develop significant hypophosphatemia requiring large doses of phosphate replacement to maintain metabolic homeostasis. This event has previously been empirically ascribed to amplified phosphate utilization of regenerating hepatocytes, although no rigorous data attest to this postulate. Recent data identifying a novel mechanism of phosphaturia in X-linked hypophosphatemic rickets, autosomal-dominant hypophosphatemic rickets, and oncogenic osteomalacia demonstrate that elevated levels of novel circulating phosphaturic factors such as fibroblast growth factor 23 (FGF-23) and PHEX are responsible for phosphate wasting. We hypothesize that posthepatectomy hypophosphatemia reflects a derangement of normal hepatorenal messaging and is the result of a disruption of renal phosphate handling consequent on aberrations in the metabolism of an as yet unrecognized chemical messenger(s) responsible for tubular phosphate homeostasis. This postulate has not previously been proposed or examined.

Methods.—Twenty patients undergoing hepatic resection were studied prospectively with respect to serum phosphate, phosphate requirements, as well as renal phosphate handling. Fractional excretion of phosphate was calculated on a daily basis. To confirm the relationship between phosphate loss and a circulating renal-targeted messenger, the plasma levels of the circulating phosphaturic factor FGF-23 were measured using a c-terminal assay both pre- and postoperatively.

Results.—All patients developed hypophosphatemia with a nadir on postoperative day 2 (average drop of 47% despite phosphate administration). This phenomenon was associated with hyperphosphaturia (mean ± standard error) with high fractional excretion of phosphate. A consistent change in FGF-23 was not identified.

Conclusion.—Hypophosphatemia after hepatic resection is a frequent occurrence. Transient isolated hyperphosphaturia and not increased phosphate utilization is the predominant cause of this phenomenon, although the identity of the agent involved remains to be identified.

► This nonrandomized prospective study sought to evaluate a well-described fact initially presented by Keushkerian and Wade in *Current Surgery* titled, "Hyphophosphatemia After Major Hepatic Resection" in 1984. This 20-year-old finding has perplexed surgeons for some time. After major trauma or major hepatic resection, it is well-known that serum phosphate levels often significantly decrease, but the etiology of this phenomenon has never been clearly described. This untreated hypophosphatemia can lead to severe consequences for patients postoperatively. The authors of the present study observed some 20 patients undergoing major hepatic resections by first analyzing serum phosphate levels and urine excretion of phosphate and then measuring FGF-23 in 4 patients, which is thought to related to potential phosphate wasting. Each of these patients underwent major resections requiring exogenous IV phosphate administration ranging from 15 to 321 mmol during their postoperative period. These patients as a group had a mean fractional phosphate excretion of 1.86 mg/dL on day 2 and 2.8 mg/dL on day 4. The lowest serum phosphate level appeared to be on postoperative day 2 for these patients, and the average drop in serum phosphate levels was 45%, despite IV administration of phosphate. The unique finding in this study was an association between the nadir of serum phosphate level and the peak of renal hyperphosphaturia, which appeared to correlate very much with the drop in the serum phosphate level. At the same time that a maximum decrease in the serum phosphate level occurred, these patients demonstrated a maximum increase in the renal fractional excretion of phosphate; that is, the mean fractional excretion at postoperative day 2 was a high of 45% that dropped to a near postoperative low of 13% on day 4. This correlated closely with the decrease in the serum phosphate level. Not well understood and although not completely explained in this study, the well-described, fairly massive drop in serum phosphate level correlates with a concomitant severe rise in the level of renal phosphate excreted, thus creating a loss of phosphate that is increased by some 50% during the postoperative period. Now, for the first time, this fact explains the decrease in phosphate and serum phosphate levels; however, the factors that produce this phenomenon are still not clearly understood. The study did look at FGF-23 levels in patients before they underwent resection, but no consistent change was found when this marker was measured.

Finally, the authors are to be commended for furthering our understanding of this well-described but often mysterious hepatorenal syndrome by linking damage or injury to the liver with demonstrable renal physiologic effects. Obviously, this study will provide the groundwork for other studies that should identify the serum factors that lead to this massive drop in phosphate levels and the massive increase in phosphate excretion in the kidney.

S. M. Vickers, MD

H-Graft Portacaval Shunts Versus TIPS: Ten-Year Follow-up of a Randomized Trial With Comparison to Predicted Survivals

Rosemurgy AS, Bloomston M, Clark WC, et al (Univ of South Florida, Tampa)
Ann Surg 241:238-246, 2005 10–28

Objective.—To report long-term outcome of patients undergoing prosthetic 8-mm H-graft portacaval shunts (HGPCS) or TIPS and to compare actual with predicted survival data.

Methods.—A randomized trial comparing TIPS to HGPCS for bleeding varices began in 1993. Predicted survival was determined using MELD (Model for End-stage Liver Disease).

Results.—Patients undergoing TIPS (N = 66) or HGPCS (N = 66) were very similar by Child's class and MELD scores and predicted survival. After TIPS (P = 0.01) and HGPCS (P = 0.001), actual survival was superior to predicted survival. Through 24 months, actual survival after HGPCS was superior to actual survival after TIPS (P = 0.04). Compared with TIPS, survival was superior after HGPCS for patients of Child's class A and B (P = 0.07) and with MELD scores less than 13 (P = 0.04) with follow-up at 5 to 10 years. Shunt failure was less following HGPCS ($P < 0.01$).

Conclusions.—Predicted survival data for patients undergoing TIPS or HGPCS confirms an unbiased randomization. Actual survival following TIPS or HGPCS was superior to predicted survival. Shunt failure favored HGPCS, as did survival after shunting, particularly for the first few years after shunting and for patients of Child's class A or B or with MELD scores less than 13. This trial irrefutably establishes a role for surgical shunting, particularly HGPCS.

► Rosemurgy et al from the University of South Florida, Tampa, report the long-term outcomes of patients undergoing prosthetic 8-mm HGCPS or TIPS (transjugular intrahepatic portasystemic stent shunt). The authors have compared actual and predicted survival data and confirm that after TIPS (*P* = .01) and HGPCS (*P* = .001) actual survival was superior to predicted survival; through 24 months, HGPCS was superior to TIPS (*P* = .04) for actual survival. The authors note that the actual survival after either procedure is superior to the predicted survival, thus confirming an unbiased randomization in the study. It would appear that this trial irrefutably establishes a role for shunting with a superiority of the HGPCS for Child's A&B disease when compared with the TIPS procedure. The bias would have to be for TIPS, however, for the carefully selected patient rapidly in need of portal decompression, who is an unacceptable operative candidate.

As is indicated in the discussion of this article by Rosemurgy et al, this trial continues to have an open answer for who should undergo shunting. These data in this randomized study suggest that those patients with Child's Class A or B disease or with MELD (model for end-stage liver disease) scores less than 14, that small diameter prosthetic HGPCS should be utilized. However, when MELD scores are more than 14, and in whom hepatic transplantation is not probable or imminent, the HGPCS may palliate portal hypertension to conserve resources.[1] However, for MELD scores lower than 14 and in whom hepatic transplantation is imminent, TIPS should be strongly considered.

K. I. Bland, MD

Reference

1. Rosemurgy AS, Zervos EE, Bloomston M, et al: Post-shunt resource consumption favors small-diameter prosthetic H-graft portacaval shunt over TIPS for patients with poor hepatic reserve. *Ann Surg* 237:820-827, 2003.

Laparoscopic Curative Resection of Pheochromocytomas

Kercher KW, Novitsky YW, Park A, et al (Carolinas Med Ctr, Charlotte, NC; Univ of Maryland, Baltimore; Univ of Massachusetts, Worcester; et al)
Ann Surg 241:919-928, 2005 10–29

Purpose.—Pheochromocytomas are relatively uncommon tumors whose operative resection has clear medical and technical challenges. While the safety and efficacy of laparoscopic adrenalectomy are relatively well documented, few studies with extended follow-up have been conducted to measure the success of the procedure for the most challenging of the adrenal tumors. In addition, several reports question the applicability of a minimally invasive approach for sizeable pheochromocytomas. The purpose of our investigation was to assess the outcomes of laparoscopic adrenalectomy for pheochromocytomas in the largest study to date when performed by experienced laparoscopic surgeons.

Methods.—All pheochromocytomas removed by the authors from January 1995 to October 2004 were reviewed under an Institutional Review Board approved protocol. Eighty-five percent were documented in a prospective fashion.

Results.—Eighty consecutive patients underwent laparoscopic resection of 81 pheochromocytomas. Seventy-nine were found in the adrenal (42 left, 35 right, 1 bilateral); 2 were extra-adrenal paragangliomas. Eight patients had multiple endocrine neoplasia syndrome. Two lesions were malignant. There were 48 females and 32 males with a mean age of 45 years (range, 15-79 years). Mean tumor size was 5.0 cm (range, 2-12.1 cm); 41 of these lesions were 5 cm in size or larger. Average operative time and blood loss were 169 minutes (range, 69-375 minutes) and 97 mL (range, 20-500 mL), respectively. Intraoperative hypertension (systolic blood pressure, >170 mm Hg) was reported in 53% of patients and hypotension (systolic blood pressure, <90 mm Hg) in 28% of patients. There were no conversions to open surgery. Mean length of stay was 2.3 days (range, 1-10 days). There were 6 perioperative morbidities (7.5%) and no mortalities. No patient required a blood transfusion. No recurrence of endocrinopathy has been documented at a mean follow-up of 21.4 months.

Conclusion.—Laparoscopic resection of pheochromocytomas, including large lesions, can be accomplished safely by experienced surgeons. A short hospital stay with minimal operative morbidity and eradication of endocrinopathy support the minimally invasive approach for adrenalectomy in the setting of pheochromocytoma.

▶ The first laparoscopic approach for the management of pheochromocytoma occurred in 1992. Subsequently, this approach is becoming standard in most selective institutions for the management of functional and nonfunctional adrenal tumors. Kercher et al of the Carolinas Medical Center discuss the management of the relatively uncommon pheochromocytoma and the associated operative challenges related to its functional biochemical secreatogues. The authors used the procedure for right- and left-sided tumors, with an overall mean size of 4.7 ± 1.5 cm to 5.7 ± 2.1 cm.

This series of 80 consecutive, prospective, laparoscopically resected patients (n = 81 tumors) confirm that 79 were evident in the adrenal; 2 were extra-adrenal paragangliomas. There were no requirements for conversions to open procedures and the mean hospital stay of 2.3 days is commendable. The low morbidity (7.5%) and the absent mortality are laudable.

This article depicts the significant progress made in flexible endoscopic and laparoscopic approaches and the diminishing need for open approach in the management of functional adrenal tumors.

K. I. Bland, MD

Multivariate Analysis of Technical Variables in Pancreaticoduodenectomy: The Effect of Pylorus Preservation and Retromesenteric Jejunal Position on Early Outcome

Butler TJ, Vair DB, Colohan S, et al (Dalhousie Univ, Halifax, Nova Scotia, Canada; Univ of Western Ontario, London, Canada)

Can J Surg 47:333-337, 2004 10–30

Background.—To evaluate the effect of technical modifications to pancreaticoduodenectomy (PD) on postoperative outcome, we established a register of all patients undergoing PD at Victoria General Hospital (Queen Elizabeth II Health Sciences Centre), a tertiary care, university-affiliated hospital.

Patients and Method.—Data from 78 consecutive patients who underwent PD from January 1998 through November 2000 were collected for univariate and multivariate analyses of clinical and technical factors on early outcome after PD, including duration of gastric stasis, development of complications and length of hospital stay.

Results.—Two patients (2.6%) died; complications were recorded in 43 (55%). Upon univariate analysis, 3 factors (a diagnosis of chronic pancreatitis, pylorus preservation, and route of the jejunal limb) significantly affected duration of gastric stasis; but on multivariate analysis, only pylorus preservation and jejunal-limb route remained significant. Retromesenteric jejunal-limb placement was associated with longer periods of gastric stasis (mean 11.9 d, standard deviation [SD] 8.1 d) than the antemesenteric (retrocolic) route (mean 7.2, SD 3.6 d; $p < 0.05$); likewise pyloric preservation (mean gastric stasis 10.4 d, SD 5.9 d) compared with resection of the pylorus (mean 7.0 d, SD 3.2 d; $p < 0.05$). Pancreatic leaks occurred in 18% of retromesenteric and 8% of antemesenteric reconstructions ($p = 0.3$). Fewer patients with mucomucosal pancreaticojejunostomy suffered complications than those with invaginated anastomoses, but their hospital stays were similar in length.

Conclusion.—Route of the jejunal efferent limb and preservation of the pylorus are independent technical variables affecting early outcome after PD.

► This study addresses a common problem in pancreatic surgery. In the setting of pylorus PD, delayed gastric emptying remains a challenging complication. This also holds for those patients who have classic PDs. This study evaluated the effect of Roux-en-Y limb positioning on delayed gastric emptying. There remains a significant but small group of surgeons who place the Roux-en-Y limb under the mesenteric vessels; that is, the Roux-en-Y limb is placed in the native duodenal retromesenteric bed and then brought up to perform the anastomosis. Others routinely use a retrocolic but antimesenteric approach for the placement of this limb. Finally, some use a totally anticolic positioning of this limb. The authors conclude that delayed gastric emptying was significantly increased in those patients who had the limb placed in the retromesenteric position or in the native duodenum channel. Their findings support the conclusion that delayed gastric emptying remains a significant challenge in the management of these patients but also that limb placement may play some role in the risk as well as the frequency of this common complication. Therefore, the authors urge, and I would be in agreement, that the retromesenteric channel should not be used as a placement for this limb and can increase the risk of delayed gastric emptying.

S. M. Vickers, MD

Surgical Treatment for Anomalous Arrangement of the Pancreaticobiliary Duct With Nondilatation of the Common Bile Duct

Iwai N, Fumino S, Tsuda T, et al (Kyoto Prefectural Univ of Medicine, Japan)
J Pediatr Surg 39:1794-1796, 2004 10–31

Background/Purpose.—For anomalous arrangement of the pancreaticobiliary duct (AAPBD) with nondilatation of the common bile duct (CBD), the optimal surgical procedure remains controversial. The authors investigated which procedure would be most effective for AAPBD with nondilatation of the CBD.

Methods.—The authors encountered 60 children with AAPBD in our institution between 1979 and 2002. Six of the 60 were classified as the nondilated type (CBD diameter; less than 8 mm), whereas the other 54 were classified as the dilated type (CBD diameter; more than 9 mm). Amylase levels in serum, CBD, and gallbladder were examined. Cellular activity of the resected gallbladder was examined for the incidence of hyperplasia and Ki-67 labeling index (Ki-67 LI).

Results.—The amylase level in the nondilated type was elevated as in the dilated type. Epithelial hyperplasia of the gallbladder was present in 4 of the 6 with the nondilated type (67%). 10 of the 20 with the dilated type (50%), and none of the 6 controls (0%). The Ki-67 LI of the dilated type was significantly higher than that of control.

Conclusions.—A free reflux of pancreatic juice into the biliary system was found regardless of dilatation, and cellular proliferative activity of the gallbladder mucosa was increased in both the nondilated and dilated type. Therefore, excision of the extrahepatic bile duct including cholecystectomy is recommended for AAPBD with nondilatation of the CBD.

► These authors sought to answer the question of what is the appropriate treatment for patients who have an anomalous connection between their pancreatic duct and their CBD in the face of a nondilated CBD. In most cases, patients who have choledochal cysts in AAPBD often receive excision of the extrahepatic biliary tree because of the risk of gallbladder cancer. This type of cancer is believed to be due to an uncontrolled reflux of pancreatic enzymes within the biliary tree creating a carcinogenic environment. This study nicely documents the challenge in patients (primarily pediatric but applicable to adults as well) who are seen with an anomalous arrangement; that is, the pancreatic duct connects to the bile duct in a much higher position than at the ampulla, which allows an uncontrolled reflux of pancreatic juices into the biliary tree. The controversy remains, then, about how patients should be treated if they do not have a dilated CBD. In this study, 6 patients with nondilated CBDs of the 60 who had anomalous pancreaticobiliary duct connections were also at risk of potential gallbladder cancer or cholangiocarcinoma. The study demonstrated that the level of Ki-67, which is a proliferation marker, appeared to be significantly elevated in the epithelial mucosal cells in 67% of patients with nondilated biliary ducts. It also correlated with an increased serum amylase level in this group of patients, which points to concurrent biliary-induced pancreatitis. This increased proliferation probably increased the risk of carcinogenesis in the biliary tree (ie, the CBD and the gallbladder). Thus, AAPBD appears to cause a brief reflux of bile into the pancreatic duct as well as pancreatic juice within the biliary tree and puts these patients, as expected, at an increased risk of carcinogenesis due to hyperproliferation of cholangeocytes both in the biliary tree as well as in the gallbladder. Thus, the recommendation, appropriately so, is that these young patients should also have cholecystectomy and excision of the extrahepatic biliary tree.

S. M. Vickers, MD

Acute Pancreatitis Induces FasL Gene Expression and Apoptosis in the Liver

Gallagher SF, Yang J, Baksh K, et al (James A Haley Veterans Affairs Med Ctr, Tampa, Fla; Univ of South Florida, Tampa)

J Surg Res 122:201-209, 2004 10–32

Background.—Liver injury is an important prognostic indicator in acute pancreatitis. We previously demonstrated that Kupffer cell-derived cytokines mediate liver injury. In this work, we sought to characterize the role of Fas Ligand (FasL) in liver injury during acute pancreatitis.

Methods.—Acute pancreatitis was induced in mice using cerulein; serum FasL, AST, ALT, liver FasL, p38-MAPK, and caspase-3 were measured. FasL mRNA and protein and its receptor (Fas) were determined in rat Kupffer cells treated with elastase (1 U/ml) to mimic acute pancreatitis. Apoptosis was measured by flow cytometry.

Results.—Cerulein-induced pancreatitis increased serum AST, ALT, and FasL and up-regulated liver FasL (1315 ± 111 versus 310 ± 164 pg/ml, P = 0.002 versus sham), while inducing p38-MAPK phosphorylation ($P < 0.01$ versus sham) and cleavage of caspase-3 ($P < 0.04$ versus sham); all were attenuated by pretreatment with the Kupffer cell inhibitor, gadolinium (all $P <$ 0.003). In vitro, elastase induced a time-dependent increase in Kupffer cell FasL protein (FasL = 404 ± 94 versus 170 ± 40, P = 0.02, versus control), a 100-fold increase in FasL mRNA, and up-regulated Fas (FasL receptor). Gadolinium significantly attenuated the elastase-induced increase in FasL and FasL mRNA (FasL = 230 ± 20 versus 404 ± 94, P = 0.01, versus elastase) but had little effect on Fas. Additionally, elastase-primed Kupffer cell media induced apoptosis in hepatocytes (29 ± 1 versus 16% ± 1%; versus control, $P < 0.001$).

Conclusions.—Acute pancreatitis induces liver injury and hepatocyte death while up-regulating FasL, p38-MAPK, and caspase-3. Fas is up-regulated within Kupffer cells, suggesting that FasL may autoregulate its production by inducing its originator-cell death. The ability to manipulate interactions between Kupffer cells and hepatocytes may have important therapeutic implications.

► This article has used a well-established liver injury model of cerulein-induced acute pancreatitis. The authors have focused on the potential control and modulation of macrophages, specifically Kupffer cells, which reside in the liver, and their critical role in liver injury that is associated with acute pancreatitis. The authors have provided novel information about levels of FasL, standard liver enzymes, and the Fas death receptor.

This study nicely demonstrates that a significant correlation may exist between the expression of FasL and the creation of an autocrine effect due to upregulation of FasL in stable expression of the Fas death receptor. This upregulation of FasL may provide a means of creating a liver injury in the setting of acute pancreatitis. The article also demonstrates potential means of mediating this cell interaction by the in vitro and in vivo use of gadolinium, which is a Kupffer cell inhibitor. Gadolinium is a standard infusion used in MRI evaluation and can provide a chemotherapeutic effect in certain tumor models. It may also have a regulatory effect in preventing end organ injury and acute pancreatitis by downregulating FasL and preventing its activation of the Fas death receptor.

Thus, this article nicely demonstrates a potential basis for multiple organ failure seen in acute pancreatitis through upregulation of a death receptor ligand, which may allow for increased cell death within the liver as well as associated pancreatitis.

S. M. Vickers, MD

A Prospective Comparison of the Yield of EUS in Primary vs Recurrent Idiopathic Acute Pancreatitis

Yusoff IF, Raymond G, Sahai AV (Hopital Saint Luc, Montreal; Univ of Western Australia, Perth)

Gastrointest Endosc 60:673-678, 2004 10–33

Background.—It is uncertain whether EUS should be performed after a single episode of idiopathic pancreatitis vs. recurrent episodes or if clinical factors can predict positive EUS findings.

Methods.—Consecutive patients with a single episode of idiopathic pancreatitis or with recurrent episodes underwent EUS (with analysis of bile for bilirubinate and cholesterol crystals, when possible). The diagnostic yield was compared for patients with a single episode of idiopathic pancreatitis and recurrent episodes (stratified by cholecystectomy status). Predictors of positive EUS findings were sought. EUS was considered "positive" if it identified any possible cause of pancreatitis other than chronic pancreatitis.

Results.—A total of 370 patients were studied (246 no-cholecystectomy group [134 single episode of idiopathic pancreatitis, 112 recurrent episodes] and 124 post-cholecystectomy group [67 single episode of idiopathic pancreatitis, 57 recurrent episodes]). Overall, EUS yielded a positive finding in 29.2%. For patients in the no-cholecystectomy group, positive EUS findings were not significantly more frequent in those with a single episode of idiopathic pancreatitis vs. those with recurrent episodes (31.3% vs. 32.1%; p = 0.89). In the post-cholecystectomy group, the yield was not significantly different for single episode of idiopathic pancreatitis (29.9%) vs. recurrent episodes (17.5%) (p = 0.15). Chronic pancreatitis was the only abnormality identified in 30.9% of patients in the no-cholecystectomy group vs. 26.6% of those in the post-cholecystectomy group (p = 0.24). It was the most common abnormality found in all 4 subgroups (range 16.4%-42.0%) and was approximately twice as frequent in patients with recurrent episodes vs. a single episode of idiopathic pancreatitis (no-cholecystectomy: 42.0% vs. 21.6%, p = 0.0008; post-cholecystectomy: 38.6% vs. 16.4%, p = 0.008). Analysis of bile revealed crystals in 38/80 (47.5%) patients in whom it could be performed. Patients with positive EUS findings tended to be older.

Conclusions.—In patients with idiopathic pancreatitis, the yield of EUS is not significantly different after an initial attack or after recurrent attacks. Therefore, it is reasonable to perform EUS after an initial attack of idiopathic acute pancreatitis, especially in older patients.

▶ Understanding the cause of pancreatitis continues to be a challenge in patients who do not have evidence of gallstones or a significant history of alcohol disease. After individuals have had these 2 causes excluded, as well as hypertriglyceridemia and certain drugs such as azathioprine, patients are often categorized with the diagnosis of idiopathic acute pancreatitis. This usually occurs in 10% to 30% of all patients, who are seen and then left with this diagnosis of no clear etiology for their attack of pancreatitis. The standard evaluation often includes an ERCP with aspiration for biliary sludge or crystals. The ERCP may often entail sphincter of Oddi measurements in select cases to help determine the cause of the pancreatitis. The advent of EUS has provided a new opportunity to determine whether this examination may provide more insight into the diagnosis of patients who are labeled with idiopathic pancreatitis. In this study, patients with this diagnosis were assessed, and the question of whether value was gained in proceeding with an EUS for a patient who had acute pancreatitis without a perceived or clear diagnosis was determined. The study demonstrated uniquely that about one third (29.2%) of patients who did not have a diagnosis of acute pancreatitis were found to have positive results from the EUS test, which provided significant information for the management, prognosis, and outcome of acute pancreatitis in these patients. For patients, particularly elderly patients, who have the diagnosis of idiopathic acute pancreatitis, these findings demonstrate that EUS could potentially play a significant role in the management of their disease, not only by excluding the possibility of a small periampullary malignancy but also by providing a more sensitive insight into the biliary tree contents, such as adenomas, sludge, or biliary crystal concentration. The reported risk of pancreatitis from EUS, which includes a biopsy, in most series is less than 2% and, therefore, is a further argument for the use of this test in patients who have idiopathic acute pancreatitis.

S. M. Vickers, MD

A Comparison of the Ranson, Glasgow, and APACHE II Scoring Systems to a Multiple Organ System Score in Predicting Patient Outcome in Pancreatitis

Taylor SL, Morgan DL, Denson KD, et al (Univ of Oklahoma, Oklahoma City)
Am J Surg 189:219-222, 2005 10–34

Background.—Systems for evaluating acute pancreatitis are useful in hospitalized patients. Traditional systems of evaluation are well established but might be outdated. We propose a Multiple Organ System Score (MOSS) containing data that are more consistently collected and which are accurate in predicting patient outcome.

Methods.—A retrospective chart review of 49 patients was completed. We determined if the physician obtained all of the variables necessary to calculate Ranson, Glasgow, or APACHE II scores, if these scores were predictive of patient outcome in the form of length of hospital stay (LOS), and if new, more frequently evaluated variables could be used.

Results.—None of the patients could be assigned complete scores. According to Spearman rank correlation, both Glasgow and MOSS showed correlation with patient outcome when APACHE II and Ranson did not.

Conclusions.—Although larger studies should be performed, the MOSS is useful in predicting outcomes of patients with acute pancreatitis.

► These authors retrospectively sought to evaluate 4 scoring systems of pancreatitis. The study included 49 patients who were admitted with the diagnosis of pancreatitis. Their outcomes were compared on the basis of the use of criteria for the APACHE II injury severity system, Ranson's criteria, and modified Glasgow criteria at 0 hours and at 48 hours. The novel system that was developed by the authors was called the MOSS. The 4 scoring systems were evaluated for their predictive value with regard to LOS and severity of illness for patients with acute pancreatitis. The authors' challenge is that the Glasgow score had more data collected for its determination than did the APACHE II and the Ranson system. The modified Glasgow and the MOSS appeared to have 98% to 100% of the patients who had fewer than 3 variables missing for the scoring scheme. However, these data are somewhat concerning in that only 2 patients required an ICU admission. Although the sensitivity for the MOSS was 86%, the specificity was quite low at 50%; its positive predictive value was only 61%, and its negative predictive value was 81%. This is a reasonable attempt in the determination of a new scoring system for pancreatitis, but it lacks both positive predictive value and significant specificity.

Finally, the study does propose a novel scoring system scale for pancreatitis. However, the critical issues are as follows: (1) only 2 patients required ICU admissions; thus, the severity of the conditions in the patients in this scoring scheme is low; (2) the majority of the values of the other scoring systems were not collected; (3) the lack of collected data severely limits a full evaluation of the scoring scheme in comparison with the other well-recognized pancreatitis scoring systems. To conclude that the MOSS provides a novel and superior evaluation of outcomes in pancreatitis is probably incorrect because the authors designed the study using patients in their institution; therefore, the study was designed on the data routinely collected in that single institution. Thus, the study, unfortunately, provides little evidence that the MOSS will provide greater insight than either Ranson or APACHE II in the determination of the outcomes of pancreatitis.

S. M. Vickers, MD

The Optimal Timing of Laparoscopic Cholecystectomy in Mild Gallstone Pancreatitis

Taylor E, Wong C (Kern Med Ctr, Bakersfield, Calif)

Am Surg 70:971-975, 2004 10–35

Introduction.—The optimal timing of laparoscopic cholecystectomy (LC) in patients with biliary pancreatitis is not standardized. Our objective was to determine if patients with mild gallstone pancreatitis (three or fewer Ranson's criteria) can safely proceed to LC as soon as serum amylase is decreasing and abdominal tenderness is improving. We reviewed the charts of all adults admitted to our institution with gallstone pancreatitis from January 1999 until June 2002 who had LC performed by either surgeon 1 (group 1) or surgeon 2 (group 2). Surgeon 1 preferred to delay surgery until normalization of amylase and complete resolution of abdominal tenderness, whereas surgeon 2 preferred to proceed to LC as soon as serum amylase was decreasing and abdominal tenderness was improving. The two groups were well matched for sex, age, Ranson's criteria, and percentage requiring endoscopic retrograde cholangiopancreatography. Average total hospital stay was 4.7 days in group 1 versus 3.5 days in group 2 ($P = 0.01$). There was no statistical difference in complication rate between the two groups (10% in group 1 vs 11% in group 2, $P = 0.12$). The data suggest that hospital stay can be shortened with no increased complication rate if patients with mild biliary pancreatitis proceed to LC as soon as serum amylase is decreasing and abdominal tenderness is improving.

► This study answers an age-old question: what should be the timing for LC in patients with gallstone pancreatitis? The authors wisely evaluated this question only in patients who had mild gallstone pancreatitis (often these patients are grouped and treated with those who have severe gallstone pancreatitis). Because of the definition used in this study for mild pancreatitis, the majority of these patients most likely did not have pancreatic necrosis. These patients also tended to have a limited amount of inflammation identified by a CT scan. Nearly 38,000 of 500,000 annual cholecystectomies are performed because of gallstone pancreatitis. This accounts for nearly 50% of all episodes of pancreatitis in America. These findings have significant implications for costs and are important because they enlighten us about what is safe, practical management for these patients. Although the patients were not randomly assigned to groups, the data help us to understand when patients with pancreatitis can be operated on. Thus, the information gained from this study, based simply on the criteria of decreasing amylase levels and improving abdominal pain, gives us a tremendous opportunity for decreasing the length of stay for patients with gallstone pancreatitis.

S. M. Vickers, MD

A National Comparison of Surgical Versus Percutaneous Drainage of Pancreatic Pseudocysts: 1997-2001

Morton JM, Brown A, Galanko JA, et al (Stanford School of Medicine, Calif; Univ of North Carolina, Chapel Hill)

J Gastrointest Surg 9:15-21, 2005 10–36

Introduction.—Case series results indicate that a surgical approach is superior to percutaneous drainage of pancreatic pseudocysts. To determine if this surgical advantage is persistent, national outcomes for both approaches were compared from 1997 through 2001. The National Inpatient Sample, a 20% sample of all nonfederal hospital discharges, was searched for patients who had a pancreatic pseudocyst diagnosis, an ICD-9 diagnosis code 577.2, and an ICD-9 procedure code of 52.01 for percutaneous drainage (PD) or 52.4 and 52.96 for the surgical approaches. Variables were compared by using either t test or χ^2 analysis. Confounding variables were controlled for by linear or logistic regression models. No clinically significant demographic, comorbidity, and disease-specific severity-of-illness differences existed between the two groups. Significant differences in complications, length of stay (15 ± 15 versus 21 ± 22 days, $P < 0.0001$), and inpatient mortality (5.9% versus 2.8%, $P < 0.0001$) favored the surgical approach. In addition, endoscopic retrograde cholangiopancreatography use had a protective effect on mortality (odds ratio, 0.7), whereas percutaneous drainage had an increased risk of mortality (odds ratio, 1.4). This population-based study suggests that surgical drainage of pancreatic pseudocysts, particularly when coupled with use of endoscopic retrograde cholangiopancreatography, leads to decreased complications, length of stay, and mortality in comparison with percutaneous drainage.

▶ This comparative study by experienced clinicians is important because of the study arms: PD is a newer technique that can be used earlier in pseudocyst evaluation than surgical drainage (SD) and may be used to supplant SD as a short-term solution. This study is retrospective but reviews a large number of patients (15,000) with pancreatic pseudocysts over 4 years. The advantages of a shorter length of stay and reduced morbidity and mortality rates associated with SD are clear. Endoscopic retrograde cholangiopancreatography plays a complimentary role with SD in reducing the length of stay and mortality rate; its place otherwise as a separate definitive option for pseudocyst drainage is dependent on anatomy and specialized expertise, which markedly limit its usefulness.

The authors conclude by proposing certain treatment strategies: (1) observation of small cysts is safe, (2) endoscopic retrograde cholangiopancreatography can predict treatment success, does not exacerbate existing pancreatitis, and has both diagnostic and therapeutic use, and (3) SD should be used more frequently as a safe and enduring treatment modality. The authors suggest that PD might better be used as a bridge procedure for patients who have an infected pseudocyst, are malnourished, or are a poor surgical risk.

J. J. Gleysteen, MD

Randomized Clinical Trial of Laparoscopic *Versus* Open Appendicectomy for Confirmed Appendicitis

Moberg A-C, Berndsen F, Palmquist I, et al (Univ Hosp of Malmö, Sweden)

Br J Surg 92:298-304, 2005 10–37

Background.—Laparoscopy is safe for diagnostic and therapeutic purposes in patients with suspected acute appendicitis. This study compared recovery after laparoscopic (LA) and open appendicectomy (OA) for confirmed appendicitis, carried out by experienced surgeons in an educational setting.

Methods.—One hundred and sixty-three patients with laparoscopically confirmed appendicitis suitable for LA were randomized prospectively to either LA or OA in a blinded fashion (Table 1). The primary endpoint was time to full recovery. Secondary endpoints were operating time, complications, hospital stay and functional status.

TABLE 1.—Demographic of the 163 Randomized Patients

	Laparoscopic (n = 81)	Open (n = 82)	*P*
Age (years)*	31 (15-71)	31 (15-83)	*ns*
Sex ratio (M:F)	46:35	58:24	*ns*
Body mass index*	24 (17-34)	25 (17-43)	*ns*
Type of work			
Sedentary	14	15	
Light	16	16	
Heavy	9	10	
Not working	29	24	
Missing information	13	17	

*Values are median (range).

(Courtesy of Moberg A-C, Berndsen F, Palmquist I, et al: Randomized clinical trial of laparoscopic *versus* open appendicectomy for confirmed appendicitis. *Br J Surg* 92:298-304, 2005, Blackwell Science Ltd.)

TABLE 3.—Complications within 3 months

	Laparoscopic (n = 81)	Open (n = 82)
Minor complications		
Fever with prolonged hospital stay	4	4
Wound infection with drained pus	1	1
Urine infection or urine retention	1	2
Major complications		
Deep abdominal infection	0	1*
Operation for bowel obstruction	1†	1†

*Patient readmitted for drainage of a deep abdominal infection.
†During hospital stay for primary surgery.
(Courtesy of Moberg A-C, Berndsen F, Palmquist I, et al: Randomized clinical trial of laparoscopic *versus* open appendicectomy for confirmed appendicitis. *Br J Surg* 92:298-304, 2005, Blackwell Science Ltd.)

Results.—There was no significant difference between LA and OA in time to full recovery (9 and 11 days respectively; $P = 0.225$). Operating time was 55 min in the LA group and 60 min in the OA group ($P = 0.416$). The complication rate was 8.6 and 11.0 per cent respectively ($P = 0.696$) (Table 3), and median hospital stay was 2 days in both groups ($P = 0.192$). Functional status was significantly better in the LA group 7-10 days after operation ($P = 0.045$).

Conclusion.—There was no difference in time to full recovery after LA and OA in patients with laparoscopically confirmed appendicitis. A trend towards better physical activity was noted after the laparoscopic procedure.

▶ Previous meta-analyses have confirmed that LA is safe and had results that confirm a faster return to normal activity with fewer wound complications, despite the added expense of longer operating times.[1-5] As many such studies have been performed during their learning curve for laparoscopic appendectomy, Moberg et al of the University Hospital of Malmv, Sweden, compared recovery after LA versus OA for confirmed appendicitis conducted by experienced surgeons in a university environment. As is evident in the article (after demographic randomization of both cohorts), the complications evident within 3 months of operation note no differences in the LA versus the open technique for minor or major complications. The authors confirm a trend toward improved physical activity after the LA.

As diagnostic laparoscopy is increasingly accurate and safe for patients with acute appendicitis, the acceptance of LA is evident internationally. The conclusions that there are no differences in time to full recovery regarding the technique are important. Although LA extends operating time, such an approach does enhance the thoroughness of the examination of the abdominal cavity, more so than the OA, which is otherwise limited by visibility of remote structures.

K. I. Bland, MD

References

1. Chung RS, Rowland DY, Li P, et al: A meta-analysis of randomized controlled trials of laparoscopic versus conventional appendectomy. *Am J Surg* 177:250-256, 1999.
2. Garbutt JM, Soper NJ, Shannon WD, et al: Meta-analysis of randomized controlled trials comparing laparoscopic and open appendectomy. *Surg Laparosc Endosc* 9:17-26, 1999.
3. Golub R, Siddiqui F, Pohl D: Laparoscopic versus open appendectomy: A metaanalysis. *J Am Coll Surg* 186:545-553, 1998.
4. Sauerland S, Lefering R, Holthausen, et al: Laparoscopic versus conventional appendectomy—A meta-analysis of randomised controlled trials. *Langenbecks Arch Surg* 383:289-295, 1998.
5. Temple LKF, Litwin DE, McLeod RS: A meta-analysis of laparoscopic versus open appendectomy in patients suspected of having acute appendicitis. *Can J Surg* 42:377-383, 1999.

Are Negative Appendectomies Still Acceptable?

Jones K, Peña AA, Dunn EL, et al (Methodist Hosps of Dallas)
Am J Surg 188:748-754, 2004 10–38

Background.—The goal was to ascertain if there was a significant change in the negative appendectomy (NA) rate in our community hospital with the increased use of computed tomography (CT).

Methods.—This was a retrospective chart review of all appendectomies for acute disease performed at our institution from January 2000 to December 2002. There is no established protocol; therefore, CT scans were performed at the discretion of the involved physicians. The results of the physical exams, CT scans and pathology were recorded.

Results.—Three hundred eighty-nine appendectomies were performed for appendicitis. There was a progressive increase in the use of CT: 52% in 2000, 74% in 2001, and 86% in 2002. There was also a decrease in the NA rate over the 3 years: 17% in 2000, 9% in 2001 and 2% in 2002. The perforated appendicitis rate decreased from 25% in 2000 to 9% in 2002.

Conclusion.—The appropriate utilization of CT scan as an aid in the diagnosis of acute appendicitis should decrease the NA rate to 2%.

► Jones et al of the Departments of Surgery and Radiology, Dallas, Texas, ascertain the significant change in NA rates in community-based hospitals with use of CT. The authors have therefore shown a progressive increase in the use of CT for diagnosis of appendicitis from 52% (2000) to 86% (2002). There was a concurrent decrease in the frequency of NA over this 3-year interval: 17% (2000) to 2% (2002). Importantly, an issue not fully emphasized was that the perforation rate of appendicitis has decreased by one third, from 25% (2000) to 9% (2002). Thus, the inverse relationship between a NA rate and the increasing use of CT is evident.

Expectedly, there is a higher frequency of NA in the female population, as they pose a greater diagnostic challenge for evaluation of tubo-ovarian and pelvic diseases. One must weigh the added cost of CT evaluation to clinical examination to justify its usage to enhance a reduction in the NA frequency. To achieve a 2% frequency in this interval from that of 17% also must reflect on the increasing utilization of CT gastrointestinal specialists with interest in resolution of this problem, regardless of the hour the appendectomy presentation occurs.

K. I. Bland, MD

Effects of Race, Insurance Status, and Hospital Volume on Perforated Appendicitis in Children

Smink DS, Fishman SJ, Kleinman K, et al (Children's Hosp Boston; Brigham and Women's Hosp, Boston; Harvard Med School, Boston)
Pediatrics 115:920-925, 2005 10–39

Objective.—Previous research suggests that perforated appendicitis is more common in Medicaid patients, but the roles of minority race and hospital volume remain largely unstudied. We sought to investigate the association of perforated appendicitis in children with minority race, insurance status, and hospital volume.

Methods.—We conducted a retrospective, population-based cohort study of 33184 children who had an International Classification of Diseases, Ninth Revision diagnosis code for acute appendicitis in The Kids' Inpatient Database, a pediatric database from 22 states in 1997. A multivariate logistic regression model was developed to determine patient and hospital characteristics predictive of perforated appendicitis.

Results.—Of 33184 children with acute appendicitis, 10777 (32.5%) were perforated. In multivariate analysis, black (odds ratio [OR]: 1.24; 95% confidence interval [CI]: 1.10-1.39) and Hispanic (OR: 1.19; 95% CI: 1.10-1.29) children were more likely to have perforated appendicitis than white children. Perforation was also more likely in Medicaid patients (OR: 1.30; 95% CI 1.22-1.39) compared with privately insured children. Annual hospital volume of cases of appendicitis was not significantly associated with perforation in multivariate analysis.

Conclusions.—Perforated appendicitis disproportionately affected both children of minority race and children insured by Medicaid. No effect of hospital volume was observed. To reduce this racial disparity, efforts should focus on the causes of delayed diagnosis and the treatment of appendicitis in children of minority race.

► This article points out the relationship among minority status, insurance status, and perforated appendicitis. The conclusion is that minority patients and patients on public assistance have less access to medical care than patients with private insurance. The study did not show any relationship between hospital volume for appendicitis and the rate of perforation in children. The article clearly shows that patients with perforated appendicitis are being treated later than those with nonperforated appendicitis. For this reason, it is important to continue these studies and focus on the precise reasons why patients on public assistance have delayed access to medical care. Are parents on public assistance not as attentive to their child's symptoms as the parents of children with private insurance? More likely, are there more roadblocks for these patients to overcome just to access the medical care system? We should redouble our efforts to improve access for patients of minority status or patients on public assistance as we continue these studies.

K. E. Georgeson, MD

Efficacy of Laparoscopic Appendectomy in Appendicitis With Peritonitis
Mancini GJ, Mancini ML, Nelson HS Jr (Univ of Tennessee, Knoxville)
Am Surg 71:1-5, 2005 10–40

Introduction.—Laparoscopic appendectomy (LA) is safe and effective in cases of peritonitis, perforation, and abscess. We investigated our conversion rate and clinical outcomes in this patient population, as well as preoperative factors that predict operative conversion. A retrospective nonrandomized cohort of 92 patients underwent LA for acute appendicitis with peritonitis, perforation, or abscess at our institution between 1997 and 2002. Thirty-six of the 92 were converted to open appendectomy (OA), yielding a conversion rate of 39 per cent. The presence of phlegmon (42%), nonvisualized appendix (44%), technical failures (8%), and bleeding (6%) were reasons for conversion. Preoperative data had no predictive value for conversion. CT scan findings of free fluid, phlegmon, and abscess did not correlate with findings at the time of surgery. Total complication rates were 8.9 per cent in the LA group as compared to 50 per cent in the converted cohort. Postoperative data showed LA patients stayed 3.2 days versus 6.9 days for converted patients ($P = 0.01$). LA patients had less pneumonia ($P = 0.02$), intra-abdominal abscess ($P = 0.01$), ileus ($P = 0.01$), and readmissions ($P = 0.01$). LA is safe and effective in patients with appendicitis with peritonitis, perforation, and abscess, resulting in shorter hospital stays and less complication.

► In the discussion of this article at the Southeastern Surgical Congress meeting, the authors reminded the audience of 2 salient points: the study concerns a select group of complex patients with appendicitis (with perforations or abscesses), and the laparoscopic approach was associated with less morbidity and a shorter hospital stay in a majority (61%) of patients. Clearly, their surgical data show enhanced efficacy of laparoscopic versus open appendectomy overall, but a failed laparoscopy is common in this select group.

At our institution, "all" suspected patients get CT scans, by which the appendicitis diagnosis often is made; in this article, more than half had a CT scan. Across the observations, they learned that a localized abscess foreshadowed a successful laparoscopic appendectomy, but otherwise, the preoperative CT had limited correlation with the operative findings.

The important conclusion to draw is that laparoscopy should be considered first in nearly all situations. Failure is seldom predictable, and success has real clinical and financial advantages.

J. J. Gleysteen, MD

Elective Intestinal Operations in Infants and Children Without Mechanical Bowel Preparation: A Pilot Study

Leys CM, Austin MT, Pietsch JB, et al (Vanderbilt Univ, Nashville, Tenn)
J Pediatr Surg 40:978-982, 2005 10–41

Background/Purpose.—Preoperative mechanical bowel preparation (MBP) for elective intestinal operations has been a long accepted practice. However, MBP is often unpleasant and time-consuming for patients, and clinical trials in adults have not shown improved outcomes. We conducted this pilot study to test whether omitting MBP before elective intestinal operations in infants and children would increase the risk of infectious or anastomotic complications.

Methods.—Retrospective review was performed of 143 patients who had an elective colon or distal small bowel procedure performed at our children's hospital between 1990 and 2003.

Results.—Thirty-three patients (No PREP) were managed by a single surgeon who routinely omitted MBP, whereas another 110 patients (PREP) were prepared with enemas, laxatives, or both. Both groups received 24 hours of preoperative dietary restriction to clear liquids and perioperative parenteral antibiotics. The No PREP group had one anastomotic leak and no wound infections, whereas the PREP group had 2 anastomotic leaks and 1 wound infection ($P = .58$). These results occurred despite greater duration of antibiotic therapy and incidence of delayed wound closures in the PREP group.

Conclusion.—The results of this pilot study suggest that omitting MBP before elective intestinal operations in infants and children carries no increased risk of infectious or anastomotic complications. Eliminating MBP may reduce health care costs and inconvenience to patients. These findings warrant a large, prospective, randomized clinical trial to validate our findings and to investigate further the necessity of MBP in the pediatric population.

▶ This article challenges the routine use of preoperative MBP for elective intestinal operations in infants and children. MBP is unpleasant for the child-patient and often requires admission before the surgical procedure. Omitting MBP is attractive. This nonrandomized pilot study suggests that MBP offers no advantages for children having intestinal surgery. A randomized study needs to be completed to confirm or refute the findings of this report. Unfortunately, such a randomized study may be difficult to complete as few parents will choose the MBP limb if given an option.

K. E. Georgeson, MD

Temporal Changes in the Management of Diverticulitis
Salem L, Anaya DA, Flum DR (Univ of Washington, Seattle)
J Surg Res 124:318-323, 2005 10–42

Purpose.—This study was designed to evaluate temporal trends in the use and type of operative and non-operative interventions in the management of diverticulitis.

Methods.—A retrospective cohort using a statewide administrative database was used to identify all patients hospitalized for diverticulitis in the state of Washington (1987-2001). Poisson and logistic regression were used to calculate changes in the frequency of hospitalization, operative and percutaneous interventions, and colostomy over time.

Results.—Of the 25,058 patients hospitalized nonelectively with diverticulitis (mean age 69 ± 16, 60% female) there were only minimal changes in the frequency of admissions over time (0.006% increase per year-IRR 1.00006 95% CI 1.00004, 1.00008). The odds of an emergency colectomy at initial hospitalization decreased by 2% each year (OR 0.98 95% CI 0.98, 0.99) whereas the odds of percutaneous abscess drainage increased 7% per year (OR 1.07 95% CI 1.05, 1.1). Among patients undergoing percutaneous drainage, the odds of operative interventions decreased by 9% compared to patients who did not have a percutaneous intervention (OR 0.91 95% CI 0.87, 0.94). The proportion of patients undergoing colostomy during emergency operations remained essentially stable over time (range 49-61%), as did the proportion of patients undergoing prophylactic colectomy after initial non-surgical management (approximately 10%).

Conclusions.—There was a minimal increase in the frequency of diverticulitis admissions over time. A rise in percutaneous drainage procedures was associated with a decrease in emergency operative interventions. The proportion of patients undergoing colostomy remained stable, and there does not seem to be a significant increase in the use of one-stage procedures for diverticulitis.

▶ This article from a retrospective analysis of a statewide (Washington) administrative database on the frequency of diverticulitis and changes in the clinical management of diverticulitis is one of several published by this group in recent years. Each article has been analyzed carefully. In this case, the initial search of the database began with ICD-9 codes for colectomies and colostomies and was then narrowed to diverticulitis rather than starting with the latter diagnostic ICD-9 code. Thus, the database was launched with surgical patients only. Covering 14 years overall, it was divided into 5-year segments for comparative univariate analyses.

The results are nicely described in the abstract. The frequency of disease did not change, but the use of percutaneous drainage (a result of CT availability) avoided increasing numbers of urgent surgical interventions. The authors showed that the frequency of colectomy with urgent/emergent operations was stable at 50% to 60% but were surprised to note the unchanged use of colostomy over the time periods (10%-20%) with the later elective operations.

The surprise was related to the existence of several publications advocating the safety of primary anastomosis with diverticulitis, even in the presence of peritonitis. This is another area for clinical trials.

J. J. Gleysteen, MD

Mechanical Bowel Preparation for Elective Colorectal Surgery: A Meta-Analysis

Bucher P, Mermillod B, Gervaz P, et al (Geneva Univ, Switzerland)

Arch Surg 139:1359-1364, 2004 10–43

Hypothesis.—There is little scientific evidence to support the routine practice of mechanical bowel preparation (MBP) before elective colorectal surgery in order to minimize the risk of postoperative septic complications.

Data Sources.—Trials were retrieved using a MEDLINE search followed by a manual search of the bibliographic information in select articles. Languages were restricted to English, French, Spanish, Italian, and German. There was no date restriction.

Study Selection.—Only prospective randomized clinical trials (RCTs) evaluating MBP vs no MBP before elective colorectal surgery were included.

Data Extraction.—Outcomes evaluated were anastomotic leakage, intra-abdominal infection, wound infection, reoperation, and general and extra-abdominal morbidity and mortality rates. Data were extracted by 2 independent observers.

Data Synthesis.—Seven RCTs were retrieved. The total number of patients in these RCTs was 1297 (642 who had received MBP and 655 who had not). Among all the RCTs reviewed, anastomotic leak was significantly more frequent in the MBP group, 5.6% (36/642), compared with the no-MBP group, 2.8% (18/655) (odds ratio, 1.84; $P = .03$). Intra-abdominal infection (3.7% for the MBP group vs 2.0% for the no-MBP group), wound infection (7.5% for the MBP group vs 5.5% for the no-MBP group), and reoperation (5.2% for the MBP group vs 2.2% for the no-MBP group) rates were nonstatistically significantly higher in the MBP group. General morbidity and mortality rates were slightly higher in the MBP group.

Conclusions.—There is no evidence to support the use of MBP in patients undergoing elective colorectal surgery. Available data tend to suggest that MBP could be harmful with respect to the incidence of anastomotic leak and does not reduce the incidence of septic complications.

▶ Bucher et al of the Clinic of Visceral and Transplantation Surgery, and the Division of Medical Statistics, Geneva, Switzerland, completed a meta-analysis using a MEDLINE search of prospective randomized clinical trials that evaluate MBP before elective colorectal surgery versus no MBP before the elective procedure. The purpose of the MBP was the reduction of risk of post-operative septic complications related to bowel content spillage, intraabdominal infections, and anastomotic leaks.

The accompanying editorial by an experienced surgeon, Dr Pickleman, properly relates my own concern, in that the generalization of the outcomes of 7 "studies" conducted as prospective randomized trials may stretch the belief for limits of safety and common practicality. To come to the conclusion evident in the report cannot provide comfort or solace to practicing surgeons in an attempt to avoid a stoma-formation or perform a primary anastomosis in the patient having an emergency procedure. Most surgeons will continue to favor MBP to the mild discomfort and slight expense for the patient and hospital to provide this important physiological "prep."

K. I. Bland, MD

Is Mechanical Bowel Preparation Mandatory for Elective Colon Surgery? A Prospective Randomized Study

Ram E, Sherman Y, Weil R, et al (Tel Aviv Univ, Israel)

Arch Surg 140:285-288, 2005 10–44

Background.—Bowel preparation prior to colonic surgery usually includes antibiotic therapy together with mechanical bowel preparation (MBP). Mechanical bowel preparation may cause discomfort to the patient, prolonged hospitalization, and water and electrolyte imbalance. It was assumed that with the improvement in surgical technique together with the use of more effective prophylactic antibiotics, it was possible that MBP would no longer be necessary.

Hypothesis.—There is no statistical difference in the postoperative results of patients who undergo elective colon resection with MBP as compared with those who have no MBP.

Design and Patients.—The study includes all patients who had elective large bowel resection at Campus Golda between April 1, 1999, and March 31, 2002. Emergency operations were not included. The patients were randomly assigned to the 2 study groups (with or without MBP) according to identification numbers. All patients were treated with intravenous and oral antibiotics prior to surgery. The patients in the MBP group received Soffodex for bowel preparation.

Results.—A total of 329 patients participated in the study, 165 without MBP and 164 with MBP. The 2 groups were similar in age, sex, and type of surgical procedure. Two hundred sixty-eight patients (81.5%) underwent surgery owing to colorectal cancer and 61 patients (18.5%) owing to benign disease. The hospitalization period was longer in the bowel-prepared group (mean ± SD, 8.2 ± 5.1 days) as compared with the nonprepared group (mean ± SD, 8.0 ± 2.7 days). However, this difference was not statistically significant. The time until the first bowel movement was similar between the 2 groups: a mean ± SD of 4.2 ± 1.3 days in the nonprepared group as compared with a mean ± SD of 4.3 ± 1.1 days in the prepared group (P = NS). Four patients (1.2%) died in the postoperative course owing to acute myocardial infarction and pulmonary embolism. Sixty-two patients (37.6%) of the non-

MBP group suffered from postoperative complications as compared with 77 patients (46.9%) of the MBP group.

Conclusion.—Our results suggest that no advantage is gained by preoperative MBP in elective colorectal surgery.

► The authors are to be commended for conducting outstanding clinical research in the form of a prospective randomized study. This group, like many others in the past 2 to 3 years, sought to demonstrate the significance of as well as the requirement for having chemical preparation of the bowel or MBP in elective colorectal surgery. This study included a total of 329 patients: 164 with MBP and 165 without MBP. The groups did not differ in age, sex, or type of surgical procedure. Regarding mortality, wound dehiscence, wound infection, anastomotic breakdown, anastomotic bleeding, pulmonary complications, and ileus, no statistically significant differences were determined in patients who either received an MBP or did not receive an MBP. Two deaths occurred in each group. In addition, 2 anastomotic breakdowns occurred in the group with no MBP, and 1 occurred in the group with MBP, but this was not statistically different. Thus, in each of the categories, having an MBP does not seem to convey any clear advantage. However, most surgeons still use MBPs for colorectal surgery. Some positive factors relate to the aim of MBP, which is to rid the colon of solid stool, thus reducing the bacteria load and minimizing the risk of infection. An MBP allows surgeons to perform an intraoperative colonoscopy, allows them to palpate the entire colon, and allows them to produce a bowel preparation with minimal contamination. However, the negative aspects of an MBP are that it can cause a significant electrolyte imbalance, dehydration, abdominal pain, bloating, and fatigue. In addition, it can also increase the risk of perforation before surgery from enemas.

This study does promote the benefit of prophylactic antibiotic therapy in the setting of surgery; however, it clearly questions the need and the persistence for MBP. It is the second study[1] to be published with more than 300 participating patients demonstrating no clear advantage of MBP but promoting safe, elective primary anastomosis with antibiotic prophylaxis at the time of surgery. Neither study has shown a significant added value for MBP or a difference in outcomes or complications.

S. M. Vickers, MD

Reference

1. Fa-Si-Oen P, Roumen R, Buitenweg J, et al: Mechanical bowel preparation or not? Outcome of a multicenter, randomized trial in elective open colon surgery. *Dis Colon Rectum* 48:1509-1516, 2005.

Diagnosis-Related Group Assignment in Laparoscopic and Open Colectomy: Financial Implications for Payer and Provider

Senagore AJ, Brannigan A, Kiran RP, et al (Cleveland Clinic Found, Ohio)

Dis Colon Rectum 48:1016-1020, 2005 10–45

Purpose.—In carefully matched patients, the length of hospital stay after laparoscopic colectomy is shorter than after open surgery. Higher operating room costs for laparoscopic surgery are offset by lower costs for hospitalization because of less utilization of pharmacy, laboratory, and nursing services. Clinical outcome is comparable. We examined the effect of the surgical approach for colectomy (open vs. laparoscopic) regarding the reasons for disease-related group assignment to disease-related group 148, and institutional cost under Part A of the U.S. Medicare system.

Methods.—Colectomy patients were assigned to either disease-related group 148 (colorectal resection with complications) or disease-related group 149 (colorectal resection without complications) with significant institutional reimbursement implications (disease-related group 149, \$8,310; disease-related group 148, \$20,291). A total of 100 consecutive disease-related group 148 patients undergoing laparoscopic colectomy from July 2000 to September 2002 were identified from a prospective database and case-matched with 100 patients undergoing open colectomy. Patients were matched for gender, age, operative procedure, and pathology. A certified coder determined the reason(s) for disease-related group 148 assignment, which were grouped into: preoperative comorbidity, a combination of preoperative comorbidity/postoperative complications, or postoperative complications alone.

Results.—Significantly more lapararoscopy patients were assigned to disease-related group 148 solely because of preoperative comorbidities (62 percent *vs.* 21 percent; $P < 0.0001$). Significantly more patients in the open surgery group were classified as disease-related group 148 solely because of postoperative complications (22 percent *vs.* 42 percent; $P < 0.0001$). An additional group of patients were assigned to the disease-related group 148 category based on a combination of preoperative and postoperative diagnoses (16 percent *vs.* 37 percent). The mean direct hospital costs were significantly less for laparoscopy patients (\$3971 *vs.* \$5997; $P = 0.0095$). Increased cost to Part A of Medicare for 20 open surgery patients who "migrated" to disease-related group 148 because of postoperative complications was \$239,620.

Conclusions.—Our data are the first to demonstrate that disease related group assignment can change solely because of a differential rate of postoperative complications for two competing operative techniques. This change occurred at twice the rate for open colectomy and resulted in significantly increased cost to the insurer under a prospective payment program. The savings to the institution coupled with the shortened length of stay offset the potential loss in revenue to the institution.

► This is the first study to demonstrate that disease-related group assignment (DRG) can change solely based on a differential rate of operative complications for 2 competing surgical approaches (laparoscopic vs open colectomy). It is not unexpected that the change occurs twice as frequently for open colectomy and resulted in significant increase in cost to the insurer under the prospective payment program. However, savings to the institution coupled with shortened length of stay offset the potential loss of revenue to the institution. As these data are the first to demonstrate the effects of laparoscopically assisted colectomy for cost to the prospective payment system and provider reimbursement cost, the authors emphasize the importance of assessing new technology in the light of improvements in both quality and cost for patient care. Medical centers therefore should critically assess the net reimbursement effects that use evolving technologies based on the same quality measures and total reimbursement formulas.

K. I. Bland, MD

A Prospective, Randomized, Controlled Clinical Trial of Placement of the Artificial Bowel Sphincter (Acticon Neosphincter) for the Control of Fecal Incontinence

O'Brien PE, Dixon JB, Skinner S, et al (Monash Univ, Melbourne; Caulfield Gen Med Centre, Melbourne)

Dis Colon Rectum 47:1852-1860, 2004 10–46

Background.—Severe fecal incontinence remains a disabling condition for the patient and a major therapeutic challenge for the physician. A series of observational studies have indicated that placement of an artificial bowel sphincter is associated with marked improvement of continence and quality of life. We have performed a prospective, randomized, controlled trial to evaluate the effect of placement of an artificial bowel sphincter (Acticon Neosphincter) on continence and quality of life in a group of severely incontinent adults.

Methods.—Fourteen adults (male:female, 1:13; age range, 44-75 years) were randomized to placement of the artificial bowel sphincter or to a program of supportive care and were followed for six months from operation or entry into the study. The principal outcome measure was the level of continence, measured with the Cleveland Continence Score, which provides a scale from 0 to 20, representing perfect control through to total incontinence. Secondary outcome measures were perioperative and late complications in the artificial bowel sphincter group, and the changes in quality of life in both groups.

Results.—In the control group, the Cleveland Continence Score was not significantly altered, with an initial value of 17.1 ± 2.3 and a final value of 14.3 ± 4.6 at six months (Fig 1). The artificial bowel sphincter group showed

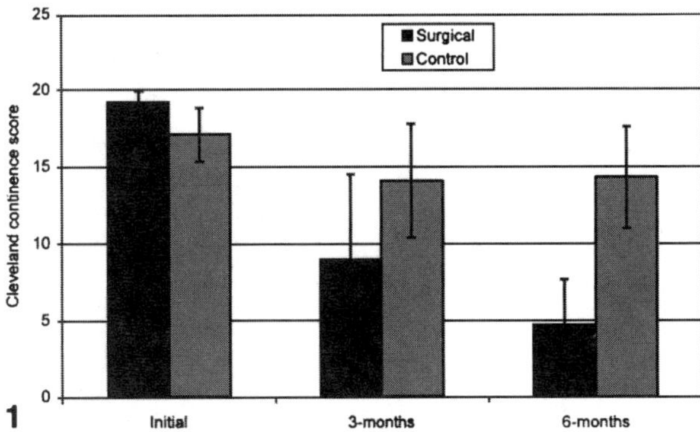

FIGURE 1.—Cleveland Continence Score (mean ± 95 percent confidence interval) for the surgical and control groups at initial assessment, and three and six months after commencing the treatment program. The difference between the groups at six months is significant ($P = 0.002$). (Courtesy of O'Brien PE, Dixon JB, Skinner S, et al: A prospective, randomized, controlled clinical trial of placement of the artificial bowel sphincter (Acticon Neosphincter) for the control of fecal incontinence. *Dis Colon Rectum* 47:1852-1860, 2004. Copyright Springer-Verlag.)

a highly significant improvement, changing from 19.0 ± 1.2 before placement to 4.8 ± 4.0 at six months after placement. One patient in the artificial bowel sphincter group had failure of healing of the perineal wound and explantation of the device (14 percent explantation rate). There were two other significant perioperative events of recurring fecal impaction initially after placement in one patient and additional suturing of the perineal wound in another. There were major improvements in the quality of life for all measures in the artificial bowel sphincter group (Table 5). There was significant improvement in all eight subscales of the Medical Outcome Study Short Form-36 measures. The American Medical Systems Quality of Life score was raised from 39 ± 6 to 83 ± 14 (Fig 2) and the Beck Depression Inventory showed reduction from a level of mild depression (10.8 ± 9.3) to a normal value (6.8 ± 8.7). No significant changes in any of the quality of life measures occurred for the control group.

Conclusions.—Through a prospective, randomized trial format, we have shown that placement of an artificial bowel sphincter is safe and effective when compared with supportive care alone. Perioperative and late problems are likely to continue to occur and between 15 percent and 30 percent of patients may require permanent explantation. For the remainder, the device is easy and discrete to use, highly effective in achieving continence, and able to generate a major improvement in the quality of life.

► The major morbidity evident with severe fecal incontinence includes disabling cosmetic and hygienic issues for the patients involved. This major therapeutic challenge for the surgeon often follows the labor of childbirth, major pelvic trauma, and surgical intervention for pelvic/rectal neoplasms.

In this carefully studied group of 14 patients by O'Brien et al of Monash University of Melbourne, Australia, patients were randomly assigned to place-

TABLE 5.—Changes in Outcome Measures for Control and Artificial Bowel Sphincter Patients During Six-Month Follow-Up

	Control Initial	Control 1 Final	*P* Value	Surgical Initial	Surgical Final	*P* Value	Final Control *vs.* Surgical
Cleveland Continence Score	17.4 (2.3)	14.3 (4.6)	0.21	19 (1.2)	4.8 (4.0)	0.001	0.002
AMS QOL score	42.5 (22)	54.7 (26)	0.25	38.8 (6)	82.7 (14)	0.003	0.04
SF-36 physical component summary	41.6 (13)	41 (11)	0.90	37 (10)	45 (7)	0.26	0.43
SF-36 mental component summary	40.3 (10)	44.4 (5)	0.27	45 (9)	52 (4)	0.25	0.02
Beck Depression Inventory	7.3 (2)	.3 (10)	0.38	10.8 (9)	6.8 (9)	0.78	0.65

Data are mean (standard deviation). Comparison is by paired *t* -test (two-tailed). The last column provides *P* values for comparison of the final value for the control group *vs.* the final value for the artificial bowel sphincter group. Mean (SD), *P* value determined by unpaired *t* -test (two-tailed).

(Courtesy of O'Brien PE, Dixon JB, Skinner S, et al: A prospective, randomized, controlled clinical trial of placement of the artificial bowel sphincter (Acticon Neosphincter) for the control of fecal incontinence. *Dis Colon Rectum* 47:1852-1860, 2004. Copyright Springer-Verlag.)

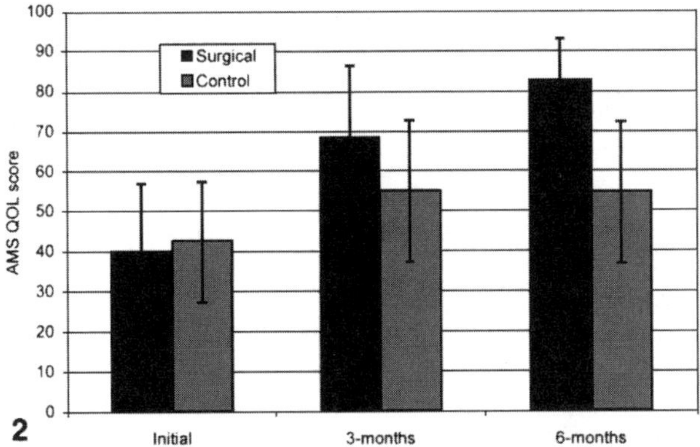

FIGURE 2.—American Medical Systems (AMS) quality of life (QOL) score (mean ± 95 percent confidence interval) for the surgical and control groups at initial assessment, and three and 6-months after commencing the treatment program. The difference between the groups at six months is significant (P = 0.04). (Courtesy of O'Brien PE, Dixon JB, Skinner S, et al: A prospective, randomized, controlled clinical trial of placement of the artificial bowel sphincter (Acticon Neosphincter) for the control of fecal incontinence. *Dis Colon Rectum* 47:1852-1860, 2004. Copyright Springer-Verlag.)

ment of an artificial bowel sphincter (ABS) or to only supportive care, and thereafter, followed for 6 months after operation and entry into the study.

As is evident in the abstract, The Cleveland Continence Score at the initial 3- and 6-month follow-up, statistical differences are seen at 6 months with the advantage of the surgical arm. In addition, with the American Medical Systems Quality Of Life (QOL) Score, a statistical advantage (P = .04) at 6 months was evident in the surgical patient using the ABS. No statistical advantage in the physical or mental component summaries or in the Beck Depression Inventory are suggested. However, the Beck Depression Inventory confirms reductions from a level of mild depression to a normal value. No significant changes were evident in the QOL measures for the control group.

Although this prospective study confirms a significant enhancement in anal continence and QOL after placement of the Acticon Neosphincter ABS, the interpretation and long-term follow-ups of this study must be assured before its general recommendation to the general surgical workforce. Other options for correction of incontinence continue to be the dynamic graciloplasty and colostomy for severe levels of this disability. The major limiting factor of this study is the power of the statistical evidence which is due to the size of the small study group expected. However, in support of this device, a small sample of patients is required to demonstrate its effectiveness that appears to be substantial. The ABS appears to be a safe bioartificial device and is effective in controlling severe fecal incontinence. Long-term outcomes with follow-up are essential to make final recommendations.

K. I. Bland, MD

Loop Ileostomy Closure After Restorative Proctocolectomy: Outcome in 1,504 Patients

Wong K-S, Remzi FH, Gorgun E, et al (Cleveland Clinic Found, Ohio)
Dis Colon Rectum 48:243-250, 2005 10–47

Purpose.—Routine use of a temporary loop ileostomy for diversion after restorative proctocolectomy is controversial because of reported morbidity associated with its creation and closure. This study intended to review our experience with loop ileostomy closure after restorative proctocolectomy and determine the complication rates. In addition, complication rates between handsewn and stapled closures were compared.

Methods.—Our Department Pelvic Pouch Database was queried and charts reviewed for all patients who had ileostomy closure after restorative proctocolectomy from August 1983 to March 2002.

Results.—A total of 1,504 patients underwent ileostomy closure after restorative proctocolectomy during a 19-year period. The median length of hospitalization was three (range, 1-40) days and the overall complication rate was 11.4 percent. Complications included small-bowel obstruction (6.4 percent), wound infection (1.5 percent), abdominal septic complications (1 percent), and enterocutaneous fistulas (0.6 percent). Handsewn closure was performed in 1,278 patients (85 percent) and stapled closure in 226 (15 percent). No significant differences in complication rates and length of hospitalization were found between handsewn and stapled closure techniques (Tables 3, 4, and 6).

Conclusions.—Our results demonstrated that ileostomy closure after restorative proctocolectomy can be achieved with a low morbidity and a short hospitalization stay. In addition, we found that complication rates and length of hospitalization were similar between handsewn and stapled closures.

► These authors from the Cleveland Clinic Foundation retrospectively evaluated 1504 patients who had undergone ileostomy closure after restorative proctocolectomy over a 19-year interval. The authors confirm low morbidity

TABLE 3.—Incidence of Small-Bowel Obstruction by Incision Type

Incision	No Small-Bowel Obstruction (n = 1,407)	Small-Bowel Obstruction (n = 97)	*P* Value[a]
Midline (n = 80)	73 (91.3)	7 (8.87)	0.23
Circumstomal (n = 1,214)	1,132 (93.3)	82 (6.8)	
Extended circumstomal (n = 201)	193 (96)	8 (4)	

Data are numbers with percentages in parentheses unless otherwise indicated.
[a]Chi-squared test.
(Courtesy of Wong K-S, Remzi FH, Gorgun E, et al: Loop ileostomy closure after restorative proctocolectomy: outcome in 1,504 patients. *Dis Colon Rectum* 48:243-250, 2005. Copyright Springer-Verlag.)

TABLE 4.—Complication Rates for Handsewn and Stapled Ileostomy Closures After Restorative Proctocolectomy

Complication	Handsewn (n = 1,278)	Stapled (n = 226)	*P* Value
Bowel obstruction	85 (6.7)	12 (5.2)	0.45[b]
Wound infection	20 (1.6)	3 (1.3)	0.99[a]
Anastomotic complications	22 (1.7)	2 (0.9)	0.56[a]

Data are numbers with percentages in parentheses unless otherwise indicated.
[a]Fisher's exact test.
[b]Chi-squared test.
(Courtesy of Wong K-S, Remzi FH, Gorgun E, et al: Loop ileostomy closure after restorative proctocolectomy: outcome in 1,504 patients. *Dis Colon Rectum* 48:243-250, 2005. Copyright Springer-Verlag.)

and mortality and a short hospital stay, and importantly, length of hospital stay is similar between handsewn and stapled closure. Moreover, as is indicated, there is no statistical difference between the type of incision for absence or presence of small bowel obstruction. Of importance, however, is the time of closure of the ileostomy to diminish small bowel obstruction, enterocutaneous fistula, abdominal septic complications, and wound infections. The odds ratio of developing wound infection of the ileostomy closure at or after 3.2 months confirms substantial differences. The infection rate was 2.2%, with closures less than 3.2 months (early closure) versus 0.7% 3.2 or more months (late closure) (*P* = .01. The authors confirm an overall complication rate of 11% with a short median hospital stay of 3 days, especially if there is a delay in the ileostomy closure of 3+ months. This objective evidence should be considered strongly by the general surgeon in practice who is inquiring about the timing of closure of a loop ileostomy after proctocolectomy.

K. I. Bland, MD

TABLE 6.—Wound Infection Rate in Early and Late Ileostomy Closure Using Median Time of Closure (3.2 months) as a Cutoff

Time of Closure	No Wound Infection (n = 1,481)	Wound Infection (n = 23)	*P* Value[a]
$<$3.2 months (n = 799)	781 (97.8)	18 (2.2)	0.015
$\geq$3.2 months (n = 705)	700 (99.3)	5 (0.7)	

Data are numbers with percentages in parentheses unless otherwise indicated.
[a]Chi-squared test
(Courtesy of Wong K-S, Remzi FH, Gorgun E, et al: Loop ileostomy closure after restorative proctocolectomy: outcome in 1,504 patients. *Dis Colon Rectum* 48:243-250, 2005. Copyright Springer-Verlag.)

Hand-Assisted Laparoscopic Versus Open Restorative Proctocolectomy With Ileal Pouch Anal Anastomosis: A Randomized Trial

Maartense S, Dunker MS, Slors JF, et al (Academic Med Ctr, Amsterdam; Vrije Universiteit, The Netherlands; VU Univ, Amsterdam)

Ann Surg 240:984-992, 2004 10–48

Objective.—The aim of the study was to evaluate postoperative recovery after hand-assisted laparoscopic or open restorative proctocolectomy with ileal pouch anal anastomosis for ulcerative colitis and familial adenomatous polyposis in a randomized controlled trial.

Methods.—Sixty patients were randomized for hand-assisted laparoscopic (n = 30) or open surgery (n = 30). Primary outcome parameter was postoperative recovery in the 3 months after surgery, measured by quality of life questionnaires (SF-36 and GIQLI). Secondary parameters were postoperative morphine requirement and surgical parameters, viz. operating time, morbidity, hospital stay, and costs.

Results.—There was no difference between the 2 procedures in quality of life assessment in the 3 months after surgery. There was a significant decline in quality of life on all scales of the SF-36 ($P < 0.001$) and total GIQLI score ($P < 0.001$) in the first 2 weeks in both groups (no significant difference between the groups). Quality of life returned to baseline levels after 4 weeks. Operating times were longer in the laparoscopic group compared with the open group (210 and 133 minutes, respectively; $P < 0.001$). No significant differences were found in morphine requirement. Neither morbidity nor postoperative hospital stay differed between the laparoscopic and open group (20% versus 17%, in 10 versus 11 days, respectively). Median overall costs were 16.728 for the hand-assisted laparoscopic procedure and 13.406 for the open procedure ($P = 0.095$).

Conclusions.—Recovery measured using quality of life questionnaires is comparable for hand-assisted laparoscopic or open restorative proctocolectomy with ileal pouch anal anastomosis. The laparoscopic approach is as safe, but more costly than the open procedure.

▶ This randomized prospective trial by Maartense et al of the Academic Medical Center of Amsterdam, Departments of Surgery and Gastroenterology, evaluates postoperative recovery after hand-assisted laparoscopy versus open restorative proctocolectomy with ileal pouch for ulcerative colitis and familial adenomatous polyposis. For 30 patients randomly assigned to either the laparoscopic versus the open technique, proper randomization of demographics confirmed that the open procedure would provide a shorter operating time ($P < .001$), whereas no other statistical advantages were evident regarding blood loss, need for protective loop ileostomy, hospital stay length, minor or major complications, or re-operation ($P < .72$). Moreover, relative to postoperative recovery in terms of narcotic requirement and return to diet, no statistical variant was evident with the open versus the laparoscopic approach. Thus, quality of life questionnaires confirm comparability for the hand-assisted laparoscopy versus the open restorative approach, and further conclude that the laparoscopic approach is as safe, but is more costly than the open technique.

Since the first report by Schmitt et al,[1] comparing open versus closed procedures with proctocolectomy with ileal pouch anal anastomosis provided disappointing results for the laparoscopic advantage. It is possible, as indicated by the authors, that these results were due to the significant learning curve effect, whereas more recent case reports confirm an advantage of the laparoscopic procedure with earlier return of bowel function, shorter length of stay, and complications rates that were similar to open techniques.[2-4] There is no question that the current study provides an outcome with similar expectations to that of the open procedure, although more costly. It is possible that with long-term follow-up that centers with expertise in the laparoscopic approach may confirm a reduction in small bowel obstruction and incisional hernia. But as confirmed by the authors, such data must be awaited in future prospective randomized trials.

K. I. Bland, MD

References

1. Schmitt SL, Cohen SM, Wexner SD, et al: Does laparoscopic-assisted ileal pouch anal anastomosis reduce the length of hospitalization? *Int J Colorectal Dis* 9:134-137, 1994.
2. Marcello PW, Milsom JW, Wong SK, et al: Laparoscopic restorative proctocolectomy: Case-matched comparative study with open restorative proctocolectomy. *Dis Colon Rectum* 43:604-608, 2000.
3. Santoro E, Carlini M, Carboni F, et al: Laparoscopic total proctocolectomy with ileal J pouch-anal anastomosis. *Hepatogastroenterology* 46:894-899, 1999.
4. Seshadri PA, Poulin EC, Schlachta CM, et al: Does a laparoscopic approach to total abdominal colectomy and proctocolectomy offer advantages? *Surg Endosc* 15:837-842, 2001.

Clinical Outcome of Laparoscopically Assisted Endorectal Pull-Through in Hirschsprung's Disease: Comparison of Abdominal and Perineal Approaches

Kubota A, Kawahara H, Okuyama H, et al (Research Inst for Maternal and Child Health, Osaka, Japan)

J Pediatr Surg 39:1835-1837, 2004 10–49

Background/Purpose.—Laparoscopically assisted endorectal pull-through (EPT) via a perineal approach using a prolapsing technique (PA) for Hirschsprung's disease (HD) has been reported. However, the clinical outcome after this approach has not been reported. The purpose of this study was to compare the clinical outcome of PA and the conventional transabdominal approach (TA).

Methods.—In the period between 1990 and 2001, 20 cases of HD underwent EPT with TA (group O), and 21 underwent EPT with PA (group L). There was no difference in age and weight distribution between the 2 groups. Clinical outcome was assessed 3 years after surgery.

Results.—The operation time was comparable in the 2 groups (4.9 ± 0.8 *v* 5.2 ± 0.8 hr), whereas blood loss (98 ± 52 *v* 36 ± 30 mL) and postoperative complications requiring surgical intervention (26% *v* 0%) were significantly lower in group L. The incidence of postoperative enteritis (27% *v* 28%) and voluntary defecation (more than once every/2 days) were compatible in the 2 groups (70% *v* 87%). Soiling (small amount of involuntary stooling; >1 per month) was significantly less frequent in group L (45% *v* 14%).

Conclusions.—Laparoscopically assisted ETP with PA is less invasive and can provide a better clinical outcome compared with TA in terms of postoperative soiling.

► This article focuses on an issue that has been largely ignored in pediatric surgical circles: the potential of inflicted trauma to the anal sphincter complex caused by the surgical repair of HD. The traction required to perform open mucosectomy was shown to be greater than the damage caused by trauma during a perineal approach for the endorectal dissection. Unfortunately, the number of patients in each group in this report is so small that definitive conclusions cannot be supported statistically. However, this article does put a focus on the potential for injury to the anal sphincter mechanism depending on the amount of surgical trauma delivered by the surgical procedure. The continence mechanism can be injured by careless operative technique, whether the operation is performed transabdominally or transanally. Patients with soiling after endorectal pull-through appear to have a wider than normal anorectal angle. This angle can be widened either by tethering of the pull-through segment from above or stretching of the levator ani muscles and external sphincter mechanisms during the operative procedure. The quality of fecal control after HD surgery is not as good as many pediatric surgeons think. Emphasis on refinements in technique, including adequate dissection of the restraining ligaments of the colon to avoid tethering of the neorectum from above along with care to avoid stretching of the levator ani and external sphincter muscles during the endorectal dissection, may improve the quality of continence after surgery for patients with HD.

K. E. Georgeson, MD

Randomized Controlled Trial to Compare the Early and Mid-term Results of Stapled Versus Open Hemorrhoidectomy

Bikhchandani J, Agarwal PN, Kant R, et al (Maulana Azad Med College, New Delhi, India)

Am J Surg 189:56-60, 2005 10–50

Background.—The new technique of circular stapler for the treatment of hemorrhoids has shown early promise in terms of minimal or no postoperative pain, early discharge from hospital, and quick return to work. This study was designed to compare stapled technique with the well-accepted conventional Milligan Morgan hemorrhoidectomy.

Methods.—After fulfilling the selection criteria, 84 patients were randomly allocated to the stapled (n = 42) or open group (n = 42). All patients were operated on under spinal anesthesia. The 2 techniques were evaluated with respect to the operative time, pain scores, complications, day of discharge, return to work, and level of satisfaction.

Results.—The mean age of patients was 46.02 years (SD, 12.33) in the stapled group and 48.64 years (14.57) in the open group. Grade III or IV hemorrhoids were more common in men (ie, 80.9% and 85.7% in the stapled and open group, respectively). The mean operative time was shorter in the stapled group 24.28 minutes (4.25) versus 45.21 minutes (5.36) in the Milligan-Morgan group ($P < .001$). The blood loss, pain scores and requirement of analgesics was significantly less in the stapled group. Mean hospital stay was 1.24 days (0.62) and 2.76 days (1.01) ($P < .001$) in the stapled and open group, respectively. The patients in the stapled group returned to work or routine activities earlier (ie, within 8.12 days [2.48]) as compared with 17.62 (5.59) in the open group. Only 88.1% of patients were satisfied by the open method compared with 97.6% after the stapled technique. The median follow-up period was 11 months with a maximum follow-up of 19 months (range 2-19 months).

Conclusions.—Stapled hemorrhoidectomy is a safe and effective day-care procedure for the treatment of grade III and grade IV hemorrhoids. It ensures lesser postoperative pain, early discharge, less time off work, complications similar to the open technique, and in the end a more satisfied patient with no perianal wound. However, more such randomized trials are essential to deny any long-term complication.

▶ This randomized controlled trial of open versus stapled hemorrhoidectomy compares the Milligan-Morgan technique with the Longo-Milito technique, which is the open procedure versus the circular staple procedure. The authors of this study are to be commended because they have performed a proper clinical trial evaluating 2 standardized procedures. The newer one involving a circular staple device is potentially a wider application of a technique previously described in gastrointestinal surgery for both esophageal varices and anorectal anastomosis.

This study demonstrates some significant findings as they relate to both outcomes and the initial management of patients with this disease. Of the 84 patients included in this randomized controlled trial, 42 were assigned to each group, and 80% of each group were men. The majority of these patients had grade III hemorrhoids: 85% and 83% in the stapled and the open groups, respectively. The other presenting symptoms were primarily bleeding and prolapse, as well as itching and constipation, which were not significantly different in either group. However, the outcomes were significantly different in each group. Blood loss was significantly less in the stapled group ($P < .001$). The operative time for the stapled group was nearly half of that for the open group, and the pain at 12 hours through a time period of 15 days was significantly improved in the stapled group as compared with that in the open group. In the group that received the staples, a significant decrease was seen in the requirement for analgesia, and the time to the first bowel movement was also earlier. Finally, as would be expected, the hospital stay was half of that in the open group, and the amount of time before a return to work was possible was likewise almost half of that in the open group: 8 days versus 17 days.

This technique provides a standardized approach to hemorrhoidectomy that may allow significant changes in the outcomes and management of these patients. However, the approach must be used with caution because it is invasive, requires general anesthesia, and requires a significant level of training for appropriate performance of the procedure. Inappropriately performed staple techniques can lead to disastrous outcomes in the rectum. Therefore, significant monitoring as well as training is required for the proper application of this device. Nonetheless, for the experienced colorectal or general surgeon, this technique is a new and important adjunct in the management of patients with hemorrhoids—a common problem that often requires a fairly extensive surgical procedure with often undesirable results and significant postoperative pain and recovery.

S. M. Vickers, MD

The Role of Antibiotic Prophylaxis in Prevention of Wound Infection After Lichtenstein Open Mesh Repair of Primary Inguinal Hernia: A Multicenter Double-blind Randomized Controlled Trial

Aufenacker TJ, van Geldere D, van Mesdag T, et al (Onze Lieve Vrouwe Gasthuis, Amsterdam; Amstelveen Hosp, The Netherlands; West-Fries Gasthuis, Hoorn, The Netherlands; et al)

Ann Surg 240:955-961, 2004 10–51

Objective.—To determine whether the use of prophylactic antibiotics is effective in the prevention of postoperative wound infection after Lichtenstein open mesh inguinal hernia repair.

Summary Background Data.—A recent Cochrane meta-analysis (2003) concluded that "antibiotic prophylaxis for elective inguinal hernia repair cannot be firmly recommended or discarded."

Methods.—Patients with a primary inguinal hernia scheduled for Lichtenstein repair were randomized to a preoperative single dose of 1.5 g intravenous cephalosporin or a placebo. Patients with recurrent hernias, immunosuppressive diseases, or allergies for the given antibiotic were excluded. Infection was defined using the Centers for Disease Control and Prevention criteria.

Results.—We included 1040 patients in the study between November 1998 and May 2003. According to the intention-to-treat principle, 1008 patients were analyzed. There were 8 infections (1.6%) in the antibiotic prophylaxis group and 9 (1.8%) in the placebo group ($P = 0.82$). There was 1 deep infection in the antibiotic prophylaxis group and 2 in the placebo group ($P = 0.57$). Statistical analysis showed an absolute risk reduction of 0.19% (95% confidence interval, −1.78%-1.40%) and a number needed to treat of 520 for the total number of infections. For deep infection, the absolute risk reduction is 0.20% (95% confidence interval, −0.87%-0.48%) with a number needed to treat of 508.

Conclusions.—A low percentage (1.7%) of wound infection after Lichtenstein open mesh inguinal (primary) hernia repair was found, and there was no difference between the antibiotic prophylaxis or placebo group. The results show that, in Lichtenstein inguinal primary hernia repair, antibiotic prophylaxis is not indicated in low-risk patients.

▶ This multicenter, double-blind, randomized trial evaluated the effectiveness of prophylactic antibiotics in the prevention of postoperative wound infection after Lichtenstein open-mesh inguinal hernia repair. As indicated, mesh repair in the majority of Western surgical clinics has become the most popular technique for repair of inguinal hernia.[1-4] As described, the Lichtenstein technique is based on a tension-free repair of the diminished strength of the inguinal floor and requires use of polypropylene mesh.[4] The postoperative wound complications in more than 1000 patients randomly assigned in this study after primary inguinal repair between the antibiotic prophylactic and placebo groups had no variance in postoperative wound infection rates. Moreover, there is no difference in superficial or deep wound infection statistically and the overall complication rate was essentially identical: 3.6% versus 3.4%, in the antibiotic versus placebo groups, respectively.

This randomized study is an important contribution that confirms no benefit for the use of antibiotic prophylaxis in low-risk patients, and its use is not cost-effective. The authors have estimated that 10 to 15 million dollars would be saved in the United States and Europe for these low-risk patients (70% of all hernias) if antibiotic prophylaxis is not used and is only reserved for high-risk patients.

K. I. Bland, MD

References

1. Bay-Nielsen M, Kehlet M, Strand L, et al: Quality assessment of 26304 herniorrhaphies in Denmark: A prospective nationwide study. *Lancet* 358:1124-1128, 2001.
2. Nyhus LM, Alani A, O'Dwyer PJ, et al: The problem: How to treat a hernia, in Schumpelick V, Nyhus LM, (eds): *Meshes: Benefits and Risks*, ed 1. Berlin, Springer-Verlag, 2004, pp 3-30.
3. EU Hernia Trialists collaboration: Mesh compared with non-mesh methods of open groin hernia repair: Systematic review of randomized controlled trials. *Br J Surg* 87:854-859, 2000.
4. Lichtenstein IL, Shulman AG, Amid PK, et al: The tension-free hernioplasty. *Am J Surg* 157:188-193, 1989.

Randomized Clinical Trial Assessing Impact of a Lightweight or Heavyweight Mesh on Chronic Pain After Inguinal Hernia Repair

O'Dwyer PJ, Kingsnorth AN, Molloy RG, et al (Western Infirmary, Glasgow, Scotland; Deeriford Hosp, Plymouth, England; Sunderland Royal Hosp, England; et al)

Br J Surg 92:166-170, 2005 10–52

Background.—Severe chronic pain is a long-term problem that may occur after inguinal hernia repair. The aim of this randomized study was to compare pain of any severity at 12 months after inguinal hernia repair with a partially absorbable lightweight mesh (LW group) or with a non-absorbable heavyweight mesh (HW group).

Methods.—Patients were assessed for pain at 1, 3 and 12 months by questionnaire, and were examined clinically at 12 months.

Results.—Some 321 patients were included in an intention-to-treat analysis, 162 in the LW group and 159 in the HW group. At 12 months, significantly fewer patients in the LW group than in the HW group had pain of any severity: 39.5 *versus* 51.6 per cent (difference −12.1 (95 per cent confidence interval −23.1 to −1.0) per cent; $P = 0.033$) (Tables 3 and 4). The recurrence rate was higher in the LW group (5.6 *versus* 0.4 per cent; $P = 0.037$) (Table 6). Five of eight recurrences in LW group were associated with a single participating centre.

Conclusion.—Use of lightweight mesh was associated with less chronic pain but an increase in hernia recurrence after inguinal hernia repair. The latter may be related to technical factors associated with fixation of such meshes rather than any inherent defect in the mesh.

▶ The authors emphasize that population-based studies and randomized clinical trials confirm that approximately 30% of patients have some variant of pain, and 3% report severe pain at 1 year after inguinal hernia repair.[1,2] The common explanation of such chronic pain is principally related to tissue necro-

TABLE 3.—Pain at 1 and 3 Months After Hernia Repair

	LW Group (n = 162)*	HW Group (n = 159)†	P‡
Pain at 1 month			
Yes	133 (82·1)	130 (81·8)	1·000
No	29 (17·9)	29 (18·2)	
Pain at 3 months			
Yes	92 (56·8)	90 (56·6)	1·000
No	70 (43·2)	69 (43·4)	

Values in parentheses are:
*Percentages or
†95 per cent confidence intervals.
‡Fisher's exact test.
Abbreviations: LW, Lightweight mesh; *HW,* heavyweight mesh.
(Courtesy of O'Dwyer PJ, Kingsnorth AN, Molloy RG, et al: Randomized clinical trial assessing impact of a lightweight or heavyweight mesh on chronic pain after inguinal hernia repair. *Br J Surg* 92:166-170, 2005, Blackwell Science Ltd.)

TABLE 4.—Visual Analogue Pain Scores at 1 and 3 Months

	Pain Score (Visual Analogue Scale)		
	LW Group (n = 162)	HW Group (n = 159)	P*
At rest			
Preoperative	10·1 (17·1)	10·3 (16·4)	
1 month	8·3 (12·0)	9·7 (16·9)	0·440
3 months	5·2 (11·4)	6·6 (16·7)	0·857
When moving			
Preoperative	17·1 (22·4)	17·9 (21·6)	
1 month	13·4 (16·7)	14·8 (20·5)	0·941
3 months	8·2 (15·1)	8·7 (17·3)	0·921

Values are mean(s.d.).
*Mann-Whitney *U* test.
Abbreviations: LW, Lightweight mesh; *HW,* heavyweight mesh.
(Courtesy of O'Dwyer PJ, Kingsnorth AN, Molloy RG, et al: Randomized clinical trial assessing impact of a lightweight or heavyweight mesh on chronic pain after inguinal hernia repair. *Br J Surg* 92:166-170, 2005, Blackwell Science Ltd.)

sis, neurovascular injury, and/or the applications of bio-synthetic repair mesh. This study was implemented by O'Dwyer et al of the UK and Germany to resolve the prevailing question for type of material (rigid vs smooth) and its effect on postoperative pain and recovery following laparoscopic inguinal hernia repair.

This randomized clinical trial compared outcome after inguinal hernia repair using absorbable-lightweight mesh or non-absorbable-heavyweight mesh. The article suggests that at 1 month and 3 months, there is no statistical variance of the pain experienced between the 2 types of mesh repairs. Moreover, the visual analogue pain scores at 1 and 3 months were not different at rest or in motion between the 2 groups. However, between the 2 group repairs, LW had a higher statistical recurrence rate (5.6 vs 0.7%; P = .037).

The authors support the hypothesis that a reduction in the total volume of mesh left in situ after the repair will reduce chronic inguinal pain. It is important, as emphasized by the authors, that the increasing rate of hernia recurrence with use of the LW warrants further research. It would appear, and we agree, that this higher recurrence rate may be related to the size of the suture

TABLE 6.—Clinical Outcome at 12 Months

	LW Group (n = 142)	HW Group (n = 142)	P†
Recurrence*	8 (5·6)	1 (0·7)	0·037
Contralateral hernia	2 (1·4)	4 (2·8)	0·684
Testicular atrophy	2 (1·4)	0 (0)	0·246
Wound sinus	0 (0)	0 (0)	—

Values in parentheses are percentages.
*Analysis performed with respect to numbers who completed postoperative assessment.
† Fisher's exact test.
Abbreviations: LW, Lightweight mesh; *HW,* heavyweight mesh.
(Courtesy of O'Dwyer PJ, Kingsnorth AN, Molloy RG, et al: Randomized clinical trial assessing impact of a lightweight or heavyweight mesh on chronic pain after inguinal hernia repair. *Br J Surg* 92:166-170, 2005, Blackwell Science Ltd.)

purchase within the mesh rather than to any inherent defects in the biosynthetic material used.

K. I. Bland, MD

References

1. Bay-Nielsen M, Perkins FM, Kehlet H: Pain and functional impairment 1 year after inguinal herniorrhapy: A nationwide questionnaire study. *Ann Surg* 233:1-7, 2001.
2. MRC Laparoscopic Groin Hernia Trial Group: Laparoscopic versus open repair of groin hernia: A randomised comparison. *Lancet* 354;185-190, 1999.

A Prospective, Randomized, Double-Blind Comparison of Unilateral Spinal Anesthesia With Hyperbaric Bupivacaine, Ropivacaine, or Levobupivacaine for Inguinal Herniorrhaphy

Casati A, Moizo E, Marchetti C, et al (Vita-Salute Univ of Milano, Italy; Univ of Parma, Italy)

Anesth Analg 99:1387-1392, 2004 10–53

Introduction.—In 60 patients undergoing inguinal hernia repair, we compared the clinical profile of unilateral spinal anesthesia produced with either 8 mg of hyperbaric bupivacaine 0.5% ($n = 20$), 8 mg of hyperbaric levobupivacaine 0.5% ($n = 20$), or 12 mg of hyperbaric ropivacaine 0.5% ($n = 20$). The study drug was injected slowly through a 25-gauge Whitacre directional needle and patients maintained the lateral decubitus position for 15 min. The onset time and intraoperative efficacy were similar in the three groups. The maximal level of sensory block on the operative and nonoperative sides was T6 (T12-5) and L3 (/[no sensory level detectable]-T4) with bupivacaine, T8 (T12-5) and L3 (/-T3) with levobupivacaine, T5 (T10-2) and T11 (/-T3) with ropivacaine ($P = 0.11$, $P = 0.23$, respectively). Complete regression of spinal anesthesia occurred after 166 ± 42 min with ropivacaine, 210 ± 63 min with levobupivacaine, and 190 ± 51 min with bupivacaine ($P = 0.03$ and $P = 0.04$, respectively); however, no differences were observed in time for home discharge (329 ± 89 min with bupivacaine, 261 ± 112 min with levobupivacaine, and 332 ± 57 min with ropivacaine [$P = 0.28$]). We conclude that 8 mg of levobupivacaine or 12 mg of ropivacaine are acceptable alternatives to 8 mg of bupivacaine when limiting spinal block at the operative side for inguinal hernia repair.

► The fast onset and the effective reproducible motor and sensory blockade with spinal anesthesia has gained high acceptance among surgeons in the treatment of inguinal herniorrhaphy. This is the first study conducted in a prospective, randomized, double-blind comparison to evaluate the pure S-enantiomers, ropivacaine, and levobupivacaine, as to their clinical efficacy when compared with bupivacaine. Patients receiving ropivacaine had faster resolution of spinal anesthesia compared with the other 2 analgesics; however, this drug was not associated with a significant acceleration of home discharge.

The interest in these 3 drugs occurred after the increasing evidence of transit neurologic symptoms (TNS) with spinal lidocaine.[1,2] Reducing the dosage of spinal lidocaine to 20 mg has been shown to reduce the incidence of TNS from 32% to 3.6%; however, intrathecal fentanyl was required for administration to provide adequate analgesia and results in postoperative nausea and vomiting in a significant percentage of patients.[2] Moreover, the incidence of TNS was nearly 3 times more frequent than that reported with bupivacaine.[2] Casati et al of the Departments of Anesthesiology in Milano and Parma, Italy, suggest in this double-blind study that 8 mg of levobupivacaine or 12 mg of ropivacaine are acceptable alternatives to 8 mg of bupivacaine between the surgeon and anesthesiologist to limit spinal anesthesia unilaterally for inguinal hernia repair.

K. I. Bland, MD

References

1. Pollock JE, Neal JM, Stephenson CA, et al: Prospective study of the incidence of transient radicular irritation in patients undergoing spinal anesthesia. *Anesthesiology* 84:1361-1367, 1996.
2. Freedman JM, Li DK, Drasner K, et al: Transient neurologic symptoms after spinal anesthesia: An epidemiologic study of 1,863 patients. *Anesthesiology* 89:633-641, 1998.

Randomized Clinical Trial Comparing the Prolene® Hernia System, Mesh Plug Repair and Lichtenstein Method for Open Inguinal Hernia Repair

Nienhuijs SW, van Oort I, Keemers-Gels ME, et al (Canisius-Wilhelmina Hosp, Nijmegen, The Netherlands)

Br J Surg 92:33-38, 2005 10–54

Background.—Most surgeons favour the use of a mesh for open inguinal hernia repair as it has a low recurrence rate. Procedures used most frequently are the Lichtenstein method, mesh plug repair and the Prolene Hernia System. The choice of technique may be influenced by the effects on postoperative pain and quality of life.

Methods.—A total of 334 patients were allocated blindly and at random to receive one of these three meshes for open hernia repair. Quality of life was assessed with the Short Form 36 and pain by a visual analogue scale 14 days, and 3 and 15 months after surgery.

Results.—Operative complications were rare and comparable between the groups. Long-term follow-up was completed by questionnaire in 95.8 per cent of patients. There were no significant differences in pain parameters between the three meshes; overall, 43.3 per cent of patients reported some form of groin pain. The severity of the chronic pain correlated with a higher pain score in the first 2 weeks after surgery ($P < 0.001$). A significant reduction in scores for role emotional (short term) and vitality (long term) quality of life domains was found in patients who had a Lichtenstein repair.

Conclusion.—These short- and long-term results did not show any clinically significant difference in postoperative pain and quality of life between the three types of mesh hernia repair. Severe early postoperative pain reliably predicted the likelihood of persisting chronic groin pain.

▶ The majority of inguinal hernia repairs internationally are completed with an open mesh technique, for which different prosthetic devices have been used. With the original descriptions by Lichtenstein for use of the mesh technique, additions such as Prolene Hernia System (Ethicon, Norderstedd, Germany) and mesh plug repair have been used. Each repair has a very low recurrence rate; as a consequence of these factors, the teaching hospital and the Departments of Surgery and Urology, Canisius-Wilhelmina Hospital, The Netherlands, attempted to provide a standard technique from an educational point of view. Thus, a comparison among the Prolene Hernia System, the Lichtenstein method, and mesh plug repair were simultaneously compared in a randomized clinical trial for 334 patients. These authors conclude that the short- and long-term results were equivalent statistically regarding postoperative pain and quality of life among the 3 types of repair. Of interest, early postoperative pain reliably predicts the probability of persistent chronic groin pain. In previous meta-analyses of randomized clinical trials, there were advantages for laparoscopic repair.[1] However, with laparoscopic approaches, operating times are longer, and there is a significant learning curve. The current study by Nienhuijs et al, however, confirms that reasonable results for surgeons can be achieved with a learning curve of only 5 procedures in this Netherlands teaching hospital.

K. I. Bland, MD

Reference

1. Memon MA, Cooper NJ, Memon B, et al: Meta-analysis of randomized clinical trials comparing open and laparoscopic inguinal hernia repair. *Br J Surg* 90:1479-1492, 2003.

Routine Ilioinguinal Nerve Excision in Inguinal Hernia Repairs

Dittrick GW, Ridl K, Kuhn JA, et al (Baylor Univ, Dallas)

Am J Surg 188:736-740, 2004 10–55

Background.—Chronic inguinal neuralgia is one of the most significant complications following inguinal hernia repair. Routine ilioinguinal nerve excision has been proposed as a means to avoid this complication. The purpose of this report is to evaluate the long-term outcomes of neuralgia and paresthesia following routine ilioinguinal nerve excision compared to nerve preservation.

Methods.—Retrospective chart review identified 90 patients who underwent Lichtenstein inguinal hernia repairs with either routine nerve excision (n = 66) or nerve preservation (n = 24). All patients were contacted and data were collected on incidence and duration of postoperative neuralgia and paresthesia. Comparison was made by χ^2 analysis.

Results.—The patients with routine neurectomy were similar to the group without neurectomy based on gender (male/female 51/15 vs. 19/5) and mean age (68 ± 14 vs. 58 ± 18 years). In the early postoperative period (6 months), the incidence of neuralgia was significantly lower in the neurectomy group versus the nerve preservation group (3% vs. 26%, P <0.001). The incidence of paresthesia in the distribution of the ilioinguinal nerve was not significantly higher in the neurectomy group (18% vs. 4%, P = 0.10). At 1 year postoperatively, the neurectomy patients continued to have a significantly lower incidence of neuralgia (3% vs. 25%, P = 0.003). The incidence of paresthesia was again not significantly higher in the neurectomy group (13% vs. 5%, P = 0.32). In patients with postoperative neuralgia, mean severity scores on a visual analog scale (0-10) were similar in neurectomy and nerve preservation patients at all end points in time (2.0 ± 0.0 to 2.5 ± 0.7 vs. 1.0 ± 0.0 to 2.2 ± 1.5). In patients with postoperative paresthesia, mean severity scores on a visual analog scale (0-10) were similar in the neurectomy and nerve preservation patients at 1 year (2.5 ± 2.2 vs. 4.0 ± 0.0) and 3 years (3.5 ± 2.9 vs. 4.0 ± 0.0).

Conclusions.—Routine ilioinguinal neurectomy is associated with a significantly lower incidence of postoperative neuralgia compared to routine nerve preservation with similar severity scores in each group. There is a trend towards increased incidence of subjective paresthesia in patients undergoing routine neurectomy at 1 month, but there is no significant increase at any other end point in time. When performing Lichtenstein inguinal hernia repair, routine ilioinguinal neurectomy is a reasonable option.

► Postoperative neuralgia can be a significant adverse outcome after inguinal herniorrhaphy, and it has reportedly been litigious in 5% to 7% of patients in several series. These authors demonstrate that the decision to do an ilioinguinal neurectomy at the time of operation can reduce the incidence of neuralgia significantly, without producing an increase in paresthesia in the groin. The surgeon who did neurectomies in this series did them routinely; that may not be the best decision. In a classic surgical procedure with a pristine ilioinguinal nerve coursing along the cord structures, cutting it arbitrarily seems meddlesome and unnecessary. Nonetheless, during intricate dissections with large or chronic or recurrent hernias, the election of identifying a proximal segment of the nerve and transecting it seems prudent to avoid potential injury and later neuralgia. I contest the implication of "routine" neurectomy and would agree with the authors that the issue should be addressed for the usual cases in a randomized controlled trial.

J. J. Gleysteen, MD

Preventing Parastomal Hernia With a Prosthetic Mesh: A Randomized Study

Jänes A, Cengiz Y, Israelsson LA (Umeå Univ, Sweden)

Arch Surg 139:1356-1358, 2004 10–56

Hypothesis.—Parastomal hernia is a common complication following colostomy. The lowest recurrence rate has been produced when repair is with a prosthetic mesh. This study evaluated the effect on stoma complications of using a mesh during the primary operation.

Design.—Randomized clinical study.

Methods.—Patients undergoing permanent colostomy were randomized to have either a conventional stoma or the addition of a mesh placed in a sublay position. The mesh used was a large-pore lightweight mesh with a reduced polypropylene content and a high proportion of absorbable material.

Results.—Twenty-seven patients had a conventional stoma, and in 27 patients the mesh was used. No infection, fistula formation, or pain occurred (observation time, 12-38 months). At the 12-month follow-up, parastomal hernia was present in 13 of 26 patients without a mesh and in 1 of 21 patients in whom the mesh was used.

Conclusions.—A lightweight mesh with a reduced polypropylene content and a high proportion of absorbable material placed in a sublay position at the stoma site is not associated with complications and significantly reduces the rate of parastomal hernia.

▶ After construction of a stoma, a parastomal hernia has been reported in up to half of patients regardless of the modification of the surgical technique used.[1-3] A lower frequency of stomal hernia has been reported when the stoma was created via the rectus abdominis muscle, although this has been contradicted in other studies.[4-6]

With the large frequency of recurrence rates that vary between 30% and 70%, necessity of stomal relocation, and after aponeurotic repair, some studies suggest an improvement in outcomes using prosthetic mesh repair.[7-11] As a consequence of these concerns, this study evaluates stomal complications in a randomized prospective trial receiving either a conventional stoma or the same procedure with the addition of lightweight mesh repair in a sublay position. Of importance, this mesh was trimmed to a 10×10 cm size. With the use of an absorbable stitch after transfer of the bowel via a crosscut in the center of the mesh, fixation to the lateral corners in the posterior rectus muscle sheath was assured. The mesh was placed dorsal to the rectus and anterior to the posterior rectus sheath. At 12 months of follow-up for parastomal hernia recurrence, 13 of 27 such hernias were evident in the no-mesh group, whereas 1 of 27 ($P = .001$) were evident in the mesh-applied group. Importantly, the authors have not explained in detail how there is absence of infection with placement of a prosthetic material near an open stoma. This could be explained by the inertness of the prosthetic bowel materials. Moreover, there was no fistulization and no increase in pain related to the application of the device.

Such long-term follow-up of these approaches are clearly important at 36 and 60 months to make certain that the latter 3 complications (pain, fistulization, and hernia) are not significantly increased.

K. I. Bland, MD

References

1. Birnbaum W, Ferrier P: Complications of abdominal colostomy. *Am J Surg* 83:64-67, 1952.
2. Abrams BL, Alskafi FH, Waterman NG: Colostomy: A new look at morbidity and mortality. *Am J Surg* 45:462-464, 1979.
3. Makela JT, Turko PH, Laitenen ST: Analysis of late stomal complications following ostomy surgery. *Ann Chir Gynaecol* 86:305-310, 1997.
4. Sjodahl R, Anderberg B, Bolin T: Parastomal hernia in relation to site of the abdominal stoma. *Br J Surg* 75:339-341, 1998.
5. Carne PW, Robertson GM, Frizelle FA: Parastomal hernia. *Br J Surg* 90:784-793, 2003.
6. Eldrup J, Wied U, Bishoff N, et al: Parakolostomihernier: Incidens og relation till stomiens placering. *Ugeskr Laeger* 144:3742-3743, 1982.
7. Martin L, Foster G: Parastomal hernia. *Ann R Coll Surg Engl* 78:81-84, 1996.
8. Rubin MS, Schoetz DJ Jr, Matthews JB: Parastomal hernia: Is stoma relocation superior to fascial repair? *Arch Surg* 129:413-418, 1994.
9. Kasperk R, Klinge U, Schumpetick V: The repair of large parastomal hernias using a midline approach and a prosthetic mesh in the sublay position. *Am J Surg* 179:186-188, 2000.
10. Stephenson BM, Phillips RK: Parastomal hernia: Local resiting and mesh repair. *Br J Surg* 82:1395-1396, 1995.
11. Amin SN, Armitage NC, Abercrombie JF, et al: Lateral repair of parastomal hernia. *Ann R Coll Sug Engl* 83:206-208, 2001.

Electron-Microscopic Alterations of the Peritoneum After Both Cold and Heated Carbon Dioxide Pneumoperitoneum

Erikoglu M, Yol S, Avunduk MC, et al (Selcuk Univ, Konya, Turkey; Ankara Univ, Turkey)

J Surg Res 125:73-77, 2005 10–57

Background.—Carbon-dioxide (CO_2) is used universally as an insufflation agent to create a laparoscopic pneumoperitoneum. In this study, we aimed to examine the electron and light microscopic alterations of the peritoneum after both cold-dry and heated-humidified CO_2 pneumoperitoneum.

Materials and Methods.—Thirty male Sprague-Dawley rats were used in this study. The rats were separated into three groups each comprising 10 rats. Group-I: (Control group): Gas insufflation was not applied to these animals. Group-II: These animals received standard cold-dry (21°C, 2% relative humidity) CO_2. Group-III: These animals received heated-humidified (40°C, 98% relative humidity) CO_2. In groups II and III, peritoneal gas was emptied 2 h after pneumoperitoneum application. All rats were killed after 12 h. Peritoneal samples were examined both by scanning electron and light microscopy by two different pathologists who were not aware of the groups.

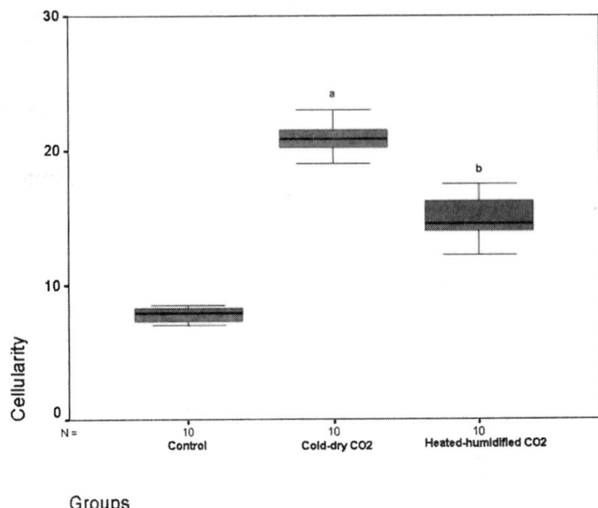

FIGURE 1.—Increased lymphocyte count significantly diminished by heated-humidified CO_2 application. (a) $P < 0.05$ according to control group, (b) P 0.05 according to group cold-dry CO_2 group. (Color version of figure is available online.) (Courtesy of Erikoglu M, Yol S, Avunduk MC, et al: Electron-microscopic alterations of the peritoneum after both cold and heated carbon dioxide pneumoperitoneum. *J Surg Res* 125:73-77, 2005. With permission from Elsevier Science.)

Results.—According to light microscopic examination; in group II and III, cellular response (increased lymphocyte) was significantly higher than the control group ($P < 0.01$). Similarly, in group II cellular response was significantly higher than group III. ($P < 0.01$). There was no difference in increased capillarity among all groups (Fig 1). ($P > 0.05$). According to scanning electron microscopic examination, in group I, normal peritoneum was covered by a sheet of flat mesothelial cells densely covered with microvilli. No intercellulary clefts and no free basal lamina were detected. In group II, drastic alterations of the surface layer were seen. The mesothelial cells had extreme desquamation, and the basal membrane was clearly visible. In group III, the mesothelial cells had bulged up to the surface layer and retracted. Intercellulary clefts become visible, but the basal lamina was not seen.

Conclusions.—Electron and light microscopic examination revealed that heated-humidified CO_2 results in less peritoneal alteration than cold-dry CO_2. Accordingly, we believe that heated-humidified CO_2 is more suitable for pneumoperitoneum application in laparoscopic surgery especially in selected cases.

► The increasing use of laparoscopy for both pediatric and adult patients is a world-wide movement and not one limited to Western economies. This article documents the diminished harmful effects of warm and humidified gas for the pneumoperitoneum when compared with cool, dry gas. The study shows that warming and humidifying the gases used for pneumoperitoneum cause less microscopic alterations in the peritoneum when evaluated by electron-microscopy than after the use of cool, dry gases. Heating and humidifying the infused gases is more costly. However, if it can be documented that the microscopic changes caused by dry air are associated with other negative effects such as the formation of intra-abdominal adhesions or increased third-space fluid losses or even hypothermia, the trouble and cost of humidifying and warming the gasses for pneumoperitoneum are worthwhile. Other questions that need to be answered are the effects of time. Is insufflation of less than 45 minutes as traumatic to the peritoneal tissues as the 2 hours of pneumoperitoneum as documented in this study? It does seem prudent for laparoscopic surgeons to consider the potential benefits of the use of warm and humidified CO_2 in preference to cool, dry CO_2 that is most commonly used for the development of a pneumoperitoneum.

K. E. Georgeson, MD

Simulator Training for Laparoscopic Suturing Using Performance Goals Translates to the Operating Room

Korndorffer JR Jr, Dunne JB, Sierra R, et al (Tulane Univ, New Orleans, La)

J Am Coll Surg 201:23-29, 2005 10–58

Background.—The purpose of this study was to develop a performance-based laparoscopic suturing curriculum using simulators and to test the effectiveness (transferability) of the curriculum.

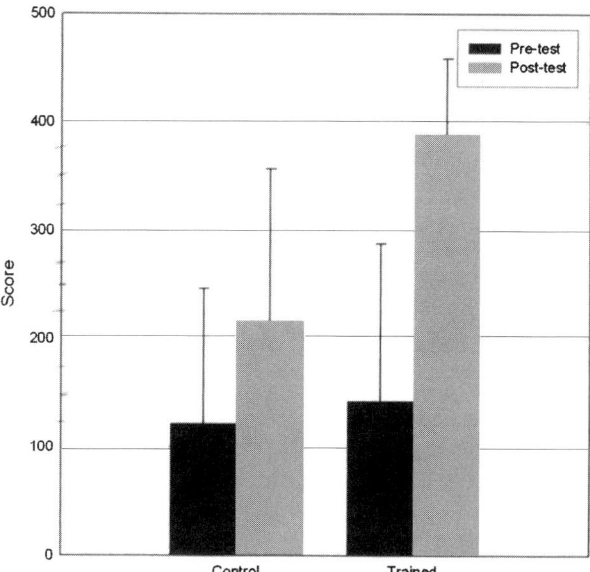

FIGURE 6.—Overall score (higher score indicates superior performance). Intragroup comparisons: Control pretest versus posttest, $p < 0.003$. Trained pretest versus posttest, $p < 0.001$. Intergroup comparisons: Pretest control versus trained, p = ns. Posttest control versus trained, $p < 0.001$. (Courtesy of Korndorffer JR Jr, Dunne JB, Sierra R, et al: Simulator training for laparoscopic suturing using performance goals translates to the operating room. *J Am Coll Surg* 201:23-29, 2005. By permission of the Journal of the American College of Surgeons.)

Study Design.—Surgical residents (PGY1 to PGY5, n = 17) proficient in basic skills, but with minimal laparoscopic suturing experience, were enrolled in an IRB-approved, randomized controlled protocol. Subjects viewed an instructional video and were pretested on a live porcine laparoscopic Nissen fundoplication model by placing three gastrogastric sutures tied in an intracorporeal fashion. A blinded rater objectively scored each knot based on a previously published formula (600 minus completion time [sec] minus penalties for accuracy and knot integrity errors). Subjects were stratified according to pretest scores and randomized. The trained group practiced on a videotrainer suturing model until an expert-derived proficiency score (512) was achieved on 12 attempts. The control group received no training. Both the trained and control groups were posttested on the porcine Nissen model.

Results.—For the training group, mean time to demonstrate simulator proficiency was 151 minutes (range 107 to 224 minutes) and mean number of attempts was 37 (range 24 to 51 attempts). Both the trained and control groups demonstrated significant improvement in overall score from baseline. But the trained group performed significantly better than the control group at posttesting (389 ± 70 versus 217 ± 140, $p < 0.001$), confirming curriculum effectiveness (Fig 6).

Conclusions.—These data suggest that training to a predetermined expert level on a videotrainer suture model provides trainees with skills that translate into improved operative performance. Such curricula should be further developed and implemented as a means of ensuring proficiency.

▶ This represents an important and confirmatory article that advocates a performance-based laparoscopic suturing protocol that uses simulators to test effectiveness and transferability of the curriculum to the operating room. After viewing an instructional video with pretesting in a live porcine laparoscopic Nissen fundoplication model with placement of 3 gastrogastric sutures in this model allowed evaluation of pretesting and posttesting proficiency. As one would expect, training to a predetermined expert level on a video trainer suture model enhances trainee performance with skills that translate into improvement in operation proficiency. Such curricula should be further developed and implemented as a measure of ensuring proficiency.

As indicated in the article, there is an overall score enhancement that is statistically significant in the posttest setting for both the control as well as the trained surgeon. Moreover, there is a significant difference in the posttest control versus trained surgeon, suggesting enhancement of technical proficiency. This proficiency-based curriculum will almost certainly be increasingly supported by universities and the American College of Surgeons for developing laparoscopic intracorporeal suturing skills for transfer to the operating room. One will expect many software and equipment companies to enhance the surgeon's proficiency after development of future teaching aids.

K. I. Bland, MD

Brief Communication of the Residency Review Committee–Surgery (RRC-S) on Residents' Surgical Volume in General Surgery

Bland KI, for the Members of the Residency Review Committee–Surgery (Univ of Alabama at Birmingham; et al)

Am J Surg 190:345-350, 2005 10–59

Background.—The Residency Review Committee–Surgery (RRC-S), 1 of 10 surgical specialties of the Accreditation Council for Graduate Medical Education (ACGME) has monitored the surgical volume of all general surgical residents closely. As a consequence of the reduction of duty hours with the limitation of an 80-hour work-week (averaged over 4 weeks), we were interested in the impact of these restrictions on surgical (volume) experience since its first year of implementation (2003-2004). Therefore, we evaluated the surgical volume of general surgical services since the implementation of the ACGME duty-hour restrictions and compared this volume with that of previous years without these duty limits.

Methods.—The Biostatistical Management Section of the ACGME implemented prospective analysis of categorized data for total surgical procedures and Chief Resident cases. The study interval included all resident surgical procedures completed from 1997 to 2004. We were interested particularly in evaluating trends and outcomes after the first year of successful full compliance of the 80-hour work week. Specific evaluations included the impact on surgical programs for total major procedures and Chief Resident cases requisite for application to the American Board of Surgery.

Results.—The average number of total major procedures for both resident and program averages were noted to increase steadily through the academic years of evaluation (1997-2001). A sharp decrease was evident in the

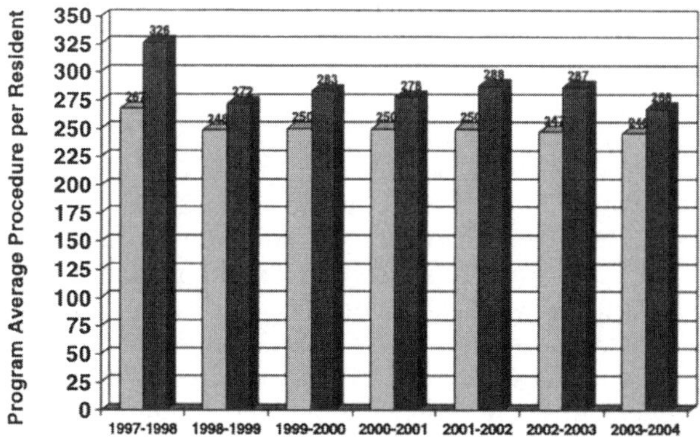

FIGURE 5.—Evaluation of the average (per resident) of surgical procedures completed as Chief Resident surgeon in the specialty of general surgery (1997-1998 through 2003-2004). These data have simultaneous comparisons for programs that were allowed ACGME-approved exemptions for duty-hour requirements (88 h/wk averaged over 4 weeks). The data suggest that for these limited evaluation parameters, no statistical differences are noted for the exempt programs from year to year, inclusive of the academic year 2003-2004. (Reprinted from Bland KI, for the Members of the Residency Review Committee–Surgery: Brief Communication of the Residency Review Committee–Surgery (RRC-S) on residents' surgical volume in general surgery. *Am J Surg* 190:345-350, 2005, with permission from Excerpta Medica Inc.)

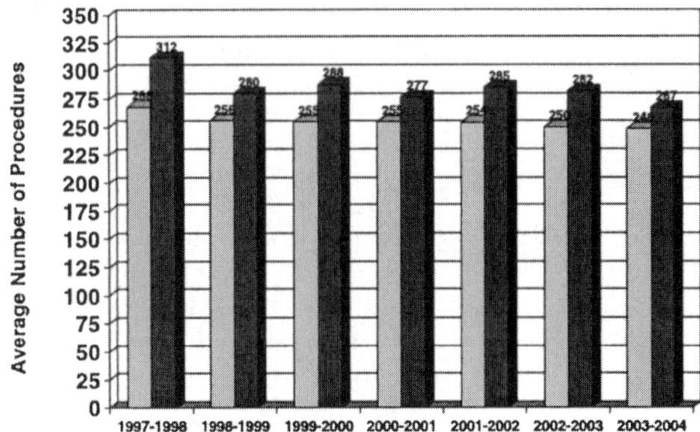

FIGURE 6.—Average (per program) of resident surgical procedures as chief surgeon in general surgery for the academic years 1997-1998 through 2003-2004. these datasets provide side-by-side comparisons of duty-hour exception versus nonexception programs. Greater numbers of cases were performed for the programs in which exemption for the 88-hour work week was granted by the RRC-S. Since the implementation of the duty-hour restrictions in July of 2003, these exceptions have not indicated a reduction in Chief Resident cases for the academic year 2003-2004. (Reprinted from Bland KI, for the Members of the Residency Review Committee–Surgery: Brief Communication of the Residency Review Committee–Surgery (RRC-S) on residents' surgical volume in general surgery. *Am J Surg* 190:345-350, 2005, with permission from Excerpta Medica Inc.)

total major procedures for the academic year 2001-2002 that relates to a correction of the biostatistical database implemented by the ACGME to correct a system conversion that began in the academic year 2001-2002. Despite significant changes to the system data mappings, beginning in the academic year 2001, this reduction is explained by the total counted surgeries as major that were eliminated in a revised counting methodology. It was evident on evaluation of the average (of averages) for major surgical procedures per resident (per program) in academic years 1997 to 2004 that the number of procedures was not statistically different in the academic years evaluated when compared with the year for implementation of duty-hour standards (2003-2004). Data analysis further indicates that the average procedures (per resident) performed as Chief Resident in general surgery remained stable from 1997 to 2004; the use of tiered *t* tests comparing Chief Resident averages (per program) for the academic years 2002-2003 versus 2003-2004 indicated that data remained consistent and confirmed no statistical variance in volumes during this interval (P = 0.43). Because some general surgery programs have exceptions for duty-hour requirements (n = 15) to allow an 88-hour week averaged over 4 weeks, these differences were of interest to evaluate programs with and without these duty-hour exceptions. Preliminary data with these limited parameters of evaluation suggest no detrimental outcomes related to the duty-hour restrictions for total major procedures per resident or for surgical procedures as Chief Residents for programs with and without these approved exceptions (Figs 5 and 6).

Conclusions.—RRCs that evaluate general surgery and surgical specialties have responded aggressively and professionally to implement the duty-hour standards per the ACGME. This brief report should be considered an interim communication to evaluate the surgical experience impact for programs currently under the restriction of duty-hour limits. The data provided in the first year of evaluation since the implementation of the 80-hour work-week restriction policy suggest that there has been no significant change in the overall surgical experience for major procedures (per resident), nor has there been a negative impact on Chief Resident surgical experience. A continuum of the prospective evaluation process is required by the RRC-S and other surgical specialties to ensure that requisite surgical volume is maintained throughout the entire 5 years of clinical surgery.

► The RRC-S is 1 of the 10 surgical subspecialties of the ACGME and monitors surgical operative volume of all general surgical residents. This communication by Bland and members of the RRC-S implemented a prospective analysis of categorized data for total surgical procedures and chief resident cases. This brief report should be considered only an interim communication to evaluate surgical experience, and is the first to evaluate surgical experience impact on programs currently under the 80-hour restriction duty-hour limit. These data suggest in the first year of evaluation since implementation of the 80-hour week requirement that there was no significant change in overall surgical experience for major procedures (per resident), nor has there been a negative impact for the average (per resident) number of surgical procedures completed as chief resident surgeon (1997-1998 through 2003-2004). The authors emphasize that a continuum of this prospective evaluation process will be required by the RRC-S and other surgical specialties to ensure that requisite surgical volume is maintained throughout the entire 5 years of clinical surgery. Such variance in these numbers could possibly affect competence if there is limitation of case numbers based on reduction of time on service with the 80-hour policy limits.

K. I. Bland, MD

11 Oncology

Introduction

This year has seen several important paradigm shifts in the therapy for surgical oncology patients. We have seen an ever-growing trend for identifying either genes or molecular markers to more accurately stage patients or select them for appropriate therapies. Additionally, we have seen a very important trend toward more minimal surgeries and/or more emphasis on multidisciplinary approaches that allow patients to receive a combination of modalities usually with reduced toxicity. These trends will only continue and, in fact, accelerate over the next several years. The challenge for the practicing surgeon will be the continuing medical education necessary to stay up with these new trends, as well as learning the newer, more minimal invasive technical procedures.

In the area of breast cancer, these paradigms are very evident. In a paper from the National Surgical Adjuvant Breast and Bowel Project, investigators defined an algorithm to calculate the recurrence score utilizing 16 cancer related genes and 5 reference genes. Patients were stratified into risk groups, and the recurrence score was validated as quantifying the likelihood of distant recurrence in Tamoxifen-treated patients. Not all recurrence, however, is necessarily related to gene panels. In a paper from the British Columbia Cancer Agency, the authors studied a cohorts group of woman looking at lymphovascular invasion (LVI). LVI was found to be an adverse prognostic factor for relapse and survival in node-negative patients treated with mastectomy and systemic therapy. LVI, particularly when combined with premenopausal status, grade III histology, or estrogen receptor–negative tumors, identified patient subsets that had particularly high risk of local regional recurrence. Clearly, these patients will benefit from more aggressive adjuvant therapies. Immunohistochemistry is utilized as the most common test to determine estrogen receptor status and therefore predict hormone responsiveness. In a paper from Thomas Jefferson University, the authors studied GATA-3 expression to see if GATA expression influences response to estrogen. The association between GATA-3 expression and hormone responsiveness suggested GATA-3 may play an important role in the mechanism controlling response to estrogen. We've also seen the importance of careful clinical studies determining important paradigms for the management of patients with breast cancer. For example, in a study from the University of Basal, the authors studied a large group of prospective patients assessing axillary recurrence rate in breast cancer patients with negative sentinel lymph nodes or sentinel lymph nodes that had micrometastatic disease. The authors found that axillary recurrence in patients with negative sentinel lymph nodes or patients with sentinel lymph nodes who had micrometastatic disease did not occur more frequently after sentinel lymph node biopsy alone compared with results from the recent literature regarding breast cancer patients undergoing formal axillary lymph node dissection. The authors concluded that the presence of sentinel lymph node micrometastases does not seem to lead to axillary recurrence or distant disease. Their follow-up was one of the longest in the literature. Another important question that is frequently asked on the management of breast cancer patients is whether sentinel lymph node biopsy is necessary after an initial diagnosis of ductal carcinoma in situ. In a paper from the University of Texas M.D. Anderson Cancer Center, the authors concluded that sentinel lymph node biopsy should not be performed routinely for all patients with an initial diagnosis of ductal carcinoma in situ. Patients who are younger or who have large, particularly high-grade tumors might be patients who benefit from sentinel lymph node biopsy. Another important issue that faces surgeons is how to analyze the adequacy of resection intraoperatively when performing breast conserving surgery. In a paper from the University of Florida, Gainesville, the authors felt that frozen section analysis minimized the number of additional operations. Utilizing frozen sections, these authors avoided second operations and had a very high rate of breast-conserving therapy.

We are beginning to see more neoadjuvant treatment for patients with large tumors. In a study from the M.D. Anderson of patients with T3 tumors or ipsilateral supraclavicular nodal disease, the authors compared neoadjuvant chemotherapy and mastectomy with or without radiation from a group of 6 different institutional trials. The authors found that radiation therapy was not only of benefit in improving local control, but there was also an improvement in survival. Therefore, patients with large tumors, supraclavicular nodal disease, or 4 or more positive nodes are likely to benefit from adjuvant radiation therapy, even after mastectomy. A very important aspect in patients who undergo mastectomy is the current trend toward immediate reconstruction. One of the controversial areas is whether the patient should undergo definitive reconstruction, or whether an attempt at a tissue expander, which allows further treatment, should be performed. In a study from the University of California, San Francisco, the authors studied immediate transverse rectus abdominus myocutaneous breast reconstruction followed by radiation therapy. They found that radiation was safe and had minimal morbidity with no significant change in tissue volume. The authors further concluded that immediate breast reconstruction should be considered after mastectomy in spite of the need or even if the patient requires radiation therapy.

Finally, we are probably going to see new treatments for breast cancer. Already there have been some reports of cryoablation, focused ultrasound as a treatment for breast cancer. In a study from the University of Michigan Comprehensive Cancer Center, the authors studied patients after cryoablation looking specifically at the characteristics at ultrasound and mammography. They showed that the tumor size mammographic density and ultrasound characteristics may in fact all indicate the likelihood of complete cryoablation. Obviously, if these new technologies are to be utilized more in the therapy of patients with breast cancer, we will need to have a better handle on the radiographic follow-up findings.

Similar issues are important in the management of patients with colorectal cancer. In a manuscript from the Taipei Veterans General Hospital in Taiwan, the authors attempted to evaluate the possibility of adding carcinoembryonic antigen and carbohydrate antigen 19-9 into the current staging system by analyzing prognostic significance. These authors found that elevation of both antigens significantly worsened prognosis. The recommendation was that these antigens be added to the follow-up of colorectal cancer patients. In another study from Indiana University, the authors studied abnormal DNA in stool samples with the Hemoccult II fecal occult blood test. While the authors found that the majority of neoplastic lesions identified by colonoscopy were not detected by either occult blood or fecal DNA, they were able to show that fecal DNA detected a greater proportion of important colorectal neoplasia compared with fecal occult blood and did so without compromising the specificity of their test.

The role of laparoscopy in the management of colorectal cancer patients remains to be fully defined. In a study from St James University Hospital in Leeds, England, the authors compared short term endpoints of conventional versus laparoscopically assisted surgery. The authors concluded that laparoscopic-assisted surgery for carcinoma of the colon was as effective as open surgery. They raised an important cautionary note, however, that laparoscopic assisted anterior resection in rectal cancer was not fully justified. This has now become the basis of a consensus statement that laparoscopic-assisted rectal surgery should be performed in the context of clinical studies only, so that further evaluation can be performed before making any more definitive recommendation. In another paper from the University of Leeds, England, the authors studied bladder and sexual dysfunction after laparoscopic surgery. Laparoscopic rectal resection did not appear to adversely affect bladder function in these experts' hands. However, there didn't seem to be a trend toward worse male sexual function and was undoubtedly related to the rate of total mesorectal excision.

In patients who are present with a large rectal cancer, preoperative chemoradiation is usually recommended. In a study from the John Radcliffe Hospital in Oxford, England, the regimen utilized by the authors showed a high degree of regression of tumor. Overall survival was associated with down staging of tumor. In patients with sterilized tumors after preoperative surgery, local recurrence was not seen.

Another important question yet to be given a definitive answer in the management of rectal cancers is the role of transanal excision. In a paper from the Cleveland Clinic Foundation, the authors showed that there was a high rate of recurrence even in patients with T1 rectal tumors who had low-grade malignancies. The authors questioned the role of transanal excision alone and whether it would need to be combined with adjuvant therapies or whether resective surgery is a better alternative. These issues were also raised in a study from the Mayo Clinic where all locally excised rectal cancers (with a curative intent) that required radical surgery within 30 days were reviewed. The authors found that nodal involvement was quite common. The authors felt that radical surgery within 30 days did not appear to compromise outcome compared with primary radical surgery. Once again, this points up the very important aspect of preoperative staging. Radiographic means of evaluating will continue to improve; however, combining radiographic modalities with molecular and genetic staging will ultimately provide better information for surgeons determining what type of surgery to perform for rectal cancer. Finally, functional results following colonic J-pouch anastomosis after low interior resection for rectal cancer remains controversial. In a study from Kinki University in Osaka, Japan, the authors concluded that J-pouch reconstruction increased reservoir function and provided better outcome compared with a straight anastomosis. This was particularly true for the anastomoses that were very low down.

As newer chemotherapeutic agents such as irinotecan or oxaliplatin are utilized in treating patients with metastatic colorectal cancer to the liver, a major question is what impact the chemotherapy might have on the development of steatohepatitis, which could limit surgical options. This question was studied in a work by authors at Washington University School of Medicine in St Louis. Severe steatohepatitis was associated with preoperative administration of irinotecan or oxaliplatin, especially in obese patients. Certainly, in patients who have had these agents, preoperative biopsy may be indicated to rule out severe steatohepatitis that may limit contemplated resection.

Gallbladder cancer remains a difficult entity to treat, particularly when a patient presents with a large tumor. In a study from multiple centers in North America, the authors studied if increasing R0 resections resulted in improved survival. Patients who had margin-negative R0 resections did in fact have improved survival. Of course, R0 resections increased especially more recently during the time of the study. However, R0 resections were associated with higher morbidities, even in these experienced North American Centers.

Hepatocellular carcinoma has been treated with primary surgery and transplantation, yet these interventions are not uniformly successful. A multi-institution trial looked at immunotherapy directed against various antigens associated with hepatocellular carcinoma as a potential alternative treatment for this disease. The authors found an elevated frequency, a specific CD8 lymphocyte response to the vaccine antigens, suggesting that there may be a role for these antigens in a vaccine immunotherapy regimen for hepatocellular carcinoma. Further studies will be needed to optimize these vaccine regimens and establish the role of other adjuvants in making them more uniformly successful.

In a study from the University of Yamanashi, Japan, the authors determined that CD4 CD25 lymphocytes in regional lymph nodes in patients with gastric cancer were significantly higher in comparison with those in control populations of lymph nodes. The presence of these CD4+ CD25+ lymphocytes may impair cell-mediated and other immune recognition of tumor. Reducing the number of these "suppressor" lymphocytes may improve the response to other systemic therapies, especially immune therapies.

Determining metastatic from primary pancreatic lesions is difficult. In a multicenter study of EUS-guided fine-needle aspiration, the authors show that pancreatic metastases are an important cause of focal pancreatic lesions. Utilizing immunohistochemistry is important. Additionally, metastatic lesions tend to be somewhat more well-defined at the margins compared with primary pancreatic lesions.

In summary, surgeons who treat patients with solid tumors will recognize that the field is rapidly changing. Genetic diagnoses, molecular staging, and targeted therapies are all just around the corner. Surgical procedures have changed dramatically and are now more minimal invasive and placed in the context of multidisciplinary care. The surgical oncologist of the future will be comfortable in managing patients with these targeted agents and doing smaller, more focused operations. Keeping up with these changes will undoubtedly have a profound and positive impact on the patients whom we treat.

Timothy J. Eberlein, MD

Breast Cancer

A Multigene Assay to Predict Recurrence of Tamoxifen-Treated, Node-Negative Breast Cancer

Paik S, Shak S, Tang G, et al (Natl Surgical Adjuvant Breast and Bowel Project, Pittsburgh, Pa; Genomic Health, Redwood City, Calif; Univ of Pittsburgh, Pa; et al)

N Engl J Med 351:2817-2826, 2004 11–1

Background.—The likelihood of distant recurrence in patients with breast cancer who have no involved lymph nodes and estrogen-receptor-positive tumors is poorly defined by clinical and histopathological measures.

Methods.—We tested whether the results of a reverse-transcriptase-polymerase-chain-reaction (RT-PCR) assay of 21 prospectively selected genes in paraffin-embedded tumor tissue would correlate with the likelihood of distant recurrence in patients with node-negative, tamoxifen-treated breast cancer who were enrolled in the National Surgical Adjuvant Breast and Bowel Project clinical trial B-14. The levels of expression of 16 cancer-related genes and 5 reference genes were used in a prospectively defined algorithm to calculate a recurrence score and to determine a risk group (low, intermediate, or high) for each patient.

Results.—Adequate RT-PCR profiles were obtained in 668 of 675 tumor blocks. The proportions of patients categorized as having a low, intermediate, or high risk by the RT-PCR assay were 51, 22, and 27 percent, respectively. The Kaplan-Meier estimates of the rates of distant recurrence at 10 years in the low-risk, intermediate-risk, and high-risk groups were 6.8 percent (95 percent confidence interval, 4.0 to 9.6), 14.3 percent (95 percent confidence interval, 8.3 to 20.3), and 30.5 percent (95 percent confidence interval, 23.6 to 37.4). The rate in the low-risk group was significantly lower

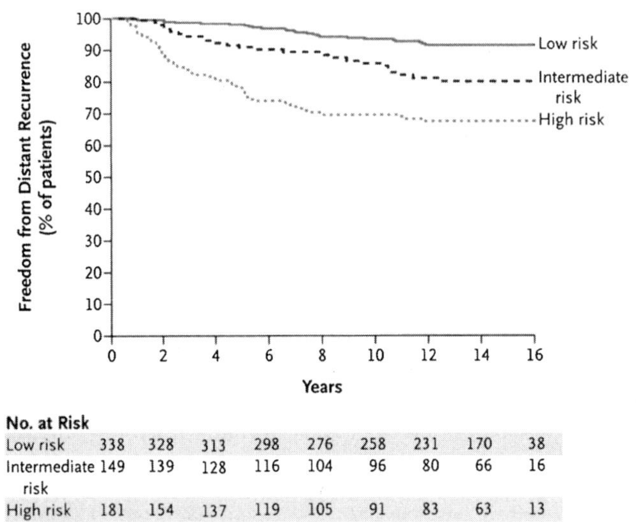

No. at Risk

Low risk	338	328	313	298	276	258	231	170	38
Intermediate risk	149	139	128	116	104	96	80	66	16
High risk	181	154	137	119	105	91	83	63	13

FIGURE 2.—Likelihood of distant recurrence, according to recurrence-score categories. A low risk was defined as a recurrence score of less than 18, an intermediate risk as a score of 18 or higher but less than 31, and a high risk as a score of 31 or higher. There were 28 recurrences in the low-risk group, 25 in the intermediate-risk group, and 56 in the high-risk group. The difference among the groups is significant (P<0.001). Reprinted by permission of The New England Journal of Medicine, from Paik S, Shak S, Tang G, et al: A multigene assay to predict recurrence of tamoxifen-treated, node-negative breast cancer. *N Engl J Med* 351:2817-2826, 2004, Copyright 2004. Massachusetts Medical Society. All rights reserved.)

than that in the high-risk group (P<0.001). In a multivariate Cox model, the recurrence score provided significant predictive power that was independent of age and tumor size (P<0.001). The recurrence score was also predictive of overall survival (P<0.001) and could be used as a continuous function to predict distant recurrence in individual patients.

Conclusions.—The recurrence score has been validated as quantifying the likelihood of distant recurrence in tamoxifen-treated patients with node-negative, estrogen-receptor-positive breast cancer (Fig 2).

► One of the most difficult issues facing the surgical oncologist is the prediction of recurrence in a patient with negative nodes and an estrogen–receptor-positive breast cancer. This study used an RT-PCR assay of 16 cancer-related and 5 referenced genes in paraffin-embedded tumor tissue. As seen in Figure 2, categorizing patients as low, intermediate, or high risk was significantly associated with prediction of recurrence. Even more importantly, the recurrence score of this panel of genes appeared to be independent of age or clinical tumor size in predicting the likelihood of recurrence.

Thus, this study was able to show in a prospectively defined gene expression assay the ability to quantify the likelihood of distant recurrence in patients treated with node-negative ER positive breast cancer who had been treated with tamoxifen. It is interesting to note that it appeared that the recurrence score was independent of tumor size. In fact, some patients with small tumors had intermediate- or high-risk recurrent scores. This kind of panel of gene analysis may be less subjective than standard tumor grading during pathologic evaluation. It is not known how the panel of 16 genes impacted the prediction of recurrence. That is, were they truly associated with the biology of breast cancer, or was the result somehow predictive of responsiveness to tamoxifen or perhaps a little of both. In the meantime, it is likely that these kinds of genetic predictive analyses will aid in selecting patients for likelihood of recurrence and, therefore, potentially more aggressive treatment.

T. J. Eberlein, MD

Lymphovascular Invasion Is Associated With Reduced Locoregional Control and Survival in Women With Node-Negative Breast Cancer Treated With Mastectomy and Systemic Therapy

Truong PT, Yong CM, Abnousi F, et al (British Columbia Cancer Agency-Vancouver Island Centre, Victoria, Canada; Univ of British Columbia, Canada; Vancouver Island Health Authority, Victoria, BC, Canada)

J Am Coll Surg 200:912-921, 2005 11–2

Background.—The impact of lymphovascular invasion (LVI) on postmastectomy locoregional relapse (LRR) and its use in guiding locoregional therapy in node-negative breast cancer are unclear. This study evaluates the association of LVI with relapse and survival in a cohort of women with early-stage breast cancer.

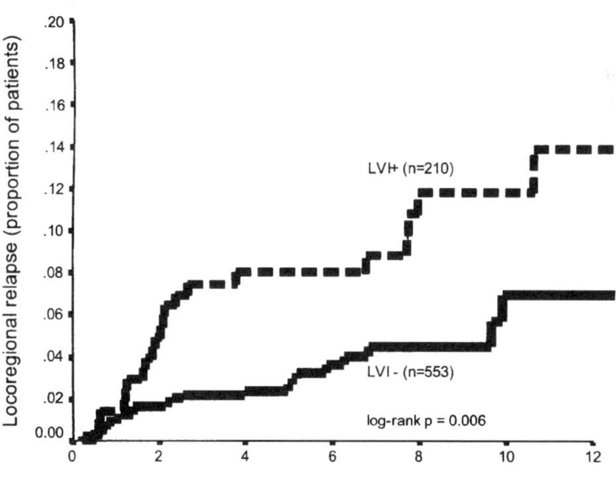

FIGURE 1.—Kaplan-Meier locoregional relapse curves stratified by lymphovascular invasion (LVI) status. (Reprinted from Truong PT, Yong CM, Abnousi F, et al: Lymphovascular invasion is associated with reduced locoregional control and survival in women with node-negative breast cancer treated with mastectomy and systemic therapy. *J Am Coll Surg* 200:912-921, 2005. Copyright 2005, with permission from the American College of Surgeons.)

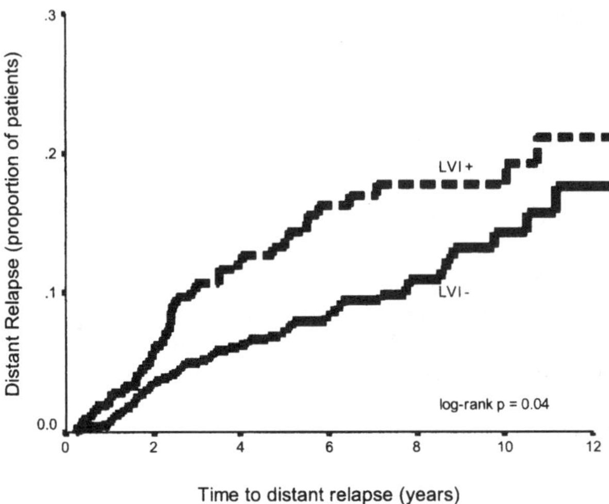

FIGURE 2.—Kaplan-Meier distant relapse curves stratified by lymphovascular invasion (LVI) status. (Reprinted from Truong PT, Yong CM, Abnousi F, et al: Lymphovascular invasion is associated with reduced locoregional control and survival in women with node-negative breast cancer treated with mastectomy and systemic therapy. *J Am Coll Surg* 200:912-921, 2005. Copyright 2005, with permission from the American College of Surgeons.)

Study Design.—The study cohort comprised 763 women with pT1-2, pN0 breast cancer referred from 1989 to 1999 and treated with mastectomy and adjuvant systemic therapy without radiotherapy. Kaplan-Meier LRR, distant relapse, and overall survival rates at 7 years were compared between

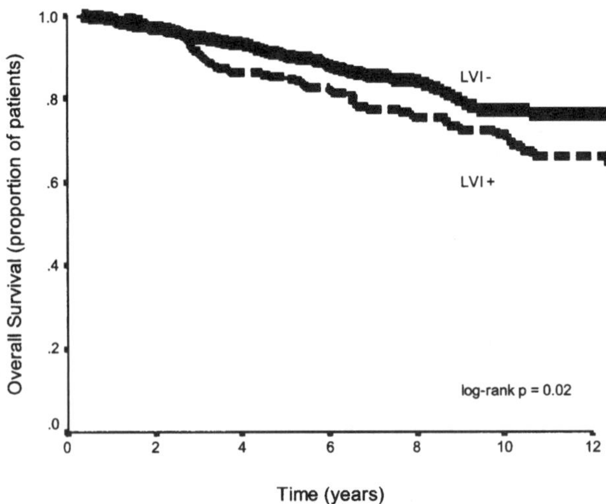

FIGURE 3.—Kaplan-Meier overall survival curves stratified by lymphovascular invasion (LVI) status. (Reprinted from Truong PT, Yong CM, Abnousi F, et al: Lymphovascular invasion is associated with reduced locoregional control and survival in women with node-negative breast cancer treated with mastectomy and systemic therapy. *J Am Coll Surg* 200:912-921, 2005. Copyright 2005, with permission from the American College of Surgeons.)

TABLE 2.—Cox Regression Analyses of Relapse and Overall Survival

	Locoregional Relapse			Distant Relapse			Overall Survival		
Variable	RR	95% CI	P Value	RR	95% CI	P Value	RR	95% CI	P Value
Age (< 50 versus ≥ 50 y)	1.44	0.49-4.22	0.51	1.67	0.74-3.79	0.22	1.38	0.65-2.94	0.40
Menopausal status (pre- versus postmenopausal)	0.95	0.32-2.88	0.93	0.69	0.30-1.57	0.38	0.37	0.17-0.80	0.01
Histology (lobular versus ductal)	2.35	0.86-6.42	0.10	0.65	0.26-1.64	0.36	0.69	0.36-1.32	0.26
T stage (T2 versus T1)	0.68	0.36-1.26	0.22	1.09	0.71-1.69	0.16	1.40	0.98-2.00	0.06
Grade (III versus I/II)	2.11	1.05-4.28	0.04	1.41	0.88-2.28	0.16	1.01	0.69-1.47	0.98
Lymphovascular invasion (present versus absent)	2.32	1.26-4.27	0.007	1.53	1.00-2.35	0.05	1.46	1.04-2.07	0.03
Estrogen receptor status (negative versus positive)	0.70	0.32-1.53	0.38	0.87	0.50-1.52	0.62	0.80	0.50-1.29	0.36
No. of nodes removed (≤10 versus >10)	1.09	0.59-2.00	0.79	0.82	0.54-1.26	0.36	0.85	0.60-1.20	0.36
Type of systemic therapy									
Chemotherapy alone versus chemotherapy and hormones	0.50	0.20-1.26	0.14	0.80	0.40-1.60	0.52	1.30	0.64-2.66	0.47
Hormone alone versus chemotherapy and hormones	0.42	0.16-1.09	0.07	0.72	0.36-1.43	0.35	1.33	0.71-2.50	0.38

Abbreviation: RR, Relative Risk.

(Reprinted from Truong PT, Yong CM, Abnousi F, et al: Lymphovascular invasion is associated with reduced locoregional control and survival in women with node-negative breast cancer treated with mastectomy and systemic therapy. *J Am Coll Surg* 200:912-921, 2005. Copyright 2005, with permission from the American College of Surgeons.)

patients with and without LVI. Cox regression analyses were performed to evaluate the prognostic significance of LVI for relapse and survival.

Results.—Median followup was 7.0 years (range 0.34 to 14.9 years). LVI was present in 210 (27.5%) patients. In log-rank comparisons of Kaplan-Meier curves stratified by LVI status, LVI-positive disease was associated with significantly higher risks of LRR (p = 0.006), distant relapse (p = 0.04), and lower overall survival (p = 0.02) (Figs 1-3). In the multivariable Cox regression analysis, LVI was significantly associated with LRR (relative risk [RR] = 2.32; 95% CI, 1.26-4.27; p = 0.007), distance relapse (RR = 1.53; 95% CI, 1.00-2.35; p = 0.05), and overall survival (RR = 1.46; 95% CI, 1.04-2.07; p = 0.03) (Table 2). In patients with one of the following characteristics: age younger than 50 years, premenopausal status, grade III histology, or estrogen receptor-negative disease, 7-year LRR risks increased threefold from 3% to 5% when LVI was absent, to 15% to 20% in the presence of LVI.

Conclusions.—LVI is an adverse prognostic factor for relapse and survival in node-negative patients treated with mastectomy and systemic therapy. LVI, in combination with age older than 50 years, premenopausal status, grade III histology, or estrogen receptor-negative disease, identified patient subsets with 7-year LRR risks of approximately 15% to 20%. Prospective research is required to define the role of adjuvant radiotherapy in these patients.

▶ An important question in the management of patients with breast cancer is the impact on LVI. This study with a median follow-up of 7 years analyzed almost 800 patients with node negative breast cancer, but with histologically positive evidence of LVI. LVI had a significant impact in LRR, distant relapse, and overall survival.

Results of this study support the hypothesis that LVI identifies patients at higher risk of relapse. While treating these patients with standard radiation techniques may increase long-term morbidity while reducing breast cancer-related deaths, new radiation therapy techniques, such as conformal radiotherapy, may minimize these long-term side effects. In addition, these patients who are LVI positive should participate in systemic trials because they clearly are at higher risk of distant relapse and would therefore benefit from adjuvant systemic therapies.

T. J. Eberlein, MD

GATA-3 Expression as a Predictor of Hormone Response in Breast Cancer

Parikh P, Palazzo JP, Rose LJ, et al (Thomas Jefferson Univ, Philadelphia)

J Am Coll Surg 200:705-710, 2005 11–3

Background.—Expression of estrogen receptor-alpha (ERα) as determined by immunohistochemistry of tumor tissue is currently the most clinically useful test to predict hormone responsiveness of breast cancer. Thirty percent of ERα-positive breast cancers do not respond to hormonal therapy.

TABLE 2.—Comparison of GATA-3 Expression in Cases (Hormone Unresponsive) and Age-Matched Controls (Hormone Responsive), Using Various Definitions of GATA-3 Positivity (Cut Points)

Positive Cut Point	Negative Cases		Negative Controls				
for GATA-3+	n	%	n	%	OR	95% CI	p Value
>10%	3	21	0	0	3.85	0.41, ∞	0.250
>20%	6	43	0	0	8.17	1.18, ∞	0.031
>30%	7	50	0	0	9.61	1.44, ∞	0.016
>40%	7	50	1	7	8.17	1.18, ∞	0.031
>50%	7	50	3	21	3.00	0.54, 30.39	0.289

Abbreviations: 95% CI, Confidence interval; *OR,* odds ratio.

(Reprinted from Parikh P, Palazzo JP, Rose LJ, et al: GATA-3 expression as a predictor of hormone response in breast cancer. *J Am Coll Surg* 200:705-710, 2005.)

GATA-3 is a transcription factor that is expressed in association with ERα and there is evidence that GATA factors influence response to estrogen. In this pilot study, we investigated whether GATA-3 expression is associated with hormone response in breast cancer.

Study Design.—Breast cancer tissue was stained for GATA-3 expression by immunohistochemistry in ERα-positive cancers from 28 patients, 14 of whom were defined as hormone unresponsive (cases) and 14 of whom were age-matched controls with hormone-responsive, ERα-positive cancers (controls).

Results.—Comparing cases and controls, there were no differences in expression of ERα; progesterone receptor, ErbB2; or tumor grade. Using 20% nuclear staining to characterize tumors as GATA-3 positive or GATA-3 negative, 6 of 14 (43%) cancers in the hormone-unresponsive group and none of the controls were classified as GATA-3 negative (odds ratio, 8.2; 95% confidence interval, 1.2-∞; $p = 0.031$) (Table 2). Using different cut points to characterize GATA-3 positivity yielded very similar results, indicating a positive association between lack of GATA-3 expression and lack of response to hormonal therapy.

Conclusions.—The study suggests that analyzing ERα-positive breast tumors for GATA-3 using immunohistochemistry might improve prediction of hormone responsiveness. The association between GATA-3 expression and hormone response suggests that GATA-3 may play a role in mechanisms controlling response to estrogen.

► In most institutions expression of ERα is determined by immunohistochemistry. Approximately 30% of ERα-positive patients do not respond to hormone therapy. GATA-3 is a transcription factor that is expressed in association with ERα and may well influence response to estrogen. These authors utilized a 20% cut-off to characterize tumors as GATA-3 positive or negative. GATA-3 expression correctly predicted 43% of the cancers in the hormone unresponsive group and none of the controls.

This study suggests that GATA-3 might improve prediction of hormone responsiveness in ERα-positive breast cancers. There are some limitations to this study, most notable of which is its relatively small sample size. No adjustments were made for other markers of hormone response. In addition, a formal determinant of optimal GATA-3 positivity was not determined in this relatively small study.

Future studies may address whether GATA-3 expression may also be used to predict hormone response among patients with ERα-negative breast cancers. Further work defining the mechanisms by which this transcription factor alters the clinical course of breast cancer has yet to be determined.

T. J. Eberlein, MD

Axillary Recurrence Rate in Breast Cancer Patients With Negative Sentinel Lymph Node (SLN) or SLN Micrometastases: Prospective Analysis of 150 Patients After SLN Biopsy

Langer I, Marti WR, Guller U, et al (Univ of Basel, Switzerland; Kantonsspital, Olten, Switzerland)

Ann Surg 241:152-158, 2005 11–4

Objective.—To assess the axillary recurrence rate in breast cancer patients with negative sentinel lymph node (SLN) or SLN micrometastases (>0.2 mm to ≤2.0 mm) after breast surgery and SLN procedure without formal axillary lymph node dissection (ALND)

Summary Background Data.—Under controlled study conditions, the SLN procedure proved to be a reliable method for the evaluation of the axillary nodal status in patients with early-stage invasive breast cancer. Axillary dissection of levels I and II can thus be omitted if the SLN is free of macrometastases. The prognostic value and potential therapeutic consequences of SLN micrometastases, however, remain a matter of great debate. We present the follow-up data of our prospective SLN study, particularly focusing on the axillary recurrence rate in patients with negative SLN and SLN micrometastases.

Methods.—In this prospective study, 236 SLN procedures were performed in 234 patients with early-stage breast cancer between April 1998 and September 2002. The SLN were marked and identified with 99m technetium-labeled colloid and blue dye (Isosulfanblue 1%). The excised SLNs were examined by step sectioning and stained with hematoxylin and eosin and immunohistochemistry (cytokeratin antibodies Lu-5 or CK 22). Only patients with SLN macrometastases received formal ALND of levels I and II, while patients with negative SLN or SLN micrometastases did not undergo further axillary surgery.

Results.—The SLN identification rate was 95% (224/236). SLN macrometastases were found in 33% (74/224) and micrometastases (>0.2 mm to ≤2 mm) in 12% (27/224) of patients. Adjuvant therapy did not differ between the group of SLN-negative patients and those with SLN micrometastases. After a median follow-up of 42 months (range 12-64 months), 99% (222/224) of evaluable patients were reassessed. While 1 patient with a negative SLN developed axillary recurrence (0.7%, 1/122), all 27 patients with SLN micrometastases were disease-free at the last follow-up control.

Conclusions.—Axillary recurrences in patients with negative SLN or SLN micrometastases did not occur more frequently after SLN biopsy alone compared with results from the recent literature regarding breast cancer patients undergoing formal ALND. Based on a median follow-up of 42 months—one of the longest so far in the literature—the present investigation does not provide evidence that the presence of SLN micrometastases leads to axillary recurrence or distant disease and supports the theory that formal ALND may be omitted in these patients.

► The status of the ALNs in breast cancer is 1 of the most important prognostic indicators and is certainly a major determinant in the recommendation of adjuvant therapies. One of the major questions is whether a negative SLN or an SLN with micrometastatic disease predicts for metastatic recurrence or is more consistent with a negatively staged axilla. This article from the Department of Surgery in Basel, Switzerland analyzes 150 prospective patients after SLN biopsy. Their follow-up—42 months—is one of the longest in the literature and shows that the presence of SNL micrometastases is not associated with an increase in axillary recurrence or distant disease.

This question will be better answered in the ACOSOG randomized prospective trial. However, in the meantime, this study suggests that in patients with micrometastatic disease in the axilla, formal ALND may be omitted. Certainly, in the patients who received radiation therapy, the port can be extended to the low axilla with relatively little morbidity. After further studies are done, perhaps all therapy to the axilla can be omitted in patients with micrometastatic disease.

T. J. Eberlein, MD

Predictors of Invasive Breast Cancer in Patients With an Initial Diagnosis of Ductal Carcinoma In Situ: A Guide to Selective Use of Sentinel Lymph Node Biopsy in Management of Ductal Carcinoma In Situ

Yen TWF, Hunt KK, Ross MI, et al (Univ of Texas MD Anderson Cancer Ctr, Houston)

J Am Coll Surg 200:516-526, 2005 11–5

Background.—The role of sentinel lymph node biopsy (SLNB) in patients with an initial diagnosis of ductal carcinoma in situ (DCIS) has not been well defined. The purpose of our study was to determine when the risk of finding invasive disease on final pathology in patients with an initial diagnosis of DCIS was sufficiently high to justify use of SLNB.

Study Design.—The records of 398 consecutive patients from our prospective database with an initial diagnosis of DCIS, treated between July 1999 and December 2002, were analyzed. Associations between clinical and pathologic factors and patient selection for SLNB and outcomes were analyzed for significance using univariate (Table 5) and multivariate analyses.

Results.—Of the 398 patients, 80 (20%) were found to have invasive disease on final pathology. Multivariate analysis revealed 4 independent predictors of invasive cancer on final pathology: 55 years of age or younger (odds ratio [OR], 2.19; $p = 0.024$), diagnosis by core-needle biopsy (OR, 3.76; $p = 0.006$), mammographic DCIS size of at least 4 cm (OR, 2.92; $p = 0.001$), and high-grade DCIS (OR, 3.06; $p = 0.002$). A total of 141 patients (35%) underwent SLNB as a component of their initial operation. Multivariate analysis revealed that the presence of comedonecrosis (OR, 2.69; p =

TABLE 5.—Predictors of a Positive Sentinel Lymph Node in Patients With an Initial Diagnosis of Ductal Carcinoma In Situ Who Underwent Sentinel Lymph Node Biopsy

Clinicopathologic Feature	Negative SLNB (n = 127)	Positive SLNB (n = 14)	*P* Value*
Median age at diagnosis (y)	53.6	49.1	0.056
Range	35–79	29–67	
Palpable lesion, n (%)	19 (15)	6 (43)	0.009
Median mammographic DCIS size (cm)	3.5	5.75	0.031‡
Range†	0.3–12 vm	1.3–13 cm	
Tumor grade, n (%)			0.652§
1	2 (1)	0	
2	44 (35)	6 (43)	
3	81 (64)	8 (57)	
Median pathologic DCIS size (cm)	2	5	0.376‡
Range‖	0.15–10	0.3–8	
Comedonecrosis, n (%)			0.794¶
Present	101 (80)	11 (79)	
Absent	23 (18)	3 (21)	
Unknown	3 (2)	0	
Final pathology, n (%)			0.001§
Invasive cancer	29 (23)	10 (71)	
DCIS with microinvasion	2 (1)	1 (7)	
DCIS	96 (76)	3 (21)	
Type of final operation, n (%)			0.958
Segmental mastectomy	28 (22)	3 (21)	
Total mastectomy	99 (78)	11 (79)	

*p value calculated by Pearson chi-square test unless otherwise noted.
†Based on 90 patients with a negative SLNB and 16 patients with a positive SLNB for whom mammographic DCIS size was known.
‡p value calculated by Mann-Whitney U test.
§p value calculated by Fisher's exact test.
‖Based on 96 patients with a negative SLNB and 7 patients with a positive SLNB for whom pathologic DCIS size was known.
¶Excludes patients with unknown values.
Abbreviations: DCIS, Ductal carcinoma in situ; *SLNB,* sentinel lymph node biopsy.
(Reprinted from Yen TWF, Hunt KK, Ross MI, et al: Predictors of invasive breast cancer in patients with an initial diagnosis of ductal carcinoma in situ: A guide to selective use of sentinel lymph node biopsy in management of ductal carcinoma in situ. *J Am Coll Surg* 200:516-526, 2005. Copyright 2005, with permission from the American College of Surgeons.)

0.007) and larger mammographic DCIS size (OR, 1.18; p = 0.0002) were independent predictors of patients' undergoing SLNB. Of these 141 patients, 103 (73%) were diagnosed by core-needle biopsy, 42 (30%) had invasive disease on final pathology, and 14 (10%) had a positive sentinel lymph node: 12 (86%) by hematoxylin and eosin staining and 2 by immunohistochemistry. The only independent predictor of a positive SLN was the presence of a palpable tumor (OR, 4.28, p = 0.042). Of these 14 patients with a positive sentinel node, only 11 (79%) had invasive cancer on final pathology.

Conclusions.—SLNB should not be performed routinely for all patients with an initial diagnosis of DCIS. Risks and benefits of SLNB should be discussed with patients who are younger, are diagnosed by core-needle biopsy, or have large or high-grade DCIS.

▶ This is a large study of 398 consecutive patients from the M.D. Anderson database. One of the important questions in surgeons who take care of patients with breast cancer, particularly DCIS, is to determine the risk of finding invasive disease on final pathology tests and whether justification of SLNB is upheld.

In this study, younger patients, those patients who had a core biopsy of infiltrating cancer, were large size of the DCIS, particularly high grade, was associated with SLNB. As seen in the article, however, a positive SLNB was particularly associated with a final pathology of invasive cancer, large size in comedo necrosis.

In the future, it will be important to have more precise predictors of potential positive SLNBs because of 141 SLNBs only 14 were positive. Until more precise markers are identified, large-sized comedo necrosis, particularly if invasive disease is documented, would seem to justify SLNB.

T. J. Eberlein, MD

Accuracy of Intraoperative Frozen-Section Analysis of Breast Cancer Lumpectomy-Bed Margins

Cendán JC, Coco D, Copeland EM III (Univ of Florida, Gainesville)

J Am Coll Surg 201:194-198, 2005 11–6

Background.—My colleagues and I have been using intraoperative frozen-section analysis (FSA) to evaluate lumpectomy margins in an attempt to reduce the number of additional operations that patients with ductal carcinoma in situ or stage I and II breast cancer would have to endure. We review our experience in breast-conservation therapy (BCT) at the University of Florida (Gainesville) to determine the effectiveness of this approach.

Study Design.—Operative reports, operative logs, and pathology reports were retrospectively reviewed for patients who had BCT from January 2001 to January 2004. Ninety-seven patients (116 operations) were reviewed.

Results.—Nineteen patients required an additional operation (19.6%). Forty-three patients had positive margins on paraffin-embedded histologic

TABLE 3.—Number of Slides Containing Tumor by Type

Pathology	Total No. of Slides	Tumor Present on FSA (n)	Tumor Present on Permanent Pathology n	%
Infiltrating ductal	374	11	16	4.2
Infiltrating lobular	45	13	18	40
DCIS	211	31	51	24.2

*Chi-square analysis reflects a difference in the anticipated distribution of these cases, $p < 0.001$, chi-square = 83.71.

Abbreviations: DCIS, Ductal carcinoma in situ; *FSA*, frozen-section analysis.

(Courtesy of Cendán JC, Coco D, Copeland EM III: Accuracy of intraoperative frozen-section analysis of breast cancer lumpectomy-bed margins. *J Am Coll Surg* 201:194-198, 2005. Reproduced by permission of the Journal of the American College of Surgeons).

analysis (44.3%). Accuracy of FSA was 84% when evaluated on a per-case basis, and 96% on a per-slide basis. False negatives were identified in 22 patients, affecting the operative pathway of 19 patients (19.6%) and were identified more frequently in cases of ductal carcinoma in situ ($p < 0.001$). There were no false positives. Additional operative time required for FSA was approximately 13 minutes per case. Eighty-four (86.6%) patients had successful BCT and 13 patients (13.4%) required mastectomy.

Conclusions.—Intraoperative analysis of margins using FSA is effective at minimizing the number of additional operations, with 19 patients benefiting from immediate intervention in this study. The authors believe that the number of second operations prevented and the high BCT rates justify performing FSA. Ductal carcinoma in situ is more difficult to identify in FSA. Preop-

TABLE 4.—Analysis of Margin Involvement Accuracy Stratified by Tumor Type

Pathology	Observed on FSA	Expected (Permanent)	Chi-Square, Two-Tailed *P* Value
Infiltrating ductal			
Tumor-bearing	11	16	0.202
No tumor	374	369	
Infiltrating lobular			
Tumor-bearing	13	18	0.128
No tumor	32	27	
DCIS			
Tumor-bearing	31	51	0.0013
No tumor	180	160	

Abbreviations: DCIS, Ductal carcinoma in situ; *FSA*, frozen-section analysis.

(Courtesy of Cendán JC, Coco D, Copeland EM III: Accuracy of intraoperative frozen-section analysis of breast cancer lumpectomy-bed margins. *J Am Coll Surg* 201:194-198, 2005. Reproduced by permission of the Journal of the American College of Surgeons).

erative discussions with the patient should reflect these findings (Tables 3 and 4).

► The gold standard in evaluating margin of breast-cancer resection is fixation and review by permanent histologic analysis. This obviously has limitations for intraoperative consultation. An alternative is to use FSA; however, adipose tissue is difficult to freeze. This report from the University of Florida is a 3-year retrospective analysis of all patients undergoing BCT. As can be seen in Table 3, the most common type of tumor with a positive margin was an infiltrating lobular cancer, followed by DCIS. Determining a positive margin by histologic analysis of both of these tumors is especially difficult if FSA is not performed. As seen in Table 4, DCIS was missed more often on FSA when compared with invasive cancers on permanent sections. The overall accuracy for FSA was 84% per case and 96% on the basis of slides.

Still, final pathologic status of margins is not known until permanent sections are available. Patients with DCIS and lobular invasive cancer are highest risk for needing an additional procedure because of a false-negative FSA.

T. J. Eberlein, MD

Postmastectomy Radiation Improves Local-Regional Control and Survival for Selected Patients With Locally Advanced Breast Cancer Treated With Neoadjuvant Chemotherapy and Mastectomy

Huang EH, Tucker SL, Strom EA, et al (Univ of Texas, Houston)
J Clin Oncol 22:4639-4647, 2004 11–7

Purpose.—To evaluate the efficacy of radiation in patients treated with neoadjuvant chemotherapy and mastectomy.

Patients and Methods.—We retrospectively analyzed the outcomes of 542 patients treated on six consecutive institutional prospective trials with neoadjuvant chemotherapy, mastectomy, and radiation. These data were compared to those of 134 patients who received similar treatment in these same trials but without radiation.

Results.—Irradiated patients had a lower rate of local-regional recurrence (LRR) (10-year rates: 11% v 22%, $P = .0001$). Radiation reduced LRR for patients with clinical T3 or T4 tumors, stage ≥ IIB disease (AJCC 1988), pathological tumor size >2 cm, or four or more positive nodes ($P \leq .002$ for all comparisons). Patients who presented with clinically advanced stage III or IV disease but subsequently achieved a pathological complete response to neoadjuvant chemotherapy still had a high rate of LRR, which was significantly reduced with radiation (10-year rates: 33% v 3%, $P = .006$). Radiation improved cause-specific survival (CSS) in the following subsets: stage ≥ IIIB disease, clinical T4 tumors, and four or more positive nodes ($P \leq .007$ for all comparisons). On multivariate analyses of LRR and CSS, the hazard ratios for lack of radiation were 4.7 (95% CI, 2.7 to 8.1; $P < .0001$) and 2.0 (95% CI, 1.4 to 2.9; $P < .0001$), respectively.

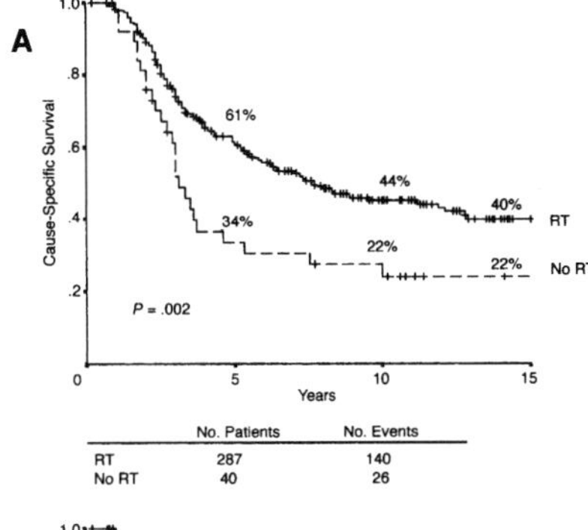

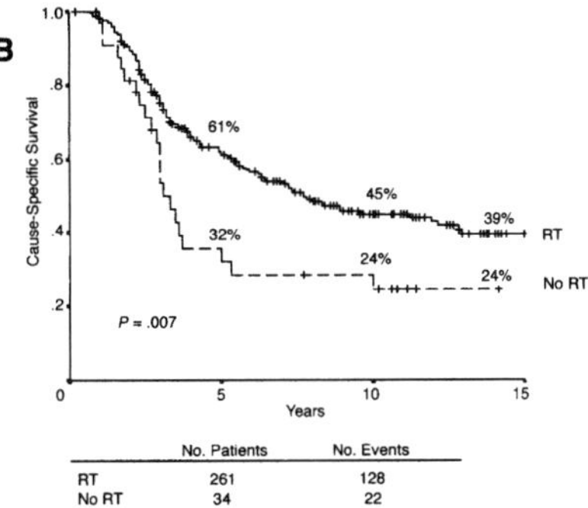

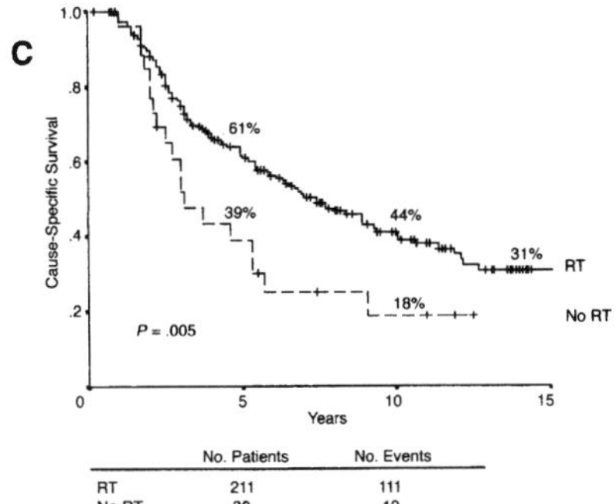

FIGURE 3.—A, Rate of cause-specific survival for patients with clinical stage IIIB to stage IV disease treated with radiation (*RT*) and without radiation (*No RT*). B, Rate of cause-specific survival for patients with clinical T4 tumors treated with RT and without. (C), Rate of cause-specific survival for patients with 4 or more positive nodes treated with and without RT. (Courtesy of Huang EH, Tucker SL, Strom EA, et al: Postmastectomy radiation improves local-regional control and survival for selected patients with locally advanced breast cancer treated with neoadjuvant chemotherapy and mastectomy. *J Clin Oncol* 22:4639-4647, 2004. Reprinted with permission from the American Society of Clinical Oncology.)

Conclusion.—After neoadjuvant chemotherapy and mastectomy, comprehensive radiation was found to benefit both local control and survival for patients presenting with clinical T3 tumors or stage III-IV (ipsilateral supraclavicular nodal) disease and for patients with four or more positive nodes. Radiation should be considered for these patients regardless of their response to initial chemotherapy (Fig 3 and Table 3).

▶ This is not a randomized prospective trial but rather a retrospective analysis of 6 different independent trials from M. D. Anderson Cancer Center. The commonality of each of these trials is that patients received neoadjuvant chemotherapy followed by mastectomy with or without radiation therapy. As seen in Table 3, large clinical stage tumors advanced nodal disease, in patients with more than 4 positive nodes tended to benefit from radiation therapy in an adjuvant setting. Once again, with a caveat that this is not a randomized trial, radiation therapy conferred CSS improvement for clinical stage IIIB (A), clinical T4 tumors (B) or 4 or more positive nodes (C) (Fig 3).

There are several limitations to this trial. The first is that it is a retrospective analysis. In addition, there is always the issue of possible postradiation morbidity. However, with increasingly more precision in modern radiation techniques, morbidity—particularly ischemic heart-related problems—should be minimized.

T. J. Eberlein, MD

TABLE 3.—Ten-Year Actuarial Rates of LRR According to Clinical and Pathological Disease Status

Factor	10-Year LRR Rate No Radiation (%)	Radiation %	*P*
Clinical T-stage			
T1	0	8	.535
T2	10	7	.408
T3	22	8	.002
T4	46	15	<.0001
Clinical N-stage			
N0	23	10	.014
N1	14	9	.062
N2-3	40	12	<.0001
Pathological tumor size, cm			
0-2	13	8	.051
2.1-5.0	31	14	.002
≥ 5.1	52	13	.001
No. of positive nodes			
0	11	4	.010
1-3	13	11	.636
≥ 4	59	16	<.0001

Abbreviation: LRR, Local-regional recurrence.

(Courtesy of Huang EH, Tucker SL, Strom EA, et al: Postmastectomy radiation improves local-regional control and survival for selected patients with locally advanced breast cancer treated with neoadjuvant chemotherapy and mastectomy. *J Clin Oncol* 22:4639-4647, 2004. Reprinted with permission from the American Society of Clinical Oncology.)

Safety of Immediate Transverse Rectus Abdominis Myocutaneous Breast Reconstruction for Patients With Locally Advanced Disease

Foster RD, Hansen SL, Esserman LJ, et al (Univ of California, San Francisco)
Arch Surg 140:196-200, 2005 11–8

Hypothesis.—Immediate transverse rectus abdominis myocutaneous breast reconstruction combined with postoperative radiation therapy after mastectomy is safe and effective.

Design.—Retrospective case series.

Setting.—University-based teaching hospital.

Patients.—From January 1, 1996, through December 31, 2003, 252 patients underwent mastectomy and immediate transverse rectus abdominis myocutaneous flap reconstruction. Of those, 35 patients received postoperative radiation therapy (stage I, n = 1; II, n = 17; III, n = 15; IV, n = 2). Age range was 29 to 72 years (mean, 49.5 years). Follow-up was 1 to 8 years (mean, 48 months).

Main Outcome Measures.—Flap loss, fat necrosis, flap volume loss, adjuvant treatment delay, and need for additional surgery.

Results.—The rate of flap survival was 100%. Median operative time was 5.5 hours. Average hospital stay was 5.2 days. Fat necrosis occurred in 3 patients, with volume loss requiring additional surgery in 2 patients (6%). Postoperative adjuvant therapy was not significantly delayed (median interval, 32 days). With a median follow-up of 48 months, local recurrence was present in only 1 patient (3%), who underwent successful local salvage, and distant metastasis occurred in 4 patients (11%).

Conclusions.—Immediate transverse rectus abdominis myocutaneous breast reconstruction followed by radiation therapy is safe, with minimal morbidity and no significant change in tissue volume. Complications tend to be minor, not delaying adjuvant therapy. Immediate breast reconstruction should be considered after mastectomy, despite the need for postoperative radiation therapy.

▶ One of the major questions regarding the patients who have a breast cancer requiring a mastectomy and possible postoperative radiation therapy is whether or not immediate reconstruction should be undertaken. This is particularly true if one contemplates utilization of immediate transverse rectus abdominis myocutaneous breast reconstruction.

Many plastic surgeons prefer to utilize a temporary tissue expander so the patient can receive radiation therapy. Then, a more definitive breast reconstruction can then be undertaken after the radiation therapy is complete.

This study from the University of California, San Francisco looks at 252 patients who underwent mastectomy and immediate reconstruction using transverse rectus abdominis myocutaneous flap reconstruction. Thirty-five received postoperative radiation therapy.

In this study, there were very few complications of the transverse rectus abdominis myocutaneous flap reconstruction. Additionally, less than 10% of the patients had fat necrosis, only 2 of whom had volume loss requiring additional surgery that consisted of an implant or mastopexy and breast reduction on the opposite breast.

Immediate transverse rectus abdominis myocutaneous flap reconstruction can be considered even in patients who require radiation therapy. This allows the treating surgeon and plastic surgeon more flexibility in treating the patient who may wish to avoid a quarantined second operation that consists of a more definitive reconstruction following radiation therapy.

T. J. Eberlein, MD

Small (<2.0-cm) Breast Cancers: Mammographic and US Findings at US-Guided Cryoablation—Initial Experience

Roubidoux MA, Sabel MS, Bailey JE, et al (Univ of Michigan Comprehensive Cancer Ctr, Ann Arbor)

Radiology 233:857-867, 2004 11–9

Purpose.—To determine the mammographic and ultrasonographic (US) findings at cryoablation of small solitary invasive breast cancers and compare them with presence of residual malignancy after treatment.

Materials and Methods.—Institutional review board approval and informed patient consent were obtained. Nine patients with small solitary invasive breast cancers diagnosed at core biopsy were treated with US-guided cryoablation and a 2.7-mm cryoprobe. Mean cancer size was 12 mm (range,

8-18 mm); four were palpable. Tabletop argon gas-based cryoablation system with a double-freeze-thaw protocol was used to treat cancers in outpatient setting. Tumor sites were excised at lumpectomy 2-3 weeks after cryoablation. Findings at mammography and US before, during, and after cryoablation were assessed to categorize densities and masses on mammograms and masses on US images with Breast Imaging Reporting and Data System (BI-RADS); maximum cancer size was measured. Imaging findings and clinical breast examination data were compared with histologic findings from lumpectomy specimens to determine presence of intraductal or invasive cancer.

Results.—With US guidance, ice balls (maximal mean size, 4.4 cm) were formed around cancers. Before excision, eight patients underwent mammography; all had new focal densities (maximum size, 2.5-5.0 cm) at cancer sites. Six patients underwent preexcisional US; 100% of them had new hyperechogenicity in tissue surrounding cancer site. Seven (78%) of nine patients had no residual cancer; specimens contained fat necrosis. One patient had a small focus of invasive cancer; one had extensive multifocal ductal carcinoma in situ. Patients with BI-RADS category 1 or 2 densities on mammograms or nonpalpable tumors had no residual malignancy. No residual invasive cancer occurred in tumors 17 mm or smaller or in cancers without spiculated margins at US.

Conclusion.—After cryoablation, there was increased echogenicity at US and increased density at mammography; these findings were observed in areas that approximated location and size of the ice ball. Tumor size, mammographic density, and US characteristics may be indicators of likelihood of complete cryoablation.

▶ Breast cancer is the most common malignancy in American women. A trend has clearly been established for less invasive surgical management. I have selected this article because it presents results from an alternative noninvasive modality for primary treatment-cryoablation. Most of the tumors were small and all were stage I cancers. All underwent excision several weeks after cryoablation. Of the patients who underwent mammography after cryoablation, all had new focal densities at the cancer site. Similarly, all had new hyperechogenicity in tissue surrounding the cancer site by US. Seven of the 9 patients had no residual cancer, however, on pathologic analysis of the excision, but the specimens did contain fat necrosis.

It will be important to study and gain experience with radiographic evaluation of tumors treated with these new technologies so that mammographic and US characteristics can become predictive of complete ablation of tumor using noninvasive methodologies.

T. J. Eberlein, MD

Colon-Rectal Cancer

Is It Reasonable to Add Preoperative Serum Level of CEA and CA19-9 to Staging for Colorectal Cancer?

Chen C-C, Yang S-H, Lin J-K, et al (Taipei Veterans Gen Hosp, Taiwan, ROC; Natl Yang-Ming Univ, Taipei, Taiwan, ROC; Koo Found, Taipei, Taiwan, ROC)
J Surg Res 124:169-174, 2005 11–10

Background.—Carcinoembryonic antigen (CEA) and carbohydrate antigen 19-9 (CA19-9) are the most common tumor markers for colorectal cancer. The aim of this study was to evaluate the possibility of adding them into the current staging system by analyzing their prognostic significance.

Materials and Methods.—The study population was patients ($n = 574$, 67.1 ± 11.3 years old, 397 males) who received potentially curative resection of colorectal adenocarcinoma (stage I-III) between January 1994 and August 2002, including preoperative measurements of CEA and CA19-9. Clinicopathological characteristics and associated follow-up data were retrospectively collected by reviewing available medical charts. CEA higher or equal to 5 ng/ml was defined as abnormal (CEA+). The CA19-9 level was set at 37 U/ml (CA19-9+). Patients were further divided into four groups (1, 2, 3, 4) according to the results of these two markers (CEA/CA19-9: −/−, −/+/−, and +/+). Survival was analyzed for AJCC staging, CEA (+) *versus(−), CA19-9 (+) versus* (−), and four groups.

Results.—CEA and CA19-9 survival curves were not significantly different. However, the combined use of the two markers revealed a significant survival benefit ($P = 0.035$) of group 1 ("−"for both markers) over 4 ("+" for both) in stage II (Table 3 and Fig 4).

Conclusions.—Patients with an elevated level of both CEA and CA19-9 in stage II of colorectal cancer have a significantly poorer prognosis than those

TABLE 3.—CEA/CA19-9 *Versus* Stages

Stage	CEA/CA19-9	Patient Number	*P* Value
Stage I	−/−	92	
	−/+	4	
	+/−	18	
	+/+	5	NS
Stage II	−/−	128	
	−/+	17	
	+/−	107	
	+/+	30	0.039*
Stage III	−/−	75	
	−/+	15	
	+/−	57	
	+/+	26	NS

* Only significant difference between CEA+/CA19-9+ *versus* CEA/CA19-9.

(Reprinted from Chen C-C, Yang S-H, Lin J-K, et al: Is it reasonable to add preoperative serum level of CEA and CA19-9 to staging for colorectal cancer? *J Surg Res* 124:169-174, 2005.)

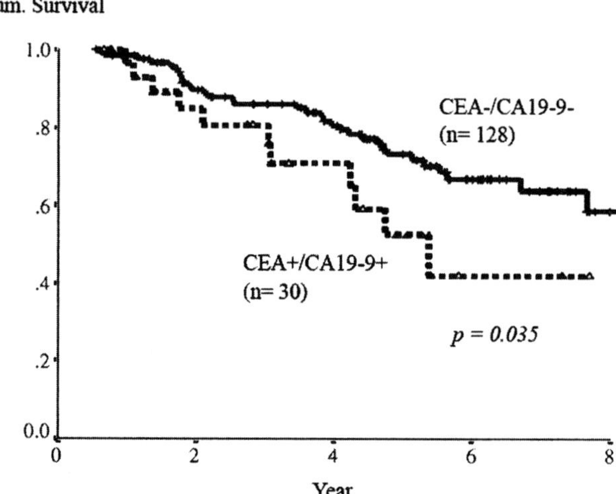

FIGURE 4.—Survival of CEA−/CA19-9− *versus* CEA+/CA19-9+ in stage II. (Reprinted from Chen C-C, Yang S-H, Lin J-K, et al: Is it reasonable to add preoperative serum level of CEA and CA19-9 to staging for colorectal cancer? *J Surg Res* 124:169-174, 2005. Copyright 2005, with permission from Elsevier Science.)

with normal levels of these markers. We recommend adding both CEA and CA19-9 to the current staging system.

▶ Traditionally, patients with stage II colon cancer do not receive adjuvant therapy beyond adequate surgery. Patients with stage III colon cancer are generally treated with adjuvant chemotherapy regimens. This article asks a provocative question. If one adds the level of CEA and CA19-9 would that be an indication for altering the staging system?

Almost 600 patients were studied in this group of patients from the Department of Surgery at the Taipei-Veterans General Hospital. As seen in the article, patients who are CEA positive and CA19-9 positive have a worse survival than patients who have both of these markers negative. What is even more provocative is if one looks at the CEA/CA19-9 positive patients in stage II colon cancer, there is clearly a worse prognosis.

Various groups are studying various gene and molecular panels in stage II colon cancer patients to try to predict those that are likely to have recurrence and therefore may benefit from adjuvant therapies. In the meantime, measurement of CEA and CA19-9 may aid those of us who take care of colorectal cancer patients. Certainly, patients with double positive levels of these antigens might be candidates for adjuvant protocols even though they are without evidence of disease.

T. J. Eberlein, MD

Fecal DNA Versus Fecal Occult Blood for Colorectal-Cancer Screening in an Average-Risk Population

Imperiale TF, for the Colorectal Cancer Study Group (Indiana Univ, Indianapolis; et al)

N Engl J Med 351:2704-2714, 2004 11–11

Background.—Although fecal occult-blood testing is the only available noninvasive screening method that reduces the risk of death from colorectal cancer, it has limited sensitivity. We compared an approach that identifies abnormal DNA in stool samples with the Hemoccult II fecal occult-blood test in average-risk, asymptomatic persons 50 years of age or older.

Methods.—Eligible subjects submitted one stool specimen for DNA analysis, underwent standard Hemoccult II testing, and then underwent colonoscopy. Of 5486 subjects enrolled, 4404 completed all aspects of the study. A subgroup of 2507 subjects was analyzed, including all those with a diagnosis of invasive adenocarcinoma or advanced adenoma plus randomly chosen subjects with no polyps or minor polyps. The fecal DNA panel consisted of 21 mutations.

Results.—The fecal DNA panel detected 16 of 31 invasive cancers (Table 2), whereas Hemoccult II identified 4 of 31 (51.6 percent vs. 12.9 percent, P=0.003). The DNA panel detected 29 of 71 invasive cancers plus adenomas with high-grade dysplasia, whereas Hemoccult II identified 10 of 71 (40.8 percent vs. 14.1 percent, P<0.001). Among 418 subjects with advanced neoplasia (defined as a tubular adenoma at least 1 cm in diameter, a polyp with a villous histologic appearance, a polyp with high-grade dysplasia, or cancer), the DNA panel was positive in 76 (18.2 percent), whereas Hemoccult II was positive in 45 (10.8 percent). Specificity in subjects with negative findings on colonoscopy was 94.4 percent for the fecal DNA panel and 95.2 percent for Hemoccult II.

Conclusions.—Although the majority of neoplastic lesions identified by colonoscopy were not detected by either noninvasive test, the multitarget analysis of fecal DNA detected a greater proportion of important colorectal neoplasia than did Hemoccult II without compromising specificity.

► Fecal occult-blood testing has limited sensitivity in detection of colorectal cancer. These authors representing the Colorectal Cancer Study Group compared fecal DNA analysis in stool samples with Hemoccult II blood test using an average risk asymptomatic population of patients age 50 years or older. Probably the most important finding was the fact that the majority of neoplastic lesions were not detected by either of these noninvasive tests. Positive fecal DNA panels appeared more likely for the detection of colorectal cancer.

One advantage of using DNA from stool is that as refinement and knowledge about tumor markers become available, these can be incorporated into the panel making it more sensitive and more specific for colorectal cancer.

There are still several caveats to this study. The first is that there are a disproportionate number of patients who were older than 65 years. Secondly, because this was a screening study, there are relatively few cancers or advanced

TABLE 2.—Most Advanced Finding at Colonscopy and Results of the Fecal DNA Panel and Occult-Blood Test in the Analyzed Subgroup*

Most Advanced Finding at Colonoscopy	Group That Could Be Evaluated (N=4404)	Analyzed Subgroup (N=2507)†	Positive Fecal DNA Panel		Positive Occult-Blood Test	
	No.		No./Total No.	% (95% CI)	No./Total No.	% (95% CI)
Adenocarcinoma	31	31	16/31	51.6 (34.8–68.0)	4/31	12.9 (5.1–28.9)
TNM stage I	15	15	8/15	53.3 (30.1–75.2)	1/15	6.7 (1.2–29.8)
TNM stage II	8	8	5/8	62.5 (30.6–86.3)	2/8	25.0 (7.1–59.1)
TNM stage III	8	8	3/8	37.5 (13.7–69.4)	1/8	12.5 (2.2–47.1)
TNM stage IV	0	0	0		0	
Adenocarcinoma + high-grade dysplasia	72	71	29/71	40.8 (30.2–52.5)	10/71	14.1 (7.8–24.6)
Advanced adenoma	426	403	61/403	15.1 (12.0–19.0)	43/403	10.7 (8.0–14.1)
High-grade dysplasia	41	40	13/40	32.5 (20.1–48.0)	6/40	15.0 (7.1–29.1)
Villous adenoma	139	133	24/133	18.0 (12.4–25.4)	13/133	9.8 (5.8–16.0)
Tubular adenoma ≥1 cm	230	214	23/214	10.7 (7.3–15.6)	22/214	10.3 (6.9–15.1)
Unspecified	16	16	1/16	6.2 (1.1–28.3)	2/16	12.5 (3.5–36.0)
Minor polyps‡	1627	648	49/648	7.6 (5.8–9.9)	31/648	4.8 (3.4–6.7)
Tubular adenoma <1 cm	762	286	23/286	8.0 (5.9–12.7)	15/286	5.2 (3.5–9.2)
Hyperplastic	633	276	17/276	6.2 (3.9–9.6)	10/276	3.6 (2.0–6.5)
Unspecified	232	86	9/86	10.5 (5.6–18.7)	4/86	4.6 (1.8–11.4)
No polyps on colonoscopy§	2318	1423	79/1423	5.6 (4.5–6.9)	68/1423	4.8 (3.9–5.8)

* The total in both the group that could be evaluated and the analyzed subgroup includes two subjects who are not included in any other category in the table; one had a rectal carcinoid, and one had cloacogenic cancer. The subject with rectal carcinoid was not identified by means of either fecal DNA or by fecal occult-blood testing. The subject with cloacogenic cancer was identified by means of fecal DNA testing, but not by fecal occult-blood testing.

† Stool specimens were selected for DNA testing on the basis of available data (i.e., polyp size and histologic findings) at the time of selection for processing. Subsequent audit of data by the clinical research organization resulted in reclassification of less than 5 percent of subjects.

‡ The fecal DNA panel had a specificity of 92.4 percent, and the occult-blood test had a specificity of 95.2 percent (95 percent confidence interval for the difference in specificity, −5.4 percent to 0.1 percent).

§ The fecal DNA panel had a specificity of 94.4 percent, and the occult-blood test had a specificity of 95.2 percent (95 confidence interval for the difference in specificity, −2.4 percent to 0.9 percent.)

(Reprinted by permission of *The New England Journal of Medicine* from Imperiale TF, for the Colorectal Cancer Study Group: Fecal DNA versus fecal occult blood for colorectal-cancer screening in an average-risk population. *N Engl J Med* 351:2704-2714, 2004.)

adenomas and in the future, the use of a more targeted higher-risk population may make analysis of confidence intervals more sensitive. Another issue is that all the DNA analyses were performed by a single laboratory. If this technology was to be adapted uniformly, multiple laboratories would need to be involved and the quality assurance issues would be important. Finally, this study does not address the issue of follow up retesting. These caveats aside, however, this type of technology, particularly when additional genes are analyzed, can provide a sensitive and relatively specific methodology for detection of early precancerous and cancerous changes in the colon.

T. J. Eberlein, MD

Short-term Endpoints of Conventional Versus Laparoscopic-Assisted Surgery in Patients With Colorectal Cancer (MRC CLASICC Trial): Multicentre, Randomised Controlled Trial

Guillou PJ, for the MRC CLASICC Trial Group (St James's Univ Hosp, Leeds, England; et al)

Lancet 365:1718-1726, 2005 11–12

Background.—Laparoscopic-assisted surgery for colorectal cancer has been widely adopted without data from large-scale randomised trials to support its use. We compared short-term endpoints of conventional versus laparoscopic-assisted surgery in patients with colorectal cancer to predict long-term outcomes.

Methods.—Between July, 1996, and July, 2002, we undertook a multicentre, randomised clinical trial in 794 patients with colorectal cancer from 27 UK centres. Patients were allocated to receive laparoscopic-assisted (n=526) or open surgery (n=268). Primary short-term endpoints were positivity rates of circumferential and longitudinal resection margins, proportion of Dukes' C2 tumours, and in-hospital mortality. Analysis was by intention to treat. This trial has been assigned the International Standard Randomised Controlled Trial Number ISRCTN74883561.

Findings.—Six patients (two [open], four [laparoscopic]) had no surgery, and 23 had missing surgical data (nine, 14). 253 and 484 patients actually received open and laparoscopic-assisted treatment, respectively. 143 (29%) patients underwent conversion from laparoscopic to open surgery. Proportion of Dukes' C2 tumours did not differ between treatments (18 [7%] patients, open *vs* 34 [6%], laparoscopic; difference −0.3%, 95% CI −3.9 to 3.4%, p=0.89), and neither did in-hospital mortality (13 [5%] *vs* 21 [4%]; −0.9%, −3.9 to 2.2%, p=0.57). Apart from patients undergoing laparoscopic anterior resection for rectal cancer, rates of positive resection margins were similar between treatment groups (Figs 3 and 4). Patients with converted treatment had raised complication rates (Table 5).

Interpretation.—Laparoscopic-assisted surgery for cancer of the colon is as effective as open surgery in the short term and is likely to produce similar long-term outcomes. However, impaired short-term outcomes after laparoscopic-assisted anterior resection for cancer of the rectum do not yet justify its routine use.

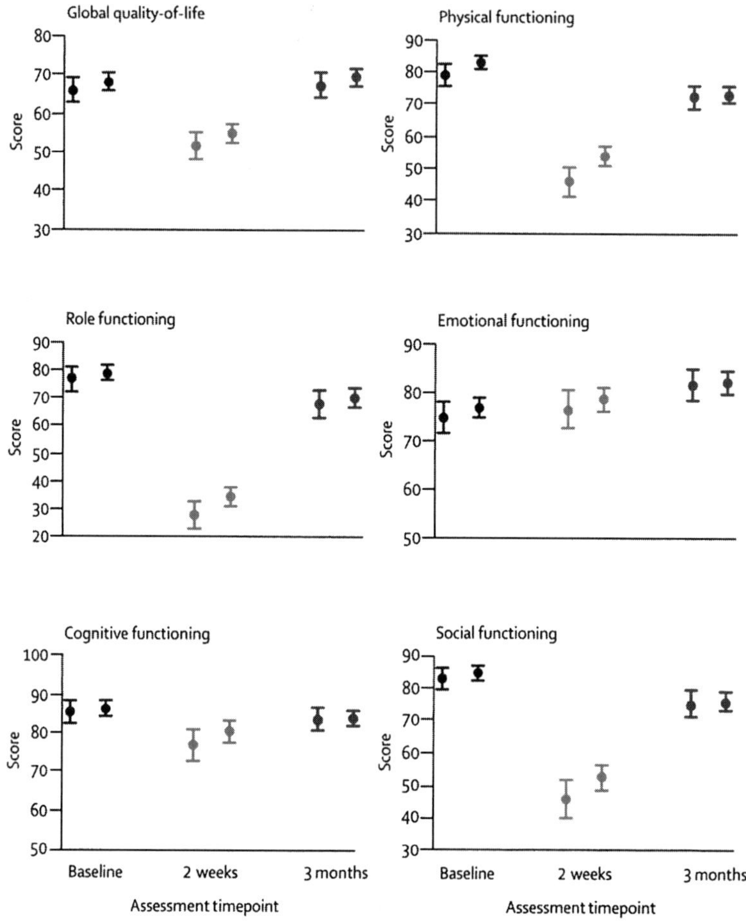

FIGURE 3.—EORTC QLQ-C30 scores for global quality-of-life and functional scales. Pairs of dots show scores for open surgery (left) and laparoscopic-assisted surgery (right). High scores indicate good functioning. (Courtesy of Guillou PJ, for the MRC CLASICC Trial Group: Short-term endpoints of conventional versus laparoscopic-assisted surgery in patients with colorectal cancer (MRC CLASICC Trial): Multicentre, randomised controlled trial. *Lancet* 365:1718-1726, 2005. Copyright 2005 by Elsevier.)

▶ This is a multicenter randomized trial involving almost 800 patients with colorectal cancer from 27 UK centers. There was an almost 2 to 1 randomization of laparoscopic-assisted versus open surgery. The patients who underwent conversion to open surgery after attempted laparoscopy tended to have higher complication rates. However, the quality of life at baseline, 2 weeks, and 3 months seem to be as good or better for laparoscopically assisted surgery.

The 1 caveat was that in patients undergoing the anterior resection a nonsignificant difference in circumferential resection margins positivity was recorded suggesting that laparoscopic procedure could be associated with a slightly raised risk of local recurrence. Therefore, these authors concluded that laparoscopically assisted anterior resection was not yet justified for rou-

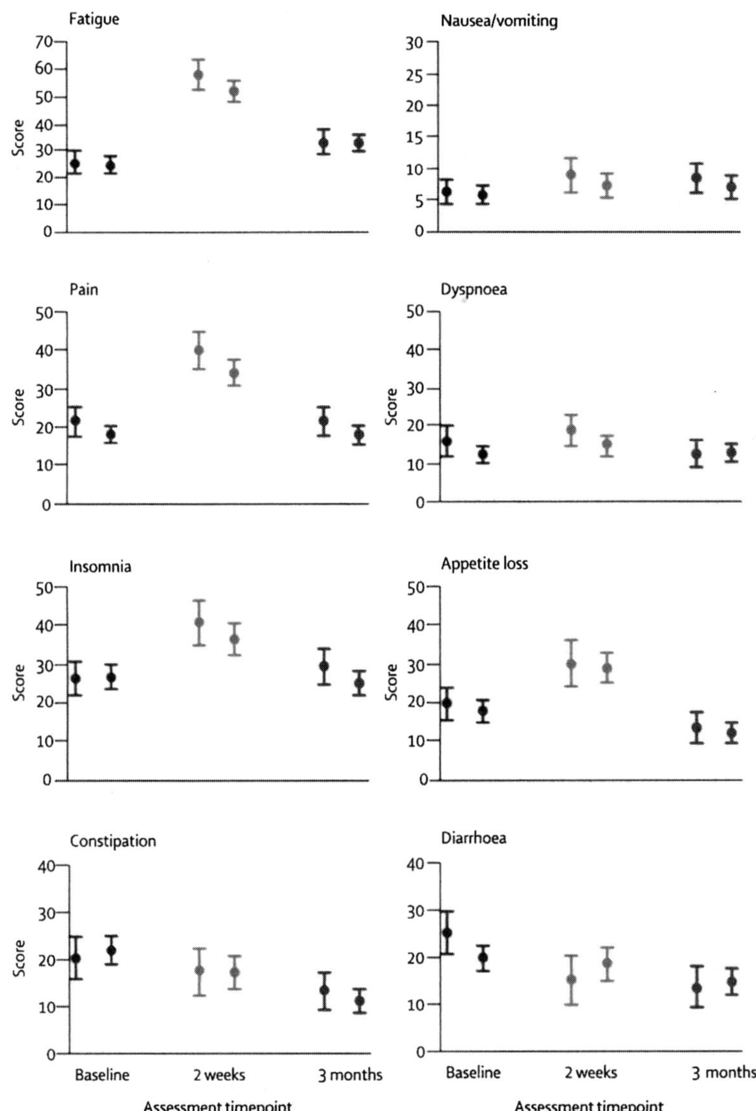

FIGURE 4.—EORTC QLQ-C30 scores for symptom scales. Pairs of dots show scores for open surgery (left) and laparoscopic-assisted surgery (right). High scores indicate severe symptoms. (Courtesy of Guillou PJ, for the MRC CLASICC Trial Group: Short-term endpoints of conventional versus laparoscopic-assisted surgery in patients with colorectal cancer (MRC CLASICC Trial): Multicentre, randomised controlled trial. *Lancet* 365:1718-1726, 2005. Copyright 2005 by Elsevier.)

TABLE 5.—30-Day Postoperative Complications

	Intention-to-Treat Population		Actual Treatment Group		
	Open	Laparoscopic	Open	Laparoscopic	Conversion
Patients with complications	85 (32%)	172 (33%)	86 (31%)	99 (29%)	64 (45%)
Colon	38 (27%)	71 (26%)	37 (26%)	48 (26%)	16 (26%)
Rectum	47 (37%)	101 (40%)	49 (37%)	51 (32%)	48 (59%)
Total complications	113 (42%)	246 (47%)	115 (42%)	133 (39%)	99 (69%)
Colon	49 (35%)	96 (35%)	48 (33%)	62 (34%)	23 (38%)
Rectum	64 (50%)	150 (59%)	67 (51%)	71 (44%)	76 (93%)
Complications (colon)					
Wound infection	7 (5%)	14 (5%)	7 (5%)	8 (4%)	5 (8%)
Chest infection	5 (4%)	18 (7%)	5 (3%)	10 (5%)	6 (10%)
Anastomotic dehiscence	4 (3%)	9 (3%)	5 (3%)	7 (4%)	1 (2%)
Deep-vein thrombosis		5 (2%)		5 (3%)	
Other	33 (24%)	50 (18%)	31 (22%)	32 (17%)	11 (18%)
Complications (rectum)					
Wound infection	15 (12%)	33 (13%)	16 (12%)	16 (10%)	16 (20%)
Chest infection	5 (4%)	25 (10%)	6 (5%)	12 (8%)	12 (15%)
Anastomotic dehiscence	9 (7%)	26 (10%)	10 (7%)	13 (8%)	12 (15%)
Deep-vein thrombosis	2 (2%)	1	2 (2%)	..	1 (1%)
Other	33 (26%)	65 (26%)	33 (25%)	30 (19%)	35 (43%)

Data are number (%).

(Courtesy of Guillou PJ, for the MRC CLASICC Trial Group: Short-term endpoints of conventional versus laparoscopic-assisted surgery in patients with colorectal cancer (MRC CLASICC Trial): Multicentre, randomised controlled trial. *Lancet* 365:1718-1726, 2005. Copyright 2005 by Elsevier.)

tine use. Otherwise in experienced hands, laparoscopically assisted surgery appeared to have as good short-term outcomes as open surgery.

T. J. Eberlein, MD

Bladder and Sexual Function Following Resection for Rectal Cancer in a Randomized Clinical Trial of Laparoscopic *versus* Open Technique

Jayne DG, Brown JM, Thorpe H, et al (Univ of Leeds, England)

Br J Surg 92:1124-1132, 2005 11–13

Background.—Bladder and sexual dysfunction are recognized complications of mesorectal resection. Their incidence following laparoscopic surgery is unknown.

Methods.—Bladder and sexual function were assessed in patients who had undergone laparoscopic rectal, open rectal or laparoscopic colonic resection as part of the UK Medical Research Council Conventional versus Laparoscopic-Assisted Surgery In Colorectal Cancer (CLASICC) trial, using the International Prostatic Symptom Score, the International Index of Erectile Function and the Female Sexual Function Index. Sexual and bladder function data from the European Organization for Research and Treatment of Cancer QLQ-CR38 collected in the CLASICC trial were used for comparison.

Results.—Two hundred and forty-seven (71.2 per cent) of 347 patients completed questionnaires. Bladder function was similar after laparoscopic and open rectal operations for rectal cancer. Overall sexual function and erectile function tended to be worse in men after laparoscopic rectal surgery than after open rectal surgery (overall function: difference −11.18 (95 per cent confidence interval (c.i.) −22.99 to 0.63), $P = 0.063$; erectile function: difference −5.84 (95 per cent c.i. −10.94 to −0.74), $P = 0.068$). Total mesorectal excision (TME) was more commonly performed in the laparoscopic rectal group than in the open rectal group. TME (odds ratio (OR) 6.38, $P = 0.054$) and conversion to open operation (OR 2.86, $P = 0.041$) were independent predictors of postoperative male sexual dysfunction. No differences were detected in female sexual function.

Conclusion.—Laparoscopic rectal resection did not adversely affect bladder function, but there was a trend towards worse male sexual function. This may be explained by the higher rate of TME in the laparoscopic rectal resection group.

► Laparoscopic surgery has been shown to reduce morbidity and expedite discharge from the hospital. This article from Leeds, England looks at patients who underwent conventional versus laparoscopic-assisted surgery and colorectal cancer. It is interesting that sexual function and erectile function tended to be worse in men after a laparoscopic surgery. Laparoscopic surgery did not seem to adversely impact bladder function. Part of the explanation for this may have been that total mesorectal excision (TME) was more commonly performed in the laparoscopic group.

It appeared to be that performing total mesorectal excision (more common when laparoscopic surgery was done) was associated with sexual dysfunction, particularly, erectile dysfunction. Conversion to open surgery also seemed to be an independent predictor of reduced postoperative male sexual function. This study was not able to draw meaningful conclusions with regard to female sexual function because of missing data.

T. J. Eberlein, MD

Preoperative Chemoradiotherapy and Total Mesorectal Excision Surgery for Locally Advanced Rectal Cancer: Correlation With Rectal Cancer Regression Grade

Wheeler JMD, Dodds E, Warren BF, et al (John Radcliffe Hosp, Oxford, England)

Dis Colon Rectum 47:2025-2031, 2004 11–14

Purpose.—Preoperative long-course chemoradiotherapy is recommended for rectal carcinoma when there is concern that surgery alone may not be curative. Downstaging of the tumor can be measured as rectal cancer regression grade (1-3) and may be of importance when estimating the prognosis. The aim of this study was to look at the long-term results of tumor regression in patients receiving long-course chemotherapy before surgical resection of rectal cancer.

Methods.—We reviewed those patients who received preoperative chemoradiotherapy followed by surgical resection for carcinoma of the mid rectum or distal rectum found to be stage T3/4 between January 1995 and November 1999. Patients received 45 to 50 Gy irradiation in 2-Gy fractions and an infusion of 5-fluorouracil. Surgical specimens were assessed for rectal cancer regression grade. Patients were followed up routinely with clinical examination, computed tomography, and colonoscopy.

Results.—Sixty-five patients with a mean age 65 (range, 32-83) years underwent chemoradiotherapy before surgical resection. Thirty patients (46 percent) were classified as rectal cancer regression Grade 1, with 9 patients (14 percent) having complete sterilization of the tumor. Fifty-three patients (82 percent) underwent a curative resection. Overall survival, with a median follow-up of 39 (range, 24-83) months, was 67 percent and was associated with tumor downstaging (Fig 1). The local recurrence rate was 5.8 percent in those patients who underwent a curative resection and was significantly lower with rectal cancer regression Grade 1 tumors ($P = 0.03$). Eight of nine

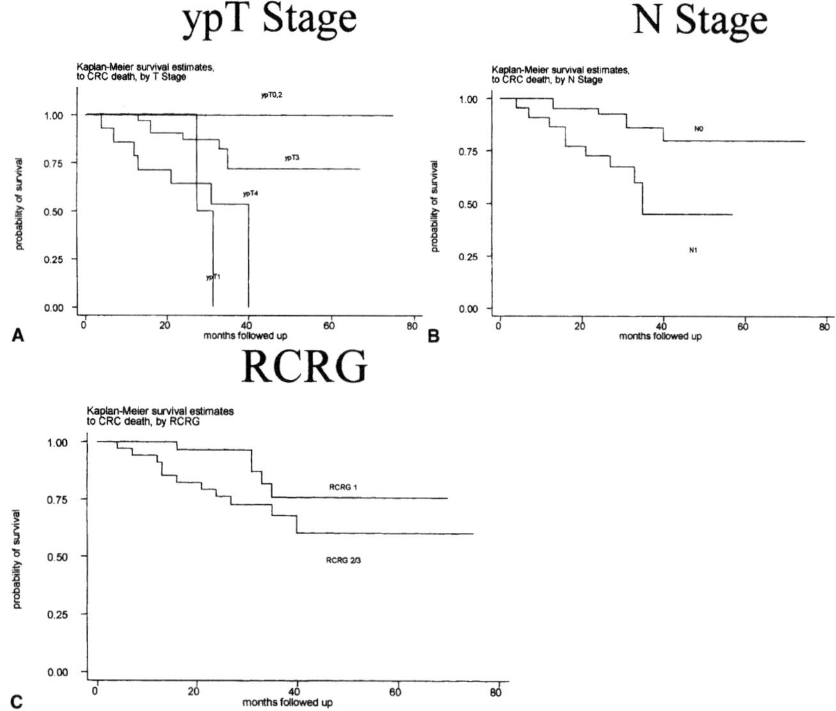

FIGURE 1.—**A.** Disease-free survival in relation to ypT stage. Only 3 of 19 patients (16 percent) with ypT0-ypT2 tumors developed metastatic disease during follow-up. This included the two patients with ypT1 tumors. **B.** Disease-free survival in relation to N stage. Histologic nodal involvement was significantly associated with decreased survival. **C.** Disease-free survival in relation to rectal cancer regression grade (RCRG). Although there was a trend toward increased survival in the 29 RCRG 1 patients, this did not reach statistical significance. (Courtesy of Wheeler JMD, Dodds E, Warren BF, et al: Preoperative chemoradiotherapy and total mesorectal excision surgery for locally advanced rectal cancer: Correlation with rectal cancer regression grade. *Dis Colon Rectum* 47:2025-2031, 2004. Copyright 2004 Springer-Verlag.)

patients (89 percent) whose tumor had been sterilized were alive and well with no recurrence of tumor at a median follow-up of 41 (range, 24-70) months.

Conclusions.—Preoperative chemoradiotherapy resulted in significant regression of tumor. Overall survival was high and was associated with downstaging of tumor. The local recurrence rate was significantly lower with rectal cancer regression Grade 1 tumors and was not seen in patients with sterilized tumors.

▶ Preoperative chemoradiotherapy is associated with downstaging of tumor and this frequently can result in better sphincter preservation as well as more improved local control and more potentially long-term survival. This single institution study from Oxford attempts to look at the long-term results from patients receiving long-course chemoradiation before surgical resection for rectal cancer. There were 65 consecutive patients studied. Only 3 of 19 patients had metastatic disease develop during follow-up. Ironically, 2 of these patients had T1 tumors. The rectal cancer regression grade tended toward increased survival but did not reach statistical significance.

One of the things that seemed more certain is that patients who had tumor that was sterilized (ypT0N0) have a very small risk of having metastatic disease develop. Perhaps in larger series the rectal cancer regression grade will be able to help identify patients who will do better after preoperative chemoradiation. Ultimately, genes will be able to identify patients who respond well to preoperative chemoradiation as well as predict patients who will not respond to neoadjuvant therapies, thereby necessitating other more aggressive approaches.

T. J. Eberlein, MD

Recurrence After Transanal Excision of T1 Rectal Cancer: Should We Be Concerned?

Madbouly KM, Remzi FH, Erkek BA, et al (The Cleveland Clinic Foundation, Ohio)

Dis Colon Rectum 48:711-721, 2005 11–15

Purpose.—Transanal excision is an appealing treatment for low rectal cancers because of its low morbidity, mortality, and better functional results than transabdominal procedures. However, controversy exists about whether it compromises the potential for cure. Several, recent reports of high recurrence rates after local excision prompted us to review our results of transanal excision alone in patients with T1 rectal cancers.

Methods.—All patients with T1 low rectal cancer undergoing local excision alone between 1980 through 1998 were reviewed for local recurrence, distant metastasis, disease-free interval, results of salvage surgery, and overall and disease-free survival. Demographics, tumor size, distance from anal verge, and preoperative endoluminal ultrasound results also were recorded.

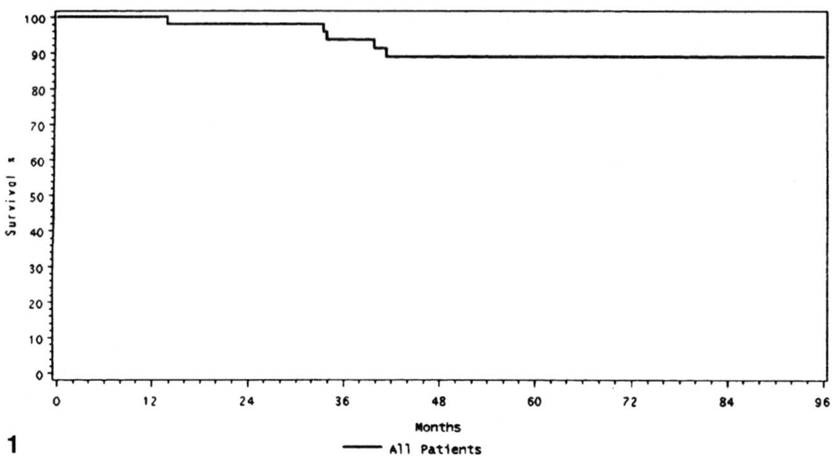

FIGURE 1.—Survival curve for death by cancer. (Courtesy of Madbouly KM, Remzi FH, Erkek BA, et al: Recurrence after transanal excision of t1 rectal cancer: Should we be concerned? *Dis Colon Rectum* 48:711-721, 2005. Copyright 2005 Springer-Verlag.)

Patients with poorly differentiated tumors, perineural or lymphovascular invasion, or with mucinous component were excluded.

Results.—Fifty-two patients underwent transanal excision during the study period. Five-year recurrence was estimated to be 29.38 percent (95 percent confidence interval, 15.39-43.48). For 52 patients, five-year, cancer-specific and overall survival rates were 89 and 75 percent respectively (Figs 1 and 2). Fourteen of 15 patients with recurrence underwent salvage treatment with 56.2 percent (95 percent confidence interval, 35.2-90) five-year survival rate (Fig 3). Gender, preoperative staging by endorectal ultrasound,

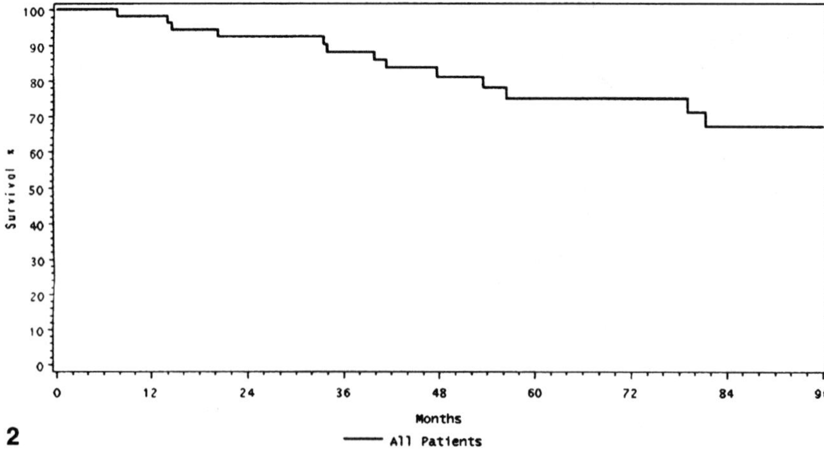

FIGURE 2.—Survival curve for death by any cause. (Courtesy of Madbouly KM, Remzi FH, Erkek BA, et al: Recurrence after transanal excision of t1 rectal cancer: Should we be concerned? *Dis Colon Rectum* 48:711-721, 2005. Copyright 2005 Springer-Verlag.)

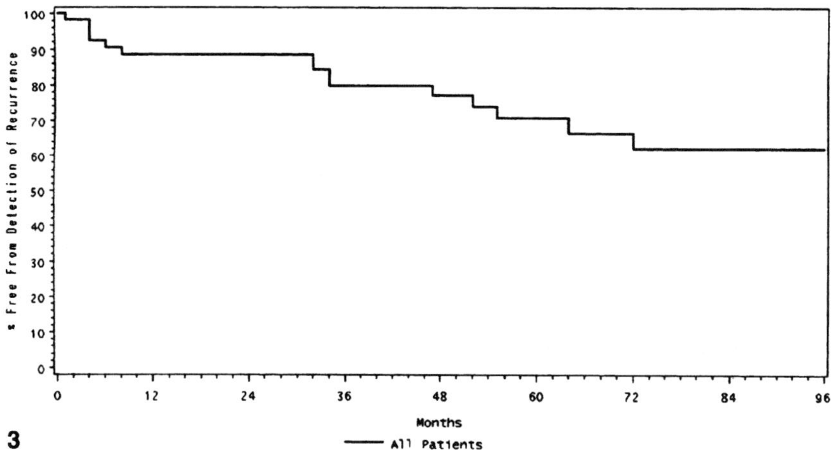

3

FIGURE 3.—Recurrence-free survival curve. (Courtesy of Madbouly KM, Remzi FH, Erkek BA, et al: Recurrence after transanal excision of t1 rectal cancer: Should we be concerned? *Dis Colon Rectum* 48:711-721, 2005. Copyright 2005 Springer-Verlag.)

distance from the anal verge, tumor size, location, and T1 status discovered after transanal excision of a villous adenoma did not influence local recurrence or tumor-specific survival.

Conclusions.—Transanal excision for T1 rectal tumors with low-grade malignancy has a high rate of recurrence. Although overall cancer survival rates might be regarded as satisfactory, this high recurrence and low salvage rate raises the issue about the role of transanal excision alone for early rectal cancer and the possible need for adjuvant therapy or increased role of resective surgery.

► This is a study from the Cleveland Clinic and demonstrates an issue in the treatment of T1 rectal cancers. By using transanal excision, the authors have carefully shown that there is significant recurrence rate. Less than half of the patients who have recurrence will be salved by radical surgery. This study points out 2 important issues. The first that preoperative radiographic evaluation of patients is necessary to select patients who are potential candidates for conservative surgery. The second issue is that there is a need to develop better validated prognostic markers, probably molecular or genetic that will better guide us to use local excision as well as to select patients for adjuvant chemotherapy and radiation therapy. In addition, these markers should help us to select patients who might appear eligible for excision alone, but because of their markers should undergo more radical intervention. In this study, tumor size, distance from anal verge, position within the anal canal, degree of differentiation did not predict for recurrence. Therefore, identification of molecular and genetic determinants will provide this information in the future. In the meantime, even T1 lesions with good histologic features can have a relatively high recurrence rate leading to diminished survival after local excision alone.

T. J. Eberlein, MD

Immediate Radical Resection After Local Excision of Rectal Cancer: An Oncologic Compromise?

Hahnloser D, Wolff BG, Larson DW, et al (Mayo Clinic, Rochester, Minn)

Dis Colon Rectum 48:429-437, 2005 11–16

Purpose.—Local excision for early-staged rectal cancers is controversial. Preoperative understaging is not uncommon and radical resection after local resection may be needed for a curative treatment. The aim of this study was to determine the frequency and outcome of radical resection (within 30 days) after local excision for rectal adenocarcinoma.

Methods.—All locally excised rectal cancers (curative intent) that required radical surgery within 30 days were reviewed (1980-2000). T2-3N0-1 stage cancers were each matched to three primary radical surgery controls for stage, age (± 5 years), gender, date (± 1 years), and type (abdominoperineal resection or low anterior resection) of operation. T1N0-1 cancers were compared with stage-matched rectal cancers treated by either primary radical surgery (n = 78) or local excision alone (n = 77).

Results.—Fifty-two locally excised rectal adenocarcinomas (29 transanal and 23 polypectomies) were followed by radical surgery (24 abdominoperineal resection and 28 low anterior resection) within 7 (range, 1-29) days. Radical surgery was performed because of a cancerous polyp (n = 42), positive margins (5), lymphovascular invasion (3), and T3-staged cancer (2). Twelve of 52 cancers (23 percent) were found to have nodal involvement and 15 of 52 (29 percent) showed residual cancer in the resected specimen. The T2-3N0-1 stage controls were well matched. No significant difference in tumor location, size, adjuvant therapy, or length of follow-up was noted. Local and distant recurrence occurred in 2 of 4 T2-3N1 tumors and in 2 of 11 T2-

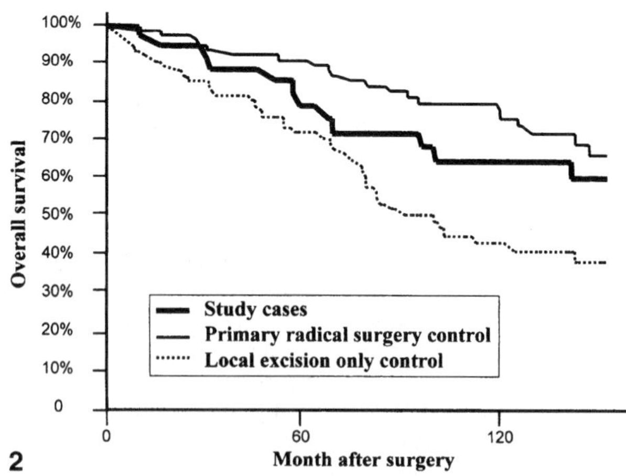

FIGURE 2.—Overall survival of T1N0-1 cases (n = 37) was comparable to overall survival of T1Nx local excision-only controls (n = 77, *P* = 0.06) and to T1N0-1 primary radical-surgery controls (n = 78, *P* 0.2). (Courtesy of Hahnloser D, Wolff BG, Larson DW, et al: Immediate radical resection after local excision of rectal cancer: An oncologic compromise? *Dis Colon Rectum* 48:429-437, 2005. Copyright 2005 Springer-Verlag.)

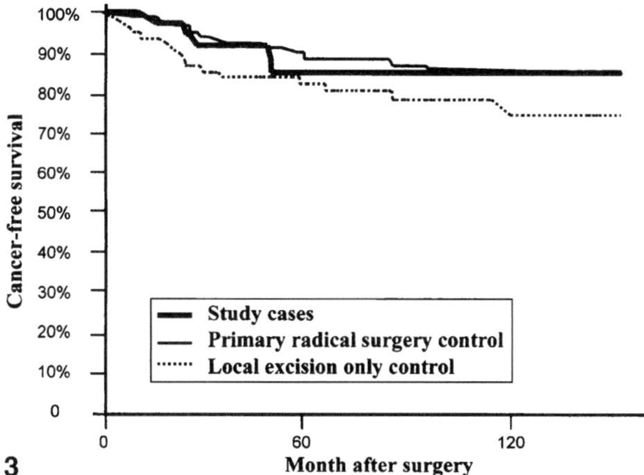

FIGURE 3.—Cancer-free survival of T1N0-1 cases (n = 37) was comparable to cancer-free survival of T1Nx local excision-only controls (n = 77, $P = 0.03$) and to T1N1-0 primary radical-surgery controls (n = 78, $P = 0.9$). (Courtesy of Hahnloser D, Wolff BG, Larson DW, et al: Immediate radical resection after local excision of rectal cancer: An oncologic compromise? *Dis Colon Rectum* 48:429-437, 2005. Copyright 2005 Springer-Verlag.)

3N0 cancers and were comparable to the matched controls, as was survival, with the exception of shorter survival in T3N1 cases, but numbers were too small for a definitive conclusion. Length of follow-up was not different. For T1 cancers, the controls were also comparable regarding patient and tumor demographics and adjuvant therapy. Nodal involvement was 21 percent in T1 study cases and 15 percent in T1 primary radical-surgery controls, with a trend toward location in the lower third of the rectum in both groups (58 percent and 50 percent, respectively). Local recurrence rates were 3 percent in the study group, 5 percent for patients undergoing primary radical surgery, and 8 percent for local excision alone. Distant metastasis (11 percent, 12 percent, and 13 percent, respectively) and overall five-year survival were also not significantly different (78 percent, 89 percent, and 73 percent, respectively) (Figs 2 and 3).

Conclusions.—Nodal involvement in attempted locally excised rectal cancers is not uncommon. Local excision of rectal tumors followed by radical surgery within 30 days in cancer patients does not compromise outcome compared with primary radical surgery. Even after radical surgery for superficial T1 rectal cancers, recurrence rates are not insignificant. Future improvements in preoperative staging may be helpful in selecting tumors for local excision only.

▶ Radical surgery is still the mainstay of treatment for rectal cancer. However, in recent years, local excision has become increasingly more practiced. Local recurrence rates, however, after local excision can be nearly 20% in T1 cancers and nearly 40% in T2 cancers. The major aim of this study was to see whether there was oncologic compromise in first attempting local excision and then proceeding with radical surgery within 30 days compared with patients who had radical surgery at the outset or who had local excision and the stage-matched fashion.

In looking at the T1 cases only, the overall survival and the cancer-free survival are comparable in the study cases compared with primary radical surgery or local excision only. Several other telling comments, however, can be made from analyzing these results. Local excision alone does not give as high survival rates when compared with these study patients or primary radical surgery. Although there is not statistical significance in cancer-free survival, there appears to be marginal difference with respect to local excision only.

All of this, of course, points to the difficulty with evaluating tumors primarily before any surgical intervention. Three-dimensional imaging is a new innovation that may improve upon MRI and endoscopic US. In the meantime, it does not appear that attempting local excision will harm the patient; if it appears local excision is inadequate, radical surgery is recommended and undertaken.

T. J. Eberlein, MD

Comparison of Long-term Functional Results of Colonic J-Pouch and Straight Anastomosis After Low Anterior Resection for Rectal Cancer: A Five-Year Follow-up

Hida J-i, Yoshifuji T, Tokoro T, et al (Kinki Univ, Osaka, Japan)
Dis Colon Rectum 47:1578-1585, 2004 11–17

Purpose.—Few reports on the long-term functional outcome of colonic J-pouch reconstruction have been published, and data comparing J-pouch and straight reconstruction are contradictory. This prospective study compares the functional outcome of colonic J-pouch and straight anastomosis five years after low anterior resection for rectal cancer.

Methods.—Functional outcome was compared in 46 patients with J-pouch reconstruction (J-group) and 48 patients with straight anastomosis (S-group). Clinical status was evaluated with a 17-item questionnaire inquiring about different aspects of bowel function. Reservoir function was evalu-

TABLE 3.—Functional Assessment

Distance of Anastomosis from Anal Verge	Functional Score Points[a] J-Pouch Group		Straight Group		*P* Value	[*P* Value]
1–4 cm No. of patients	23	[7]	24	[7]		
	2.7 ± 2.8	[3.7 ± 2.6]	7.3 ± 5.3	[8.7 ± 6.3]	0.011	[0.125]
	(0–10)	[(0–8)]	(1–19)	[(2–19)]		
5–8 cm No. of patients	23	[7]	24	[8]		
	2.1 ± 1.7	[2.0 ± 1.4]	2.7 ± 1.6	[2.3 ± 1.1]	0.198	[0.702]
	(0–6)	[(0–4)]	(0–7)	[(1–5)]		

Values are mean ± standard deviation. [ ]:subset analysis of randomized patients.
[a]Source range, 0-26; overall good function score, 0 points; overall poor function score, 26 points.
(Courtesy of Hida J-i, Yoshifuji T, Tokoro T, et al: Comparison of long-term functional results of colonic J-pouch and straight anastomosis after low anterior resection for rectal cancer: A five-year follow-up. *Dis Colon Rectum* 1578-1585, 2004. Copyright Springer-Verlag.)

TABLE 4.—Functional Results of Individual Variables in Patients With Anastomoses 1 to 4 cm From Anal Verge Five Years After Surgery

	J-Pouch Group		Straight Group			
	(n = 23) n (%)	[n = 7] n (%)	(n = 24) n (%)	[n = 7] n (%)	*P* Value	*P* Value]
No. of bowel movements						
Daytime, ≥5	1 (4.3)	0 (0)	7 (29.2)	2 (28.6)	0.028	0.231
At night, >1/week	1 (4.3)	0 (0)	8 (33.3)	2 (28.6)	0.013	0.231
No urgency (ability to defer evacuation ≥30 min)	1 (4.3)	0 (0)	8 (33.3)	2 (28.6)	0.013	0.231
Evacuation difficulty (≥15 min spent on toilet)	0 (0)	0 (0)	1 (4.2)	0 (0)	0.511	1.0
Incomplete evacuation	1 (4.3)	0 (0)	1 (4.2)	0 (0)	0.745	1.0
No. of times to attain complete evacuation, ≥3	1 (4.3)	0 (0)	2 (8.3)	1 (14.3)	0.516	0.5
Medication (laxatives or glycerine enemas)	9 (39.1)	3 (42.9)	9 (37.5)	3 (42.9)	0.573	0.704
Soiling	5 (21.7)	2 (28.6)	12 (50.0)	4 (57.1)	0.043	0.296
Protective pad use	10 (43.5)	3 (42.9)	13 (54.2)	4 (57.1)	0.33	0.5
Incontinence	2 (8.7)	1 (14.3)	6 (25.0)	2 (28.6)	0.136	0.5
No ability to differentiate between stool and flatus	6 (26.1)	2 (28.6)	10 (41.7)	3 (42.9)	0.207	0.5
No ability to release flatus safely	8 (34.8)	2 (28.6)	7 (29.2)	2 (28.6)	0.46	0.72
Perianal soreness	9 (39.1)	3 (42.9)	13 (54.2)	4 (57.1)	0.23	0.5
Dietary restrictions	10 (43.5)	3 (42.9)	11 (45.8)	3 (42.9)	0.552	0.704
Hindered leaving home	5 (21.7)	2 (28.6)	7 (29.2)	2 (28.6)	0.402	0.72
No participation in social activities	9 (39.1)	3 (42.9)	9 (37.5)	3 (42.9)	0.573	0.704
Dissatisfaction with bowel function	5 (21.7)	2 (28.6)	11 (45.8)	3 (42.9)	0.075	0.5

[ ]:subset analysis of randomized patients.

(Courtesy of Hida J-i, Yoshifuji T, Tokoro T, et al: Comparison of long-term functional results of colonic J-pouch and straight anastomosis after low anterior resection for rectal cancer: A five-year follow-up. *Dis Colon Rectum* 1578-1585, 2004. Copyright Springer-Verlag.)

TABLE 6.—Comparison of Reservoir Function Between Colonic J-Pouch and Straight Anastomosis Following Low Anterior Resection

Distance of Anastomosis from Anal Verge	J-Pouch Group		Straight Group		*P* Value	[*P* Value]
1–4 cm	n = 23	[n = 7]	n = 24	[n = 7]		
Maximum						
Tolerable Volume (ml)	101.7 ± 27.6 (60–140)	[104.3 ± 26.4] (70–140)	76.3 ± 8.8 (60–90)	[72.9 ± 11.1] (60–90)	0.004	[0.022]
Threshold Volume (ml)	46.5 ± 10.7 (30–70)	[51.4 ± 13.5] (30–70)	30.4 ± 6.2 (20–40)	[30 ± 8.2] (20–40)	<0.001	[0.011]
Compliance (ml/cm H_2O)	4.9 ± 1.7 (1.6–7.4)	[5.3 ± 1.7] (2.4–7.4)	2.5 ± 0.4 (1.8–3.1)	[2.4 ± 0.4] (1.8–2.8)	<0.001	[0.007]
5–8 cm	n = 23	[n = 7]	n = 24	[n = 8]		
Maximum						
Tolerable Volume (ml)	120.4 ± 25.5 (80–160)	[121.4 ± 24.1] (90–160)	97.9 ± 8.8 (90–110)	[98.8 ± 8.3] (90–110)	<0.001	[0.049]
Threshold Volume (ml)	58.3 ± 17.7 (40–100)	[65.7 ± 19.9] (40–100)	40.8 ± 6.5 (30–50)	[38.8 ± 8.3] (30–50)	<0.001	[0.007]
Compliance (ml/cm H_2O)	5.2 ± 1.8 (2.2–8.0)	[5.9 ± 1.8] (2.6–8.0)	3.1 ± 0.3 (2.7–3.7)	[3.0 ± 0.3] (2.7–3.5)	<0.001	[0.021]

Values are mean ± standard deviation (range).[ ]: subset analysis of the randomized patients.

(Courtesy of Hida J-i, Yoshifuji T, Tokoro T, et al: Comparison of long-term functional results of colonic J-pouch and straight anastomosis after low anterior resection for rectal cancer: A five-year follow-up. *Dis Colon Rectum* 1578-1585, 2004. Copyright Springer-Verlag.)

ated by manovolumetry. The Fisher's exact test and Wilcoxon's rank-sum test were used to compare categoric and quantitative data, respectively.

Results.—Among patients with an ultralow anastomosis ($\leq$ 4 cm from the anal verge), the number of bowel movements during the day ($\geq$5, 4.3 vs. 29.2 percent; P = 0.028) and at night (>1/week, 4.3 vs. 33.3 percent; P = 0.013) and urgency (4.3 vs. 33.3 percent; P = 0.013) and soiling (21.7 vs. 50.0 percent; P = 0.043) were less in the J-group than in the S-group. Among patients with a low anastomosis (5 to 8 cm from the verge), patients in the J-group had fewer bowel movements at night (>1/week, 0 vs. 20.8 percent; P = 0.028) and less urgency (0 vs. 20.8 percent; P = 0.028). Reservoir function was better in the J-group than in the S-group in both the ultralow (maximum tolerable volume (mean), 101.7 vs. 76.3 ml; P = 0.004; threshold volume (mean), 46.5 vs. 30.4 ml; P < 0.001; compliance (mean), 4.9 vs. 2.5 ml/cm H_2O; P < 0.001) and low-anastomosis (maximum tolerable volume, 120.4 vs. 97.9 ml; P < 0.001; threshold volume, 58.3 vs. 40.8 ml; P < 0.001; compliance, 5.2 vs. 3.1 ml/cm H_2O; P < 0.001) groups.

Conclusions.—J-pouch reconstruction increased reservoir function and provided better functional outcome than straight anastomosis, even five years after surgery, especially in patients whose anastomosis is less than 4 cm from the anal verge. (Tables 3, 4, and 6)

► This report from Osaka, Japan compared 96 patients receiving either J-pouch reconstruction or straight anastomosis after resection for rectal cancer. The authors devised a scoring systemic designed to quantify overall bowel function. As seen in Table 3 of this article, the functional assessment of the J-pouch group was statistically proved in the patients who had very low anastomoses, 1 to 4 cm from the anal verge; patients with higher anastomoses tended to do better with J-pouch, but the results were not statistically significant. J-pouch patients had fewer bowel movements, both during the day and at night and had less urgency and soiling (Table 4). This may well be due to the larger reservoir function in the J-pouch group compared to the straight group (Table 6).

T. J. Eberlein, MD

Hepatic Colorectal

Effect of Steatohepatitis Associated With Irinotecan or Oxaliplatin Pretreatment on Resectability of Hepatic Colorectal Metastases

Fernandez FG, Ritter J, Goodwin JW, et al (Washington Univ School of Medicine, St Louis; St John's Clinic, Springfield, Mo)

J Am Coll Surg 200:845-853, 2005 11–18

Background.—The objective was to evaluate the effect of preoperative administration of newer chemotherapeutic agents (irinotecan and oxaliplatin) on development of steatohepatitis, which could limit surgical options.

Study Design.—Thirty-seven patients were referred for resection of hepatic colorectal metastases. Thirteen patients received no neoadjuvant ther-

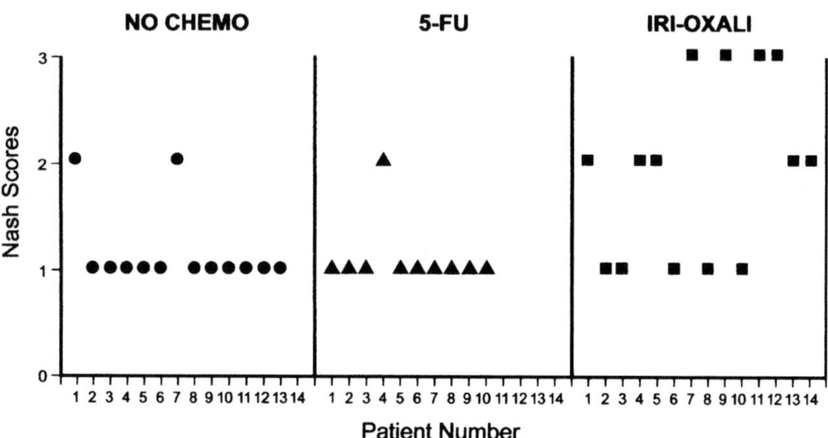

FIGURE 5.—Distribution of nonalcoholic steatohepatitis (NASH) scores in patients receiving neoadjuvant irinotecan, or oxaliplatin, or both (IR-OXALI); neoadjuvant 5-fluorouracil (5-FU) only; and no chemotherapy (NO CHEMO). There is a significant difference between the groups of patients who received no chemotherapy and the group that received irinotecan or oxaliplatin ($p < 0.003$). (Reprinted from Fernandez FG, Ritter J, Goodwin JW, et al: Effect of steatohepatitis associated with irinotecan or oxaliplatin pretreatment on resectability of hepatic colorectal metastases. *J Am Coll Surg* 200:845-853, 2005. Copyright 2005, with permission from the American College of Surgeons.)

apy (NO CHEMO group); 10 received neoadjuvant 5-fluorouracil only (5-FU group), and 14 received neoadjuvant irinotecan (n = 12), or oxaliplatin, or both (n = 4), in conjunction with 5-FU (IRI-OXALI group). Specimens were graded for the presence of nonalcoholic steatohepatitis (NASH) ac-

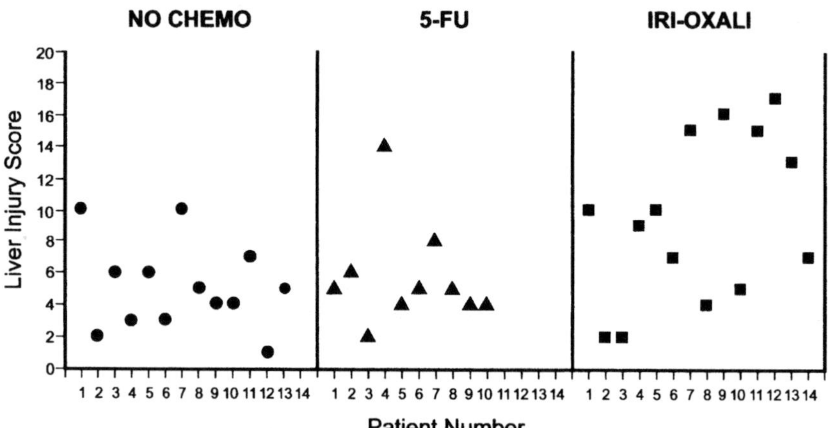

FIGURE 6.—Distribution of liver injury scores in patients receiving neoadjuvant irinotecan, or oxaliplatin, or both (IR-OXALI); neoadjuvant 5-fluorouracil (5-FU); and no chemotherapy (NO CHEMO). The difference between the groups of patients who received no chemotherapy or 5-FU and the group that received irinotecan or oxaliplatin was close to statistical significance ($p < 0.057$). (Reprinted from Fernandez FG, Ritter J, Goodwin JW, et al: Effect of steatohepatitis associated with irinotecan or oxaliplatin pretreatment on resectability of hepatic colorectal metastases. *J Am Coll Surg* 200:845-853, 2005. Copyright 2005, with permission from the American College of Surgeons.)

cording to established criteria. Specimens were also evaluated by a nine-criteria liver injury score (LIS).

Results.—Mean biopsy scores were: NO CHEMO: NASH, 1.2, LIS, 5.2; 5-FU only: NASH, 1.1, LIS 5.7; and IRI-OXALI: NASH, 1.9, LIS, 9.4. Biopsy scores were significantly worse for IRI-OXALI compared with NO CHEMO or 5-FU only for NASH score, p = 0.003 (Fig 5), and close to significantly worse for LIS score, p = 0.057 (Fig 6). A multivariate analysis showed that both being in the IRI-OXALI group and body mass index were independent risk factors for developing this type of steatohepatitis.

Conclusions.—Severe steatohepatitis can be associated with preoperative administration of irinotecan or oxaliplatin, especially in the obese. It can affect the ability to perform large liver resections. Consideration should be given to performing resections before commencing these agents and to obtaining preoperative biopsy in those who have received these agents.

▶ This is a study from Washington University School of Medicine in St Louis, Mo. It evaluates patients who are undergoing attempt at liver resection for treatment of colorectal metastases. It compares groups of patients receiving no chemotherapy versus 5-FU alone or patients who underwent neoadjuvant therapy with irinotecan or oxaliplatin. Patients who had irinotecan or oxaliplatin were more likely to statistically have nonalcoholic steatohepatitis. There were also borderline significantly worse scores for liver injury. Severe steatohepatitis appeared to be more common especially in obese patients.

Certainly in patients who have undergone neoadjuvant chemotherapy and have colorectal metastases, a liver biopsy should be evaluated preoperatively, particularly in obese patients, to determine the presence of steatohepatitis as this may limit the resectability of the patient.

T. J. Eberlein, MD

Gallbladder

An Aggressive Surgical Approach Leads to Improved Survival in Patients With Gallbladder Cancer: A 12-Year Study at a North American Center

Dixon E, Vollmer CM Jr, Sahajpal A, et al (Univ of Toronto; Univ of Calgary, Alta, Canada; Univ of Florida, Gainesville)

Ann Surg 241:385-394, 2005 11–19

Objective.—To determine if an aggressive surgical approach, with an increase in R0 resections, has resulted in improved survival for patients with gallbladder cancer.

Summary Background Data.—Many physicians express a relatively nihilistic approach to the treatment of gallbladder cancer; consensus among surgeons regarding the indications for a radical surgical approach has not been reached.

Methods.—A retrospective review of all patients with gallbladder cancer admitted during the past 12 years was conducted. Ninety-nine patients were identified. Cases treated during the 12-year period 1990 to 2002 were divided into 2 time-period (TP) cohorts, those treated in the first 6 years (TP1, N = 35) and those treated in the last 6 years (TP2, N = 64).

Results.—Disease stratification by stage and other demographic features were similar in the 2 time periods. An operation with curative intent was performed on 38 patients. Nine (26%) R0 resections were performed in TP1 and 24 (38%) in TP2. The number of liver resections, as well as the frequency of extrahepatic biliary resections, was greater in TP2 ($P < 0.04$). In both time periods, an R0 resection was associated with improved survival ($P < 0.02$ TP1, $P < 0.0001$ TP2). Overall survival of all patients in TP2 was significantly greater than in TP1 ($P < 0.03$), with a median survival of 9 months in TP1 and 17 months in TP2. The median 5-year survival in TP1 was 7%, and 35% in TP2. The surgical mortality rate for the entire cohort was 2%, with a 49% morbidity rate.

Conclusions.—A margin-negative, R0 resection leads to improved survival in patients with gallbladder cancer.

▶ Gallbladder cancer remains a disease often associated with poor survival. In addition, most centers have relatively few patients with gallbladder cancer that can be sufficiently analyzed to lead to an improved outcome.

This is a retrospective analysis of all patient treatment during the past 12 years at the University of Toronto, an outstanding hepatobiliary unit. It is interesting that the authors divided the 12-year analysis into 6-year cohorts. Even in this experienced center, the number of R0 resections increased in the later time frame as did the frequency of extra hepatic biliary resections. An R0 resection was the most important aspect associated with improved survival. However, even in an experienced center like this, these resections tended to be associated with morbidities. The presence of a drain, preoperative biliary stenting, or advanced stage or weight loss was more likely to be associated with complications after surgery for gallbladder cancer.

T. J. Eberlein, MD

Hepatocellular

The Spontaneous CD8+ T-Cell Response to HLA-A2–Restricted NY-ESO-1b Peptide in Hepatocellular Carcinoma Patients

Shang X-Y, Chen H-S, Zhang H-G, et al (Peking Univ Health Science Ctr, Beijing, People's Republic of China; Guangxi Guilin Med College, People's Republic of China; Memorial Sloan-Kettering Cancer Ctr, New York)

Clin Cancer Res 10:6946-6955, 2004 11–20

Purpose.—Hepatocellular carcinoma (HCC) can express various cancer-testis antigens including NY-ESO-1, members of the SSX family, members of the MAGE family, SCP-1, and CTP11. Immunotherapy directed against these antigens is a potential alternative treatment for HCC. To date, it remains unclear whether HCC patients have spontaneous immune responses to these tumor antigens. The objectives of this study were to measure immune responses to NY-ESO-1, a promising cancer vaccine candidate, in HCC patients using the HLA-A2-restricted NY-ESO-1b peptide (p157-165) to measure cellular responses and whole protein to measure antibody responses.

Experimental Design.—In HLA-A2$^+$ patients with NY-ESO-1$^+$ HCC, we analyzed T-cell antigen-dependent interferon (IFN)-γ and/or Granzyme B release by enzyme-linked immunospot (ELISPOT) assay and IFN-γ–producing intracellular cytokine flow cytometry (CytoSpot). As an assay independent of T-cell function, we performed tetramer staining. Antibodies to whole NY-ESO-1 were assayed by enzyme-linked immunosorbent assay.

Results.—The frequency of specific CD8$^+$ T-cell responses to NY-ESO-1b in 28 NY-ESO-1 mRNA$^+$HLA-A2$^+$ HCC patients was 35.7% (10 of 28). The average magnitude of effector CD8$^+$ T cells was 0.3% (89 ± 59 per 2.5 × 10^4 CD8$^+$ cells) and 1.2% as measured by IFN-gamma release ELISPOT and CytoSpot assays, respectively. These *in vitro* induced NY-ESO-1b–specific CD8$^+$ T cells can also recognize HepG2 cells transfected with pcDNA3.1-NY-ESO-1 in both IFN-gamma and Granzyme B ELISPOT assays. Frequencies of NY-ESO-1b–specific T cells in several patients were confirmed by tetramer staining. Nonfunctional tetramer$^+$CD8$^+$ T cells were also present. The CD8$^+$ T-cell response was apparently increased in patients with late-stage HCC. A discordance between antibody and CD8$^+$ T-cell responses in HCC patients was observed.

Conclusions.—The elevated frequency of specific CD8$^+$ T-cell responses to NY-ESO-1b in NY-ESO-1 mRNA$^+$HLA-A2$^+$ HCC patients suggests that NY-ESO-1 is appropriate for use in the immunotherapy of HCC patients.

▶ HCC is certainly 1 of the most common malignancies in the Pacific basin. In addition, it remains 1 of the more difficult to treat malignancies particularly in late stages. One methodology that has been proposed is immune therapies directed against antigens. NY-ESO-1 is 1 of the most promising cancer vaccine candidates for a variety of tumor types. Here the authors use the CD8 T-cell response to NY-ESO-1b peptide utilizing IFNγ and/or GrB release.

A cytotoxic response to this antigen is possible. However, it is not uniform. The real question is why do not all patients have this immune response and more importantly, how might one exploit this immune response to make it a more vigorous response and make it more uniform. Look for vaccine therapies to some of these difficult to treat tumors over the next year or so.

T. J. Eberlein, MD

Gastric

Distribution of CD4(+)CD25^{high} Regulatory T-Cells in Tumor-draining Lymph Nodes in Patients With Gastric Cancer

Kawaida H, Kono K, Takahashi A, et al (Univ of Yamanashi, Japan)

J Surg Res 124:151-157, 2005 11–21

Background.—Regulatory T-cells (T-regs) can inhibit the immune response mediated by T-cells. There is an increasing evidence that there is an increased proportion of T-regs in PBLs and tumor-infiltrating lymphocytes in several different human malignancies, although the mechanism remains unclear. In the present study, we evaluated the prevalence of CD4(+)CD25^{high} T-regs in tumor-draining lymph nodes in patients with gastric cancers.

Materials and Methods.—Regional lymph nodes in the stomach of the patients with gastric cancer (n = 44) were classified into N1 regional lymph nodes adjacent to the gastric tumor and N2 regional lymph nodes marginally distant from the tumor. The population of CD4(+)CD25^{high} T-cells as a percentage of total CD4(+) cells was evaluated by flow cytometric analysis with triple-color staining. Cytokine production (IL-10 and IFN-γ) was evaluated by intracellular cytokine staining and the antiproliferative function of CD4(+)CD25(+) cells positively selected by magnetic beads was measured by evaluating the proliferative activity of CD4(+)CD25(−) cells in response to anti-CD3 plus anti-CD28 in the presence of autologous CD4(+) CD25(+) cells.

Results.—The percentage of CD4(+)CD25^{high} T-cells in N1 regional lymph nodes (3.1 ± 0.3%) was significantly higher than that of control mesenteric lymph nodes (1.2 ± 0.3%, $P < 0.01$). Furthermore, a more extended area (N2) of regional lymph nodes, as well as adjacent lymph nodes (N1) to the tumors, was involved in an increased prevalence of CD4(+)CD25^{high} T-cells according to the disease progression. The functional evaluations confirmed that CD4(+)CD25^{high} T-cells derived from the lymph nodes have an inhibitory activity corresponding to T-regs.

Conclusions.—The populations of CD4(+)CD25^{high} T-cells in the regional lymph nodes in patients with gastric cancer were significantly higher in comparison to those in control lymph nodes. The increased prevalence of T-regs may be one of the explanations for impaired cell-mediated immunity in cancer-bearing hosts.

► This is a very interesting basic science publication that may have important ramifications for clinical care. It has always been puzzling how patients with malignancy are able to escape immune surveillance. Recent work in a number of laboratories have shown the importance of CD4(+)CD25(+) regulatory T cells. These cells tend to be suppressive in nature. These lymphocytes have a tendency to suppress immune surveillance functions. In the present study, lymph nodes harboring large numbers of these lymphocytes were more prevalent in regional lymph nodes in patients with gastric cancer compared with their prevalence in control lymph nodes.

Understanding the proper role of these lymphocytes in patients with malignancy will be important before having any kind of effective vaccine or gene therapy. Either elimination of these suppressor lymphocytes or neutralizing them will be important in effectively developing immune-based therapies in adjuvant or even preventative strategy.

T. J. Eberlein, MD

Pancreatic

EUS-guided FNA of Pancreatic Metastases: A Multicenter Experience

DeWitt J, Jowell P, LeBlanc J, et al (Indianapolis; Durham, NC; Mineola, NY)
Gastrointest Endosc 61:689-696, 2005 11–22

Background.—Metastatic lesions of the pancreas are a rare but important cause of focal pancreatic lesions. The purpose of this study is to describe the EUS features, cytologic diagnoses, and clinical impact of a cohort of patients with pancreatic metastases diagnosed by EUS-guided FNA (EUS-FNA).

Methods.—Over a 6-year period, in a retrospective, multicenter study, patients had the diagnosis of pancreatic metastases confirmed with EUS-FNA. All examinations were performed by one of 5 experienced endosonographers. The EUS and the clinical findings of pancreatic metastases were compared with those of a cohort with primary pancreatic malignancy.

Results.—Thirty-seven patients with possible metastases were identified, and 13 were excluded because of diagnostic uncertainty. The remaining 24 underwent EUS-FNA (mean passes 4.1) of a pancreatic mass without complications. Diagnoses included metastases from primary kidney (10), skin (6), lung (4), colon (2), liver (1), and stomach (1) cancer. In 4 (17%), 16 (67%), and 24 (100%) patients, EUS-FNA provided the initial diagnosis of malignancy, tumor recurrence, and pancreatic metastases, respectively. Four (17%) metastases initially were discovered by EUS after negative (n = 3) or inconclusive (n = 1) CT scans. Compared with primary cancer, pancreatic metastases were more likely to have well-defined margins (46% vs. 4%) compared with irregular (94% vs. 54%; $p < 0.0001$) margins. No statistically significant difference between the two populations was noted for tumor size, echogenicity, consistency, location, lesion number, or number of FNA passes performed.

Conclusions.—Pancreatic metastases are an important cause of focal pancreatic lesions and may occasionally be discovered during EUS examination after previously negative or inconclusive CT. Use of immunocytochemistry, when available, may help to confirm a suspected diagnosis. These lesions are more likely to have well-defined EUS margins compared with primary pancreatic cancer.

► One of the vexing problems in evaluating patients with a pancreatic mass is whether this is a primary tumor. CT scans are often negative or inconclusive. This article shows that endoscopic ultrasound fine needle aspiration (EUS-FNA) can lead to definitive diagnosis.

Frequently, pancreatic metastases had a different characteristic in EUS. Pancreatic metastases were more likely to have a better-defined tumor margin, whereas primary pancreatic cancers were overwhelmingly irregular in their margins. This technology can be an important way to distinguish primary metastatic lesions.

T. J. Eberlein, MD

12 Vascular Surgery

Introduction

Evolution of the role of catheter-based therapy in the management of peripheral vascular disease continues. However, as expected, with the investigation of new management approaches to any disease as more is learned, the limitations and advantages of this new, less invasive therapy become clearer.

During the past year, an increased stroke risk associated with carotid angioplasty and stenting in patients older than 80 years has been demonstrated (Abstract 12–1). Similarly, midterm results from the 2 major European randomized trials of endovascular versus open repair of infrarenal abdominal aortic aneurysms (Abstracts 12–6 and 12–7) demonstrated that the initial survival advantage associated with endovascular repair was lost by 2 years after treatment. Additionally, endovascular repair of aneurysms in patients unfit for open repair did not appear to improve survival compared with conservative therapy (Abstract 12–8). In contrast, results from the pivotal trials of endovascular repair of thoracic aortic aneurysms (including thoracoabdominal aortic aneurysms) and other thoracic aortic pathology were very encouraging (Abstracts 12–10 through 12–13), and as open surgical repair of such problems continues to be associated with high morbidity and mortality rates, endovascular treatment of these complex problems will likely be of significant patient benefit. Similarly, endovascular treatment of popliteal aneurysms now appears feasible and associated with acceptable results in properly selected patients (Abstract 12–14). Finally, the utility of endovascular techniques in patients with peripheral arterial occlusive disease sufficient to produce critical limb ischemia is becoming clearer, although the selection bias associated with the results from the retrospective studies from which these results come demonstrate the critical importance of appropriate judgment in the selection of such patients for endovascular therapy (Abstract 12–15).

While the use of endovascular techniques is certainly changing the treatment of peripheral vascular disease, advances in open surgical techniques and medical therapy also remain important. Carotid endarterectomy for now remains the mainstay of the treatment of extracranial carotid occlusive disease, and patch closure is now the standard of care for that procedure (Abstracts 12–2 and 12–3). Additionally, perioperative use of statins appears to limit the stroke risk associated with carotid endarterectomy (Abstract 12–4). Similarly, vein grafts for infrainguinal bypass procedures, arising from the most distal appropriate inflow site (Abstract 12–14), are the standard of care for symptomatic infrainguinal arterial occlusive disease not appropriate for endovascular therapy, and patients with this problem need aggressive risk factor control to limit their long-term cardiovascular morbidity. Unfortunately, this is still not done commonly enough (Abstract 12–18). Finally, the number of patients requiring access procedures for hemodialysis and surgical procedures for venous insufficiency continues to grow, and a better understanding of the outcome associated with these procedures (Abstracts 12–21 and 12–22) is making the selection of the appropriate procedure for these problems easier.

Thus, the last year has seen our knowledge base for the treatment of patients with peripheral vascular disease grow. As expected, the additions were for the most part incremental, but in most cases that is how we learn to better treat our patients. Endovascular therapy continues to be attractive because of its limited invasiveness, but open surgical procedures continue to have an important role in the care of our patients with peripheral vascular disease. The important role of medical therapy in such patients also continues to be demonstrated. The thing that we all must remember, however, is that the most difficult part of managing these complex and often frail patients is selection of the proper therapy or combination of therapies for their problems, and this selection must be based on judgment informed by knowledge.

James M. Seeger, MD

Carotid

Comparison of Angioplasty and Stenting With Cerebral Protection Versus Endarterectomy for Treatment of Internal Carotid Artery Stenosis in Elderly Patients

Kastrup A, Schulz JB, Raygrotzki S, et al (Univ of Tübingen, Germany; Univ of Jena, Germany)

J Vasc Surg 40:945-951, 2004 12–1

Purpose.—Carotid angioplasty and stenting (CAS) is being evaluated as an alternative to carotid endarterectomy (CEA) for treatment of severe carotid artery stenosis. Because CAS does not require general anesthesia and is less traumatic, it might be especially advantageous in older patients, but data comparing these 2 treatment methods in older patients are scarce.

Methods.—The periprocedural complication rates in 53 patients aged 75 years or older who had undergone protected CAS between June 2001 and April 2004 were compared with those in a group of 110 patients aged 75 years or older who had undergone CEA between January 1997 and December 2001, before widespread introduction of CAS procedures at our institution. All patients were evaluated by a neurologist both before and after surgery. According to the criteria set forth by the large trials the occurrence of minor, major, or fatal stroke, and myocardial infarction within 30 days was determined.

Results.—The demographic characteristics and indications for an intervention were similar in both treatment groups. Thirty patients (57%) in the

CAS group had symptomatic carotid stenosis, compared with 69 patients (63%) in the CEA group. In neither group was there any fatal stroke or myocardial infarction. The 30-day stroke rate was significantly higher in the CAS group (4 minor, 2 major strokes; 11.3%) than in the CEA group (no minor, 2 major strokes; 1.8%; $P < .05$). Although the 30-day major stroke rate between CAS and CEA groups was comparable (3.8% vs 1.8%; $P = 0.6$), this effect was mainly attributable to a significantly higher rate of minor stroke in the CAS group (7.5% vs 0%; $P < .05$).

Conclusion.—Despite the use of cerebral protection devices the neurologic complication rate in patients aged 75 years and older associated with CAS was significantly higher than with CEA performed by highly skilled surgeons at our academic institution. Although this finding is mainly based on a significantly higher rate of minor stroke in the CAS group, the common practice of preferentially submitting older patients to CAS is questionable, and should be abandoned until the results of further randomized trials are available.

► CAS is currently only approved for use in symptomatic patients who are high risk, and one of the defined characteristics of such high risk patients is increased age. However, this study suggests that patients aged 75 years or older have an increased risk of stroke after angioplasty and stenting compared with carotid endarterectomy, a finding that is supported by other studies as well. The reason for this increased stroke risk in elderly patients is unknown but has been suggested to possibly be a decreased tolerance for the embolic debris that occurs in all patients undergoing carotid angioplasty and stenting, even with the use of cerebral protection devices. Regardless, the precise role of this new, less-invasive technique in the treatment of carotid atherosclerosis continues to evolve, so limiting its widespread use for now seems prudent.

J. M. Seeger, MD

Systematic Review of Randomized Controlled Trials of Patch Angioplasty Versus Primary Closure and Different Types of Patch Materials During Carotid Endarterectomy

Bond R, Rerkasem K, Naylor AR, et al (Radcliffe Infirmary, Oxford, England; Southampton Gen Hosp, England; Leicester Royal Infirmary, England; et al)

J Vasc Surg 40:1126-1135, 2004 12–2

Background.—Patch angioplasty during carotid endarterectomy (CEA) may reduce the risk for perioperative or late carotid artery recurrent stenosis and subsequent ischemic stroke. We performed a systematic review of randomized controlled trials to assess the effect of routine or selective carotid patch angioplasty compared with CEA with primary closure, and the effect of different materials used for carotid patch angioplasty.

Methods.—Randomized trials were included if they compared carotid patch angioplasty with primary closure in any patients undergoing CEA or use of one type of carotid patch with another.

Results.—Thirteen eligible randomized trials were identified. Seven trials involving 1281 operations compared primary closure with routine patch closure, and 8 trials with 1480 operations compared different patch materials (2 studies compared both). Patch angioplasty was associated with a reduction in risk for stroke of any type (P = 004), ipsilateral stroke (P = .001), and stroke or death during both the perioperative period (P = .007) and long-term follow-up (P = .004). Patching was also associated with reduced risk for perioperative arterial occlusion (P = .0001) and decreased recurrent stenosis during long-term follow-up (P < 0001). Seven trials that compared different patch types showed no difference in the risk for stroke, death, or arterial recurrent stenosis either perioperatively or at 1-year follow-up. One study of 180 patients (200 arteries) compared collagen-impregnated Dacron (Hemashield) patches with polytetrafluoroethylene patches. There was a significant increase in risk for stroke (P = .02), combined stroke and transient ischemic attack (P = .03), and recurrent stenosis (P = 01) at 30 days, and an increased risk for late recurrent stenosis greater than 50% (P < .001) associated with Dacron compared with polytetrafluoroethylene.

Conclusions.—Carotid patch angioplasty decreases the risk for perioperative death or stroke, and long-term risk for ipsilateral ischemic stroke. More data are required to establish differences between various patch materials.

Primary Closure of the Carotid Artery Is Associated With Poorer Outcomes During Carotid Endarterectomy

Rockman CB, Halm EA, Wang JJ, et al (New York Univ; Mt Sinai School of Medicine, New York)
J Vasc Surg 42:870-877, 2005 12–3

Introduction.—Arterial endarterectomy and reconstruction during carotid endarterectomy (CEA) can be performed in a variety of ways, including standard endarterectomy with primary closure, standard endarterectomy with patch angioplasty, and eversion endarterectomy. The optimal method of arterial reconstruction remains a matter of controversy. The objective of this study was to determine the effect of the method of arterial reconstruction during CEA on perioperative outcome.

Methods.—A retrospective cohort study of consecutive CEAs performed by 81 surgeons during 1997 and 1998 in six regional hospitals was performed. Detailed clinical data regarding each case and all deaths and nonfatal strokes within 30 days of surgery were ascertained by an independent review of the inpatient chart, outpatient surgeon record, and the hospitals' administrative databases. Two physician investigators—one neurologist and one internist—confirmed each adverse event by independently reviewing patients' medical records.

Results.—A total of 1972 CEAs were performed. The mean age of the patients was 72.3 years, and 57.2% were male. Preoperative neurologic symptoms occurred in 28.7% of cases (n = 566), and the remaining 71.3% were asymptomatic before surgery (n = 1406). The method of arterial reconstruction was chosen by the surgeon. Primary closure was performed in 11.8% (n = 233), patch angioplasty in 69.8% (n = 1377), and eversion endarterectomy in 18.4% (n = 362). There was no significant difference in the preoperative symptom status of patients who underwent primary closure compared with the other methods of reconstruction (72.5% asymptomatic vs 71.1%, *P* = NS). Primary closure cases were significantly more likely to experience perioperative stroke compared with the other closure techniques (5.6% vs 2.2%, *P* = .006). Primary closure cases also had a higher incidence of perioperative stroke or death compared with the other closure techniques (6.0% vs 2.5%, *P* = .006). There were no significant differences with regard to either perioperative stroke, or perioperative stroke/death noted when comparing patch angioplasty with eversion endarterectomy: stroke, 2.2% vs 2.5% (*P* = NS) and stroke/death, 2.5% vs 2.5% (*P* = NS) respectively.

Conclusion.—It appears that primary closure is associated with significantly worse perioperative outcomes compared with endarterectomy with patch angioplasty and eversion endarterectomy, even when the preoperative symptom status of the patient cohorts is equivalent. Although some of its advocates have reported that they can properly select appropriate patients for primary closure based on the size of the artery and other factors, the data demonstrate that these patients have poorer outcomes nonetheless. Primary closure during carotid endarterectomy should predominantly be abandoned in favor of either standard endarterectomy with patch angioplasty or eversion endarterectomy.

► Taken together, these 2 studies (Abstracts 12–2 and 12–3) strongly support patch closure in patients undergoing carotid endarterectomy. Bond et al's systematic review of randomized trials demonstrates decreased rates of perioperative stroke, arterial occlusion, ipsilateral stroke, stroke or death, and long-term restenosis compared with primary closure. Rockman et al's retrospective study confirms these findings using real-world data from 6 hospitals in New York. Additionally, in a study by Kresowick et al cited in last year's Year Book of Surgery,[1] increased use of patch closure was associated with improved results after carotid endarterectomy, again in the real world. Thus, patch closure appears to be the standard of care for patients undergoing carotid endarterectomy, and use of primary closure especially when a complication occurs, is increasingly difficult to defend.

J. M. Seeger, MD

Reference

1. 2005 Year Book of Surgery, p 347.

3-Hydroxy-3-Methylglutaryl Coenzyme A Reductase Inhibitors Reduce the Risk of Perioperative Stroke and Mortality After Carotid Endarterectomy

McGirt MJ, Perler B, Brooke BS, et al (Johns Hopkins Med Insts, Baltimore, Md)

J Vasc Surg 42:829-836, 2005 12–4

Objective.—There is increasing evidence that 3-hydroxy-3-methylglutaryl coenzyme A reductase inhibitors (statins) reduce cardiovascular and cerebrovascular events through anti-inflammatory, plaque stabilization, and neuroprotective effects independent of lipid lowering. This study was designed to investigate whether statin use reduces the incidence of perioperative stroke and mortality among patients undergoing carotid endarterectomy (CEA).

Methods.—All patients undergoing CEA from 1994 to 2004 at a large academic medical center were retrospectively reviewed. The independent association of statin use and perioperative morbidity was assessed via multivariate logistic regression analysis.

Results.—CEA was performed by 13 surgeons on 1566 patients (987 men and 579 women; mean age, 72 ± 10 years), including 1440 (92%) isolated and 126 (8%) combined CEA/coronary artery bypass grafting procedures. The indication for CEA was symptomatic disease in 660 (42%) cases. Six hundred fifty-seven (42%) patients received a statin medication for at least 1 week before surgery. Statin use was associated with a reduction in perioperative strokes (1.2% vs 4.5%; $P < .01$), transient ischemic attacks (1.5% vs 3.6%; $P < .01$), all-cause mortality (0.3% vs 2.1%; $P < .01$), and median (interquartile range) length of hospitalization (2 days [2-5 days] vs 3 days

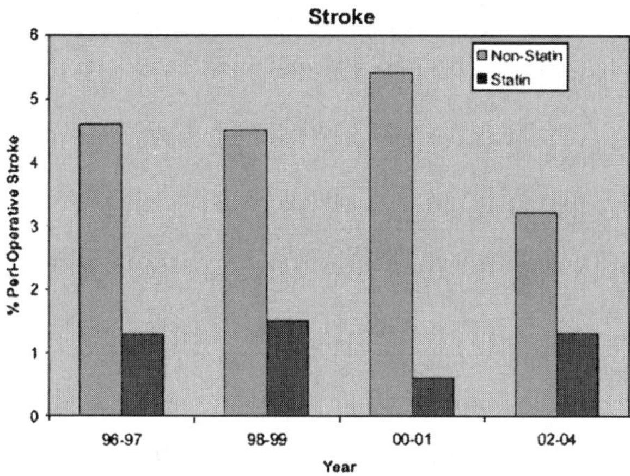

FIGURE 1.—Incidence of postoperative stroke after carotid endarterectomy as a function of statin vs no statin use over time. The postoperative stroke rate remained lower in patients receiving statins, regardless of the year of operation. (Courtesy of McGirt MJ, Perler B, Brooke BS, et al: 3-Hydroxy-3-methylglutaryl coenzyme A reductase inhibitors reduce the risk of perioperative stroke and mortality after carotid endarterectomy. *J Vasc Surg* 42:829-836, 2005. Copyright 2005 by Elsevier.)

[2-7 days]; $P < .05$). Adjusting for all demographics and comorbidities in multivariate analysis, statin use independently reduced the odds of stroke threefold (odds ratio [95% confidence interval], 0.35 [0.15-0.85]; $P < .05$) (Fig 1) and death fivefold (odds ratio [95% confidence interval], 0.20 [0.04-0.99]; $P < .05$).

Conclusions.—These data suggest that perioperative statin use may reduce the incidence of cerebrovascular events and mortality among patients undergoing CEA.

► Although a retrospective review, this study clearly demonstrates a significantly reduced risk of neurologic events and mortality after carotid endarterectomy in patients taking statin drugs. The mechanism of this reduction is likely the non–lipid-lowering effects of statins, including plaque stabilization and improved endothelial cell function. Regardless, the value of these drugs in patients with peripheral arterial disease continues to be demonstrated and likely most, if not all, of our patients should be treated with statins.

J. M. Seeger, MD

Does Carotid Endarterectomy Improve Cognitive Functioning?

Bossema ER, Brand N, Moll FL, et al (Utrecht Univ, The Netherlands; St Antonius Hosp, Nieuwegein, The Netherlands)

J Vasc Surg 41:775-781, 2005 12–5

Background.—Carotid endarterectomy (CEA) might improve cognitive functioning, but studies thus far have produced mixed results. The aim of the present study was to examine the effect of CEA on cognitive functions in a methodologically more strict design, first by testing the presumption of preoperative cognitive impairment and second through a better control for the possible influence of the nonspecific effects of practice and surgery.

Methods.—Preoperative performance on a neuropsychologic test battery of 56 patients with severe occlusive disease of the carotid artery but without history of major stroke was compared with the performance of 46 healthy control subjects and 23 patients before endarterectomy of the superficial femoral artery (remote endarterectomy). The degree of cognitive change in the 2 patient groups was compared at 3 and 12 months postoperatively. We assessed mood to control for possible momentary affective influences on cognition.

Results.—Before CEA, patients showed reduced functioning compared with that seen in healthy control subjects in terms of attention, verbal and visual memory, planning of motor behavior, psychomotor skills, and executive function. Performance of patients before remote endarterectomy was reduced as well. Improvements in several cognitive functions were observed after both types of surgical interventions and were attributed to psychologic relief from uncomplicated surgery and to practice.

Conclusions.—No specific restorative effect of CEA on cognitive functioning was observed. The preoperative impairment in several cognitive domains might be caused by factors that patients with various types of vascular disease might have in common, such as small-vessel disease or other undetected abnormalities within the brain.

▶ This well-done study should go a long way to debunk the idea that carotid endarterectomy improves cognitive function by improving cerebral blood flow. Additionally, it demonstrates that patients with significant peripheral arterial occlusive disease have decreased cognitive function compared with healthy control subjects. What is unknown is whether carotid endarterectomy stabilizes cognitive function compared with medical therapy and how appropriate medical therapy may limit cognitive decline compared with inadequate medical treatment, as many of our patients are now receiving. While we currently can't answer these important questions, it is clear that standard indications for carotid endarterectomy (stroke, transient ischemic attack, asymptomatic high-grade stenosis) remain the most appropriate.

J. M. Seeger, MD

Aneurysm

Endovascular Aneurysm Repair Versus Open Repair in Patients With Abdominal Aortic Aneurysm (EVAR Trial 1): Randomised Controlled Trial

Greenhalgh RM, for the EVAR Trial Participants (Imperial College London; et al)
Lancet 365:2179-2186, 2005 12–6

Background.—Although endovascular aneurysm repair (EVAR) has a lower 30-day operative mortality than open repair, the long-term results of EVAR are uncertain. We instigated EVAR trial 1 to compare these two treatments in terms of mortality, durability, health-related quality of life (HRQL), and costs for patients with large abdominal aortic aneurysm (AAA).

Methods.—We did a randomised controlled trial of 1082 patients aged 60 years or older who had aneurysms of at least 5.5 cm in diameter and who had been referred to one of 34 hospitals proficient in the EVAR technique. We assigned patients who were anatomically suitable for EVAR and fit for an open repair to EVAR (n=543) or open repair (n=539). Our primary endpoint was all-cause mortality, with secondary endpoints of aneurysm related mortality, HRQL, postoperative complications, and hospital costs. Analyses were by intention to treat.

Findings.—94% (1017 of 1082) of patients complied with their allocated treatment and 209 died by the end of follow-up on Dec 31, 2004 (53 of aneurysm-related causes). 4 years after randomisation, all-cause mortality was similar in the two groups (about 28%; hazard ratio 0.90, 95% CI 0.69–1.18, p=0.46), although there was a persistent reduction in aneurysm-related deaths in the EVAR group (4% vs 7%; 0.55, 0.31–0.96, p=0.04). The proportion of patients with postoperative complications within 4 years of randomisation was 41% in the EVAR group and 9% in the open repair group (4.9, 3.5–6.8, p<0.0001). After 12 months there was negligible difference in HRQL between the two groups. The mean hospital costs per patient

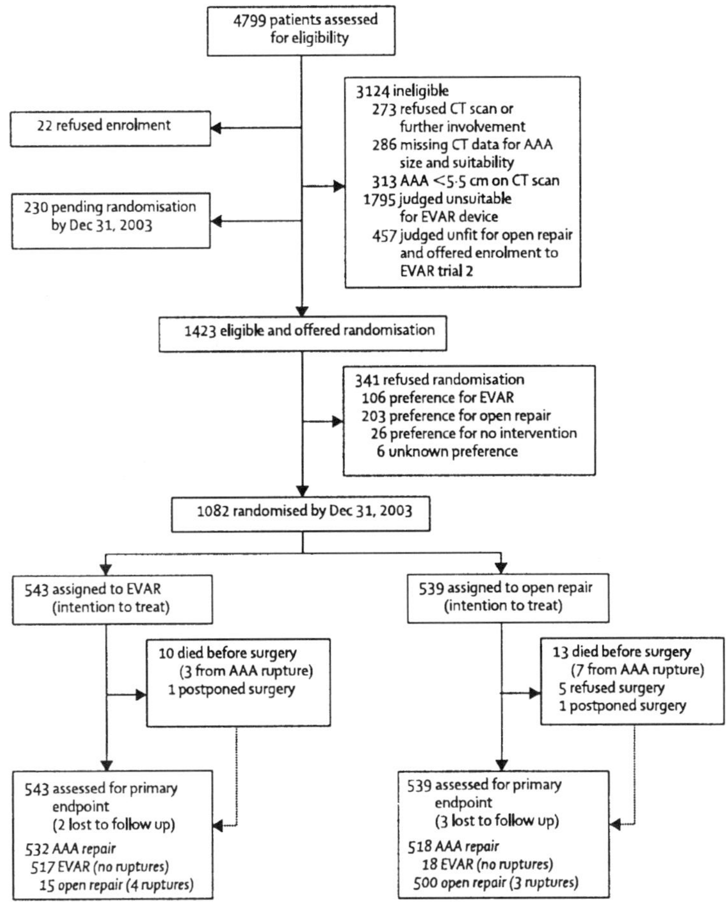

FIGURE 1.—Trial profile. (Courtesy of Greenhalgh RM, for the EVAR trial participants: Endovascular aneurysm repair versus open repair in patients with abdominal aortic aneurysm (EVAR trial 1): Randomised controlled trial. *Lancet* 365:2179-2186, 2005. Copyright by The Lancet Ltd., 2005.)

up to 4 years were UK £13,257 for the EVAR group versus £9946 for the open repair group (mean difference £3311, SE 690).

Interpretation.—Compared with open repair, EVAR offers no advantage with respect to all-cause mortality and HRQL, is more expensive, and leads to a greater number of complications and reinterventions. However, it does result in a 3% better aneurysm-related survival. The continuing need for interventions mandates ongoing surveillance and longer follow-up of EVAR for detailed cost-effectiveness assessment (Fig 1).

Two-Year Outcomes After Conventional or Endovascular Repair of Abdominal Aortic Aneurysms

Blankensteijn JD, for the Dutch Randomized Endovascular Aneurysm Management (DREAM) Trial Group (Radboud Univ, Nijmegen, The Netherlands; et al)

N Engl J Med 352:2398-2405, 2005 12–7

Background.—Two randomized trials have shown better outcomes with elective endovascular repair of abdominal aortic aneurysms than with conventional open repair in the first month after the procedure. We investigated whether this advantage is sustained beyond the perioperative period.

Methods.—We conducted a multicenter, randomized trial comparing open repair with endovascular repair in 351 patients who had received a diagnosis of abdominal aortic aneurysm of at least 5 cm in diameter and who were considered suitable candidates for both techniques. Survival after randomization was calculated with the use of Kaplan–Meier analysis and compared with the use of the log-rank test on an intention-to-treat-basis.

Results.—Two years after randomization, the cumulative survival rates were 89.6 percent for open repair and 89.7 percent for endovascular repair (difference, −0.1 percentage point; 95 percent confidence interval, −6.8 to 6.7 percentage points). The cumulative rates of aneurysm-related death were 5.7 percent for open repair and 2.1 percent for endovascular repair (difference, 3.7 percentage points; 95 percent confidence interval, −0.5 to 7.9 percentage points). This advantage of endovascular repair over open repair was entirely accounted for by events occurring in the perioperative period, with no significant difference in subsequent aneurysm-related mortality. The rate of survival free of moderate or severe complications was also similar in the two groups at two years (at 65.9 percent for open repair and 65.6 percent for endovascular repair; difference, 0.3 percentage point; 95 percent confidence interval, −10.0 to 10.6 percentage points).

Conclusions.—The perioperative survival advantage with endovascular repair as compared with open repair is not sustained after the first postoperative year.

▶ These 2 midterm reports (Abstracts 12–6 and 12–7) from randomized trials of open versus endovascular aneurysm repair from England and The Netherlands present very similar results. Previous reports from these studies established a decreased perioperative mortality rate associated with endovascular aneurysm repair, and this decrease in aneurysm-related mortality rate is preserved to 2 years in the Dutch study and to 4 years in the British study. However, overall survival was not improved in either study at 24 to 48 months and, the need for subsequent procedures was substantially higher in the endovascular repair group, which increased the cost for this group in the British study. The exact meaning of these results remains unknown, as the cause of the excess mortality rate in the endovascular group was mostly (but not entirely) cardiovascular disease, suggesting that endovascular aneurysm repair may have simply delayed death in these patients. In addition, further follow-up could actually result in the survival curves crossing if the increased rate of reintervention in the endovascular group leads to an increased incidence of complications and death. Excess mortality is known to occur in the years after aneurysm repair, likely from patient comorbidities compared with the average population, but the question remains as to how these 2 types of aneurysm treatments will influence these subsequent events. Regardless, these mid-term intervention data are valuable in better defining the place of endovascular aneurysm repair in the management of patients with aortic aneurysms. For now, high-risk patients with good anatomy can undergo endovascular repair; low-risk, young patients should probably be encouraged to undergo open repair; and average-risk patients can undergo either procedure as long as they understand the need for follow-up and potential for subsequent extra procedures associated with endovascular aneurysm repair.

J. M. Seeger, MD

Endovascular Aneurysm Repair and Outcome in Patients Unfit for Open Repair of Abdominal Aortic Aneurysm (EVAR Trial 2): Randomised Controlled Trial

Greenhalgh RM, for the EVAR Trial Participants (Imperial College London; et al)
Lancet 365:2187-2192, 2005 12–8

Background.—Endovascular aneurysm repair (EVAR) to exclude abdominal aortic aneurysm (AAA) was introduced for patients of poor health status considered unfit for major surgery. We instigated EVAR trial 2 to identify whether EVAR improves survival compared with no intervention in patients unfit for open repair of aortic aneurysm.

Methods.—We did a randomised controlled trial of 338 patients aged 60 years or older who had aneurysms of at least 5.5 cm in diameter and who had been referred to one of 31 hospitals in the UK. We assigned patients to receive either EVAR (n=166) or no intervention (n=172). Our primary endpoint was all-cause mortality, with secondary endpoints of aneurysm-related mortality, health-related quality of life (HRQL), postoperative complications, and hospital costs. Analyses were by intention to treat.

Findings.—197 patients underwent aneurysm repair (47 assigned no intervention) and 80% of patients adhered to protocol. The 30-day operative mortality in the EVAR group was 9% (13 of 150, 95% CI 5–15) and the no intervention group had a rupture rate of 9.0 per 100 person years (95% CI 6.0–13.5). By end of follow up 142 patients had died, 42 of aneurysm-related factors; overall mortality after 4 years was 64%. There was no significant difference between the EVAR group and the no intervention group for all-cause mortality (hazard ratio 1.21, 95% CI 0.87–1.69, p=0.25). There was no difference in aneurysm-related mortality. The mean hospital costs per patient over 4 years were UK £13,632 in the EVAR group and £4983 in the no intervention group (mean difference £8649, SE 1248), with no difference in HRQL scores.

Interpretation.—EVAR had a considerable 30-day operative mortality in patients already unfit for open repair of their aneurysm. EVAR did not improve survival over no intervention and was associated with a need for continued surveillance and reinterventions, at substantially increased cost. Ongoing follow-up and improved fitness of these patients is a priority.

▶ This second British randomized trial examined the value of EVAR compared with no intervention in patients considered unfit for open surgical repair. Results to 4 years showed no difference in survival or aneurysm-related mortality. However, the aneurysms of 9 patients in the endovascular repair group ruptured before repair, causing half of the aneurysm-related deaths in this group and 20% of the patients in the no-intervention group had aneurysm repair and only 1 died, both of which obviously biases the results against EVAR. Regardless, the survival improvement from EVAR in high-risk patients does not appear dramatic, and again these patients required a significant number of secondary procedures. These results certainly raise the question of whether EVAR is beneficial in such high-risk patients and suggest strongly that it should only be considered when good anatomy for such repairs is present.

J. M. Seeger, MD

The Impact of Aortic Endografts on Renal Function

Alsac J-M, Zarins CK, Heikkinen MA, et al (Stanford Univ, Calif; Henri-Mondor Univ, Creteil, France)

J Vasc Surg 41:926-930, 2005 12–9

Objective.—To determine the impact on late postoperative renal function of suprarenal and infrarenal fixation of endografts used to treat infrarenal abdominal aortic aneurysm (AAA).

Methods.—Retrospective analysis of 277 patients treated from 2000 to 2003 with three different endografts at two clinical centers. Five patients on dialysis for preoperative chronic renal failure were excluded. Group IF of 135 patients treated with an infrarenal device (Medtronic AneuRx) was compared with group SF of 137 patients treated with a suprarenal device (106 Cook Zenith and 31 Medtronic Talent). Renal function was evaluated by calculating preoperative and latest postoperative creatinine clearance (CrCl) using the Cockcroft formula. Patients who developed a >20% decrease in CrCl were considered to have significantly impaired renal function.

Results.—There were no significant differences in patient age, sex, aneurysm size, preoperative risk factors, dose of intra- and postoperative contrast, or baseline CrCl (IF: 69.3 mL/min, SF: 71.7 mL/min, $P = .4$). Follow-up time of 12.2 months was the same in both groups. CrCl decreased significantly during the follow-up period in both groups (IF: 69.3 mL/min to 61.7 mL/min, $P < .01$; SF: 71.7 mL/min to 64.9 mL/min, $P < .03$). Postoperative CrCl (IF: 61.7 mL/min, SF: 64.9 mL/min, $P = .3$), and the rate of CrCl decrease during the follow-up period (IF: −10.9%, SF: −9.5%, $P = 2$) was not different between the two groups. The number of patients with a >20%

decrease in CrCl was not different between the two groups (IF: n = 35 [25.9%], SF: n = 41 [29.9%], *P* = .46). However, the magnitude of decrease in CrCl in patients with renal impairment was greater in patients treated with suprarenal fixation endografts (SF: −39%) compared with those treated with infrarenal endografts (IF: −31%, *P* = .005). This greater degree of renal impairment was not due to identifiable differences in preoperative risk factors, age, or baseline CrCl. No patients in these series required dialysis.

Conclusions.—Regardless the type of endograft used, there is a 10% decrease in CrCl in the first year after endovascular aneurysm repair. Suprarenal fixation does not seem to increase the likelihood of postoperative renal impairment. Decline in renal function over time after endovascular aortic repair is probably due to multiple factors, and measures known to be effective in protecting kidneys should be considered for these patients. Long-term follow-up with measurement of CrCl, along with renal imaging and regular blood pressure measurements, should be performed to detect possible late renal dysfunction. Prospective studies comparing suprarenal versus infrarenal fixation are needed to confirm those results.

▶ This report suggests that concerns about the negative impact of endovascular aneurysm repair on renal function may be justified. Approximately 1 year after endovascular aneurysm repair, renal function had declined by an average of approximately 10%, and the decline in some patients was much greater. However, the location of the proximal fixation of the aortic endograft (infrarenal vs suprarenal) did not appear to influence this decline. Renal function also declines after open aneurysm repair, but not to the same degree, which may further influence long-term results for endovascular aneurysm repair compared with open repair. Although endovascular repair clearly limits the initial risks associated with aortic aneurysm repair, the long-term value of this approach remains to be determined.

J. M. Seeger, MD

Endovascular Treatment of Thoracic Aortic Aneurysms: Results of the Phase II Multicenter Trial of the GORE TAG Thoracic Endoprosthesis

Makaroun MS, for the GORE TAG Investigators (Univ of Pittsburgh, Pa; et al)

J Vasc Surg 41:1-9, 2005 12–10

Objective.—A decade after the first report of descending thoracic aortic aneurysm (DTA) repair with endografts, a commercial device is yet to be approved in the United States. The GORE TAG endoprosthesis, an investigational nitinol-supported expanded polytetrafluoroethylene tube graft with diameters of 26 to 40 mm, is the first DTA device to enter phase II trials in the United States and has been used worldwide for a host of thoracic pathologies.

Methods.—A multicenter prospective nonrandomized phase II study of the GORE TAG endoprosthesis was conducted at 17 sites. Enrollment was from September 1999 to May 2001. Preoperative workup included arteriography and spiral computed tomography scans of the chest, abdomen, and pelvis. Follow-up radiographs and computed tomography scans were obtained at 1, 6, and 12 months and yearly thereafter.

Results.—A total of 139 (98%) of 142 patients had a successful implantation of the device. Inadequate arterial access was responsible for the 3 failures. The mean DTA size was 64.1 ± 15.4 mm. Men slightly outnumbered women (57.7%), with an average age of 71 years, and 88% of the patients were white. Ninety percent were American Society of Anesthesiologists category III or IV. One device was used in 44% of patients, and 56% required two or more devices to bridge the thoracic aorta. The left subclavian artery was covered in 28 patients, with planned carotid-subclavian transposition. The procedure time averaged 150 minutes, estimated blood loss averaged 506 mL, intensive care unit stay averaged 2.6 days, and hospital stay averaged 7.6 days. Within 30 days, 45 (32%) patients had at least 1 major adverse event: 5 (4%) experienced a stroke, 4 (3%) demonstrated temporary or permanent paraplegia, 20 (14%) experienced vascular trauma or thrombosis, and 2 (1.5%) died. Mean follow-up was 24.0 months. Four patients had aneurysm-related deaths. Three patients underwent endovascular revisions for endoleak. No ruptures have been reported. Twenty wire fractures have been identified in 19 patients; 18 (90%) of these occurred in the longitudinal spine, and only 1 patient required treatment. At 2 years, aneurysm-related and overall survival rates are 97% and 75%, respectively.

Conclusions.—The GORE TAG thoracic endoprosthesis provides a safe alternative for the treatment of DTAs, with low mortality, relatively low morbidity, and excellent 2-year freedom from aneurysm-related death. Longitudinal spine fractures have so far been associated with rare clinical events.

Endovascular Repair of Thoracic Aortic Lesions With the Zenith TX1 and TX2 Thoracic Grafts: Intermediate-Term Results

Greenberg RK, O'Neill S, Walker E, et al (Cleveland Clinic Found, Ohio)
J Vasc Surg 41:589-596, 2005 12–11

Purpose.—This prospective study was designed to assess the technical success and outcome after patients with thoracic aortic pathology at high risk for conventional therapy were treated with the Zenith TX1 and TX2 endovascular graft.

Methods.—Between 2001 and 2004, patients at high risk for conventional surgical therapy presenting with chronic aortic dissections, thoracic aneurysms, or aortobronchial or aortoesophageal fistulas were treated with a single- or multiple-piece endovascular grafts. Surgical modification of proximal or distal fixation sites was performed when necessary to establish adequate regions for device landing zones. Follow-up studies included radiographic evaluation before discharge and at 1, 6, 12, and 24 months. Aortic morphologic characteristics were determined by using three-dimensional imaging studies and centerline of flow measurements. Statistical analyses were performed with Kaplan Meier analysis to assess survival, factors predictive of poor outcome, and morphologic changes, including sac shrinkage.

Results.—A total of 100 patients (42% women) were treated, including 81 aneurysms, 15 aortic dissections (with aneurysms), 2 patients with fistulous connections (1 aortobronchial and 1 aortoesophageal), 1 subclavian artery aneurysm, and 1 aortic rupture. Mean follow-up and aneurysm size were 14 months and 62 mm, respectively. Most patients (55%) had undergone prior aortic aneurysm repair. Surgical modifications were required to create adequate implantation sites in 29% patients, including 14 elephant trunk/arch reconstructions, 18 carotid-subclavian bypasses, and 4 visceral vessel bypasses. Iliac conduits were required in 19 patients. Overall mortality was 17%, and aneurysm-related mortality was 14% at 1 year. Sac regression (>5 mm maximum diameter decrease) was observed in 52% and 56% at 12 and 24 months. Growth was noted in one patient (1.6%) at 12 months. Endoleaks were detected in eight patients (8.5%) at 30 days and three patients (6%) at 12 months. Secondary interventions were required in 15 patients. Migration (>10 mm) of the proximal or distal stent was noted in three patients (6%) (two proximal and one distal), none of which required treatment or resulted in an adverse event.

Conclusions.—Acceptable intermediate-term outcomes have been achieved in the treatment of high-risk patients in the setting of both favorable and challenging anatomic situations with these devices. The complexity of the patient population, in contrast to endovascular infrarenal repair, attests to the differences in the pathophysiology aortic disease in the anatomic beds.

Repair of Thoracoabdominal Aortic Aneurysms With Fenestrated and Branched Endovascular Stent Grafts

Anderson JL, Adam DJ, Berce M, et al (Ashford Community Hosp, South Australia; Birmingham Heartlands Hosp, England; Royal Adelaide Hosp, South Australia; et al)

J Vasc Surg 42:600-607, 2005 12–12

Objective.—To report the repair of thoracoabdominal aortic aneurysms (TAAAs) with fenestrated and branched endovascular stent grafts (EVSGs).

Methods.—Four patients with asymptomatic TAAAs were treated with custom-designed Zenith fenestrated and branched EVSGs. Three patients had undergone previous open aortic aneurysm repair. Thirteen visceral vessels in four patients were targeted for incorporation by graft fenestrations and branches.

Results.—The fenestration/orifice interface was secured with balloon-expandable Genesis stents or Jostent stent grafts in 9 of 13 target vessels. Completion angiography demonstrated antegrade perfusion in 12 of 13 target vessels. One renal artery occluded because of graft rotation during deployment. There were no endoleaks. Three patients required additional surgical procedures related to access vessels. One patient required reoperation

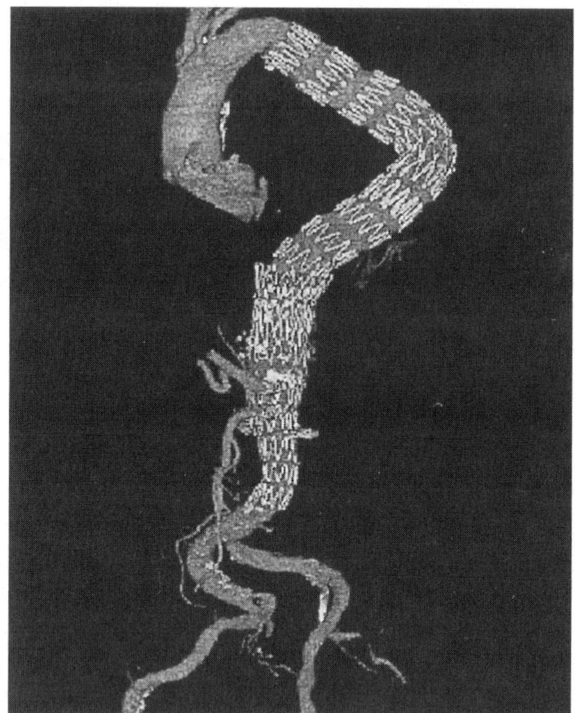

FIGURE 4.—Follow-up computed tomographic angiography in patient 2 demonstrating aneurysm exclusion and patent celiac axis, superior mesenteric artery, and both renal arteries. (Courtesy of Anderson JL, Adam DJ, Berce M, et al: Repair of thoracoabdominal aortic aneurysms with fenestrated and branched endovascular stent grafts. *J Vasc Surg* 42:600-607, 2005. Copyright 2005 by Elsevier.)

for bleeding from an extra-anatomic bypass graft and subsequently died from multisystem organ failure. Three patients made an uncomplicated recovery. No patient developed spinal cord ischemia. Computed tomography at 12 months in the 3 survivors demonstrated complete aneurysm exclusion with antegrade perfusion in all 10 target vessels (Fig 4).

Conclusions.—TAAA repair with fenestrated and branched EVSGs is feasible and provides an acceptable and promising alternative to conventional surgical repair in selected patients.

► These 3 reports (Abstracts 12–10 through 12–12) clearly demonstrate the progress in endovascular treatment of thoracic aortic pathology. Although these reports deal with early experience with this new approach to thoracic aortic disease, the potential for decreased morbidity and mortality rates in these complex patients is clear. The mortality rate appears to be significantly lower and, the incidence of spinal cord injury may be dramatically reduced. In Canada and Europe, where these devices have been available for a longer period of time, by report more than 50% of thoracic and thoracoabdominal aortic aneurysms are now repaired by using endovascular techniques alone. These reports clearly represent a glimpse into the future, and for patients with thoracic aortic disease, that glimpse is very encouraging.

J. M. Seeger, MD

Surgical Versus Endovascular Treatment of Traumatic Thoracic Aortic Rupture

Amabile P, Collart F, Gariboldi V, et al (Hôpital Sainte Marguerite, Marseille, France; Hôpital de la Timone, Marseille, France)

J Vasc Surg 40:873-879, 2004 12–13

Objectives.—Blunt traumatic thoracic aortic rupture is a life-threatening surgical emergency associated with high mortality and morbidity. The recent development of endovascular stent-graft prostheses offers a potentially less invasive alternative to open chest surgery, especially in patients with associated injuries. We sought to compare the results of conventional surgical repair and endovascular treatment of traumatic aortic rupture in a single center.

Methods.—From July 1998 to January 2004, 20 patients with acute blunt traumatic aortic rupture underwent treatment at our institution. All patients had a lesion limited to the isthmus, and associated injuries. Initial management included fluid resuscitation, treatment of other severe associated lesions, and strict monitoring of blood pressure. Eleven patients (9 men, 2 women; mean age, 32 years) underwent surgical repair, including direct suturing in 6 patients and graft interposition in 5 patients. Ten patients were operated on with cardiopulmonary support (left bypass with centrifugal pump, n = 2; extracorporeal circulation, n = 8). The delay between trauma and surgery was 2.6 days (range, 0-21 days). Nine patients (8 men, 1 woman; mean age, 32 years) underwent endovascular treatment with commercially available devices (Excluder, n = 2; Talent, n = 7). In all patients 1 stent graft was deployed. In 2 patients the left subclavian artery was intentionally covered with the device. The delay between trauma and endovascular treatment was 17.8 days (range, 1-68 days).

Results.—One patient in the surgical group (9.1%) died during the intervention. Three surgical complications occurred in 3 patients (27%), including left phrenic nerve palsy (n = 1), left-sided recurrent nerve palsy (n = 1), and hemopericardium 16 days after surgery that required a repeat intervention (n = 1). No patient in this group had paraplegia. In the endovascular group successful stent-graft deployment was achieved in all patients, with no conversion to open repair. No patient died, and no procedure-related complications, including paraplegia, occurred in this group. Control computed tomography scans obtained within 7 days after endovascular treatment showed exclusion of pseudoaneurysm in all cases. Length of follow-up for endovascular treatment ranged from 3 to 41 months (mean, 15.1 months). Computed tomography scans obtained 3 months after endovascular treatment showed complete disappearance of pseudoaneurysm in all patients.

Conclusion.—In the treatment of blunt traumatic thoracic aortic rupture, the immediate outcome in patients who receive endovascular stent grafts appears to be at least as good as observed after conventional surgical repair. Long-term follow-up is necessary to assess long-term effectiveness of such management.

▶ Although this report presents preliminary results, the value of endovascular repair of traumatic thoracic aortic disruption is clearly suggested. Patients with this problem often have several other severe injuries, and avoiding thoracotomy, anticoagulation when left heart bypass is needed, and aortic clamping—with its risk of spinal cord injury—appears clear. However, this injury usually occurs in relatively young patients, and how the thoracic stent grafts will perform long-term remains to be seen. Despite this concern, as shown in the report, the aortic injury does heal over time so that aortic integrity will not depend on the endograft beyond a few months.

J. M. Seeger, MD

Open Repair Versus Endovascular Treatment for Asymptomatic Popliteal Artery Aneurysm: Results of a Prospective Randomized Study

Antonello M, Frigatti P, Battocchio P, et al (Univ of Padua, Italy)

J Vasc Surg 42:185-193, 2005 12–14

Purpose.—The aim of this prospective randomized study was to evaluate the relative risks and advantages of using the Hemobahn graft for popliteal artery aneurysm (PAA) treatment compared with open repair (OR). The primary end point was patency rate; secondary end points were hospital stay and length of surgical procedure.

Methods.—The study was a prospective, randomized clinical trial carried out at a single center from January 1999 to December 2003. Inclusion criteria were an aneurysmal lesion in the popliteal artery with a diameter ≥ 2 cm at the angio-computed tomography (CT) scan, and proximal and distal neck of the aneurysm with a length of >1 cm to offer a secure site of fixation of the stent graft. Exclusion criteria were age <50 years old, poor distal runoff, contraindication to antiplatelet, anticoagulant, or thrombolytic therapy, and symptoms of nerve and vein compression. The enrolled patients were thereafter prospectively randomized in a 1-to-1 ratio between OR (group A) or endovascular therapy (ET) (group B). The follow-up protocol consisted of duplex ultrasound scan and ankle-brachial index (ABI) measured during a force leg flexion at 1, 3, and 6 months. Group B patients underwent an angio-CT scan and plain radiography of the knee with leg flexion (>120°) at 6 and 12 months, and then yearly.

Results.—Between January 1999 and December 2003, 30 PAAs were performed: 15 OR (group A) and 15 ET (group B). Bypass and exclusion of the PAA was the preferred method of OR; no perioperative graft failure was observed. Twenty stent grafts were placed in 15 PAAs. Endograft thrombosis occurred in one patient (6.7%) in the postoperative period. The mean follow-up period was 46.1 months (range, 12 to 72 months) for group A and 45.9 months (range, 12 to 65 months) for group B. Kaplan-Meier analysis showed a primary patency rate of 100% at 12 months for OR and 86.7% at 12 months with a secondary patency rate of 100% at 12 and 36 months for ET. No statistical differences were observed at the log-rank test. The mean operation time (OR, 155.3 minutes; ET, 75.4 minutes) and hospital stay (OR, 7.7 days; ET, 4.3 days) were statistically longer for OR compared with ET ($P < .01$).

Conclusion.—We can conclude, with the power limitation of the study, that PAA treatment can be safely performed by using either OR or ET. ET has several advantages, such as quicker recovery and shorter hospital stay (Figs 1B and 3).

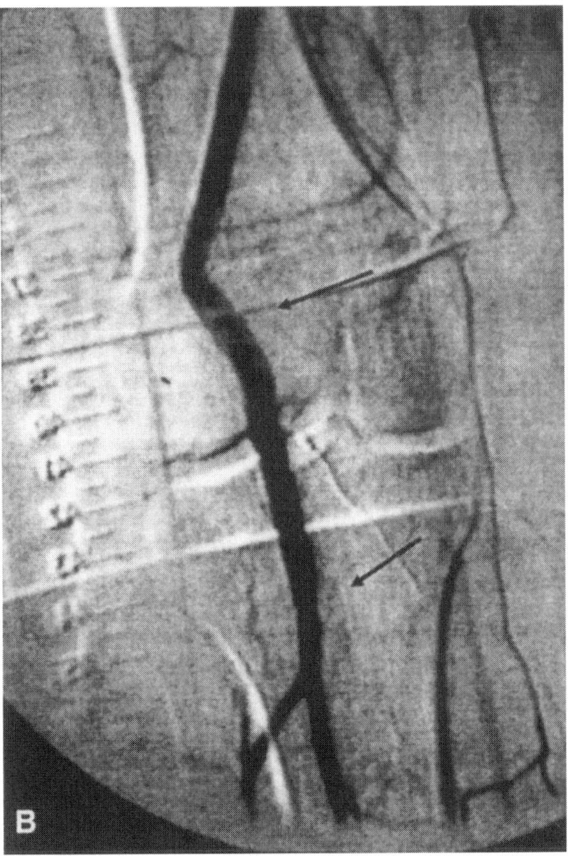

FIGURE 1B.—B, Digital subtraction angiography after coil-embolization of the collateral vessel and endograft deployment (*arrows* point to endograft location). (Courtesy of Antonello M, Frigatti P, Battocchio P, et al: Open repair versus endovascular treatment for asymptomatic popliteal artery aneurysm: Results of a prospective randomized study. *J Vasc Surg* 42:185-193, 2005. Copyright 2005 by Elsevier.)

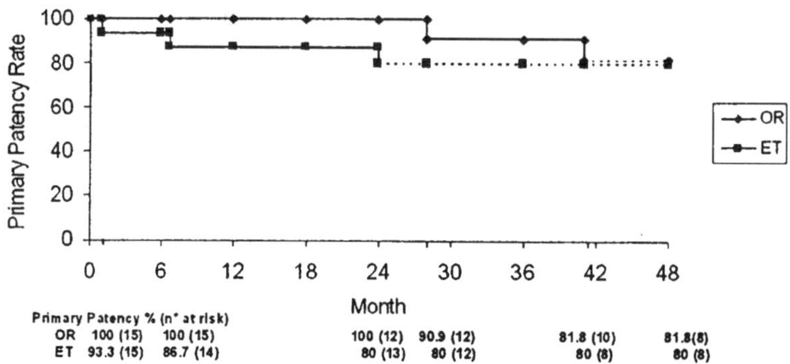

FIGURE 3.—Kaplan-Meier analysis shows the primary patency rate for open repair (*OR*) (group A) and endovascular treatment (*ET*) (group B) at 6-month intervals. Standard error is >10% after 42 months for OR and after 24 months for ET (*dashed line*) .(Courtesy of Antonello M, Frigatti P, Battocchio P, et al: Open repair versus endovascular treatment for asymptomatic popliteal artery aneurysm: Results of a prospective randomized study. *J Vasc Surg* 42:185-193, 2005. Copyright 2005 by Elsevier.)

▶ Initial attempts at endovascular treatment of popliteal aneurysms with stent grafts were plagued by graft kinking and graft thrombosis. The introduction of more flexible stent grafts has lead to better results, as reported here. However, it is important to recognize that these results were obtained in a very select group of patients with excellent popliteal artery anatomy for stent graft repair and excellent infrapopliteal run-off. Additionally, long-term results of this approach remain unknown. Thus, while these results appear good and are a significant improvement over initial reports, this approach to treatment of patients with popliteal aneurysm still cannot be considered standard of care.

J. M. Seeger, MD

Peripheral Arterial Occlusive Disease

The Effectiveness of Percutaneous Transluminal Angioplasty for the Treatment of Critical Limb Ischemia: A 10-Year Experience

Kudo T, Chandra FA, Ahn SS (Univ of California at Los Angeles)
J Vasc Surg 41:423-435, 2005 12–15

Objective.—To determine the efficacy, safety, and long-term results, including continued clinical improvement and limb salvage, of percutaneous transluminal angioplasty (PTA) in patients with critical limb ischemia (CLI).

Methods.—From August 1993 to March 2004, 138 limbs in 111 patients with CLI (rest pain in 62 [45%] and ulcer/gangrene in 76 [55%]) were treated by PTA. In iliac lesions, stents were placed selectively for primary PTA failure: residual stenosis (>30%) or pressure gradient (>5 mm Hg). Stent placement was limited in infrainguinal lesions. The most distal affected arteries treated with angioplasty were the iliac artery in 45 limbs (33%; iliac group), the femoropopliteal artery in 41 limbs (30%; FP group), and tibial arteries in 52 limbs (37%; BK group). All analysis was performed according to an intent-to-treat basis. Reporting standards of the Society for Vascular Surgery and the International Society for Cardiovascular Surgery were followed to evaluate initial success, and late follow-up status was evaluated with the Kaplan-Meier method. Patency was evaluated by using ultrasound scanning and ankle-brachial pressure index measurement.

Results.—There was one (0.9%) perioperative death. Twenty stents were placed selectively in 14 iliac arteries. Mean follow-up was 14.7 months (range, 1-75 months). Overall, initial technical and clinical success rates were 96.4% and 92.8%, respectively. The cumulative primary, assisted primary, and secondary patency; continued clinical improvement; and limb salvage rates SE at 5 years were 31.4% ± 10.4%, 75.5% ± 5.7%, 79.6% ± 5.5%, 36.1% ± 10.0%, and 89.1% ± 4.0%, respectively. In each subgroup, the primary, assisted primary, and secondary patency; continued clinical improvement; and limb salvage rates at 3 years were 51.6%, 94.7%, 97.8%, 65.1%, and 95.0%, respectively, in the iliac group; 49.4%, 72.2%, 76.4%, 57.4%, and 92.7%, respectively, in the FP group; and 23.5%, 41.8%, 46.1%, 51.1%, and 77.3%, respectively, in the BK group. Of the 12 predictable variables, hypertension, multiple segment lesions, more distal lesions, and TransAtlantic Inter-Society Consensus classification type D were significant independent risk factors for the outcomes ($P < .05$; univariate log-rank test and Cox regression multivariate analysis).

Conclusions.—PTA is a feasible, safe, and effective procedure for the treatment of CLI. The high limb salvage rate is attributed to the high assisted primary and secondary patency rates despite the low primary patency rate. Angioplasty can be the primary choice for the treatment of CLI due to iliac and infrainguinal arterial occlusive disease.

▶ The role of endovascular therapy in the management of patients with peripheral arterial occlusive disease continues to evolve. Studies such as this demonstrate acceptable clinical improvement and limb salvage rates despite poor primary patency rates when endovascular techniques (angioplasty in this study) are used to treat patients with CLI. These conclusions must be tempered by the unknown effect of the selection bias present in all retrospective studies such as this. However, it does appear that use of these techniques is associated with acceptable results as long as appropriate patient selection and careful follow-up are done. Unfortunately, we do not know exactly how the authors selected these patients to achieve these good results. Furthermore, it is unclear whether any of the patients who required amputation could have achieved limb salvage with a bypass procedure. Thus, the 2 fundamental questions concerning the use of endovascular therapy in patients with peripheral arterial occlusive disease, exactly who should be treated and who should not (because they will be hurt or achieve no benefit), remain unanswered.

J. M. Seeger, MD

Prospective Randomized Study on Reversed Saphenous Vein Infrapopliteal Bypass to Treat Limb-Threatening Ischemia: Common Femoral Artery Versus Superficial Femoral or Popliteal and Tibial Arteries as Inflow

Ballotta E, Renon L, De Rossi A, et al (Univ of Padua, Italy)
J Vasc Surg 40:732-740, 2004 12–16

Purpose.—Use of inflow sources distal to the common femoral artery (CFA) for bypass to infrapopliteal arteries is a compromise measure when the length of the vein is not adequate. The purpose of this study was to compare the clinical outcome of vein infrapopliteal bypass arising from the CFA and from the distal superficial femoral or popliteal and tibial arteries in patients with limb-threatening ischemia.

Methods.—Over 13 years, 160 vein infrapopliteal vein bypass procedures (160 patients) were randomized into 2 groups, 80 with inflow arising from the CFA (group 1) and 80 with inflow from below the CFA (group 2). Patency and limb salvage rates were assessed with the Kaplan-Meier method. All patients underwent graft surveillance at discharge and at 30 days and 6 months after surgery, then every 6 months thereafter. Follow-up ranged from 30 days to 127 months (mean, 49 months).

Results.—Groups were similar with regard to age, sex, and most atherosclerotic risk factors. Gangrene as an indication for surgery was statistically more frequent in group 1 (73.7% vs 48.7%; *P* = 002), whereas nonhealing ulcer and rest pain were statistically more frequent in group 2 (respectively, 51.2% vs 25%; *P* = .001 and 46.2% vs 28.7%; *P* = .03). No patients died during the perioperative (30 days) period. At 1, 3, and 5 years patency and limb salvage rates were comparable between groups, tending toward significance for the 5-year primary patency rate (73% vs 57%; *P* = .08).

Conclusions.—In the absence of significant proximal disease, infrapopliteal revascularization arising distal to the CFA can ensure patency and limb salvage rates statistically similar to those with use of the CFA. Moreover, procedures arising distal to the CFA required fewer graft revisions to maintain patency of failing grafts.

► This well-done, randomized trial should finally put to rest the question of the value of inflow sites distal to the CFA for infrapopliteal bypasses. The patency of such bypasses was the same or better than distal bypasses originating from the CFA, and fewer revisions were required to maintain graft patency in the shorter vein grafts (not surprising, as there was less graft length in which intrinsic graft lesions could develop). Good vein of adequate length is often problematic in patients with critical limb ischemia requiring infrapopliteal bypass and, therefore, use of distal inflow sites when appropriate will improve results in these complex patients.

J. M. Seeger, MD

Hemodynamic Changes Associated With Bypass Stenosis Regression

Taggert JB, Kupinski Am, Darling RC III, et al (Inst for Vascular Health and Disease, Albany, NY)

J Vasc Surg 41:1013-1017, 2005 12–17

Objective.—Ultrasound scanning is used to detect velocity increases indicative of a bypass stenosis. Subsequent examinations have shown regression of some stenotic lesions. This study examined hemodynamic changes that coincided with stenosis regression.

Methods.—Duplex ultrasound scans were used to record the peak systolic velocity (PSV) and volume flow from proximal and distal segments of infrainguinal bypasses. Valve remnants or other image defects were also noted. The PSV ratio (Vr) was calculated as the PSV at a stenosis divided by the PSV proximal to the lesion. A stenosis was defined as Vr ≥2.0.

Results.—An initial ultrasound scan performed 31 ± 6 days after surgery revealed a stenosis in 68 of 565 bypasses. In six bypasses, the increased PSV (272 ± 61 cm/s) and Vr (3.4 ± 1.3) were sustained during the follow-up period of 8 ± 3 months. In 27 bypasses with a PSV of 335 ± 63 cm/s and a Vr of 4.0 ± 1.6, the stenosis was repaired. In 35 bypasses with a PSV of 261 ± 82 cm/s and Vr of 3.2 ± 1.2, stenosis regression occurred with no increases in PSV observed on later scans. In this group, proximal bypass flow decreased during the follow-up interval from 247 ± 130 mL/min to 151 ± 135 mL/min and distal flow from 180 ± 102 mL/min to 103 ± 54 mL/min ($P < .05$, paired *t* test). Ultrasound image abnormalities were noted in 4 bypasses (67%) with persistent stenoses, 14 with repaired stenoses (52%), and 10 with resolved stenoses (29%).

Conclusion.—These data indicate early postoperative hyperemia is present in bypasses, demonstrating focal velocity increases. Such velocity increases may be the result of the bypass conduit acting as a flow-limiting lesion until the hyperemia subsides. As the blood flow decreases so does the PSV, giving the appearance of stenosis regression.

▶ Moderate focal graft velocity elevations (≥150 cm/s but <300 cm/s) detected by duplex US examination are relatively common and potentially indicate a developing graft stenosis. As shown in this study, some moderate velocity elevations indeed indicate a developing graft stenosis, while some are caused by limb hyperemia, which will resolve with time. Regardless, careful observation of these abnormalities appears safe, and such an approach will avoid unnecessary intervention in a significant number of patients.

J. M. Seeger, MD

Atherosclerotic Risk Factor Control in Patients With Peripheral Arterial Disease

Rehring TF, Sandhoff BG, Stolcpart RS, et al (Univ of Colorado, Denver)
J Vasc Surg 41:816-822, 2005 12–18

Background.—The presence of peripheral arterial disease (PAD), even in the absence of overt coronary artery disease (CAD), confers the same relative risk of death from a cardiovascular cause as in patients with a previous cardiovascular event. Current guidelines recommend atherosclerotic risk factor-reduction strategies in PAD patients identical to those in patients with a recent coronary event. The purpose of this study was to determine the status of atherosclerotic risk factor control in patients with PAD.

Methods.—We analyzed the records of patients treated at 2 regional clinics serving 92,940 individuals. Full examination, laboratory, and pharmacy data were available for all patients. Pharmacy data were analyzed to determine prescriptions for β-blocker therapy, angiotensin-converting enzyme inhibitors, and lipid-lowering agents. Lipid control was assessed through fasting lipid data. Glycemic control in diabetics was evaluated by using hemoglobin A_{1c} levels.

Results.—We administratively identified 2839 patients with a diagnosis of PAD. The exclusion of 1106 patients with a diagnosis of CAD or validated not to have PAD resulted in a cohort of 1733 patients. Of these, 33.1% (574/1733) were currently receiving β-blockers, 28.9% (500/1733) were receiving an angiotensin-converting enzyme inhibitor, and 31.3% (543/1733) were receiving a statin. Most patients (92%; 1594/1733) had a recent blood pressure recorded. However, 56% (893/1594) had a systolic blood pressure of 130 mm Hg or higher, 45.5% (726/1594) had a diastolic blood pressure of 80 mm Hg or higher, and 13.6% (217/1594) had a diastolic blood pressure of 90 mm Hg or higher. Screening fasting lipid profiles were found in 62.6% (1085/1733) of patients, 56% (508/912) had a low-density lipoprotein of 100 mg/dL or higher, and 21% (187/912) had a value of more than 130 mg/dL. In patients with diabetes, a hemoglobin A_{1c} level of 7.0% or higher was found in 54.2% (198/365) of patients.

Conclusions.—Despite national consensus of PAD as a CAD equivalent, patients are currently undertreated with regard to atherosclerotic risk factor modification. Until broader recognition of this disease process exists, vascular surgeons must continue to champion medical as well as surgical treatments for these patients.

► Evidence continues to accumulate demonstrating patients with PAD to be at high risk for systemic cardiovascular events and endovascular mortality. Furthermore, the effectiveness of risk factor modification using β-blockers, angiotensin-converting enzyme inhibitors, statins, and antiplatelet agents in improving outcomes in such patients has been demonstrated. Yet studies such as this continue to document significant undertreatment of patients with PAD with these medications, and guidelines for appropriate control of risk factors such as hypertension, hyperlipidemia, and even diabetes mellitus are achieved in at most 50% of such patients. Obviously, the current medical management of patients with PAD is commonly inadequate and as vascular specialists who treat such patients, we must work to improve the medical treatment of our patients with PAD.

J. M. Seeger, MD

Inflammatory Mediators Are Associated With 1-Year Mortality in Critical Limb Ischemia

Barani J, Nilsson J-Å, Mattiasson I, et al (Univ of Lund, Sweden; Malmö Univ, Sweden)

J Vasc Surg 42:75-80, 2005 12–19

Objective.—The atherosclerotic process has inflammatory features. Patients with peripheral atherosclerosis and critical limb ischemia have a poor prognosis. This study evaluated the hypothesis that inflammatory markers are associated with mortality among patients admitted to the hospital because of critical limb ischemia.

Methods.—This was a prospective, single-center, 1-year, follow-up study of 259 consecutive patients with critical limb ischemia who were admitted to a secondary referral center of vascular diseases. Interventions included evaluation of intercurrent disease, ankle and arm blood pressures, plasma glucose and lipid levels, plasma homocysteine, cardiolipin antibodies, resistance to activated protein C, plasma endothelin-1, and the inflammatory mediators tumor necrosis factor-α, interleukin-6, neopterin, high-sensitivity C-reactive protein, CD40 ligand, and 8-iso-prostaglandin F_{α} in plasma. The main outcome measure was total mortality and causes of death assessed 1 year after admission.

Results.—During the first year after admission, 61 patients (24%) died. These patients were older ($P < .0001$), showed a higher leukocyte count ($P = .0011$) and levels of serum creatinine ($P < .0001$), lower levels of high-density lipoprotein (HDL) cholesterol ($P = .003$) and frequency of active treatment ($P = .014$) than the 198 (76%) survivors. More nonsurvivors had gangrene ($P < .0001$), and fewer ($P = .004$) had lipid-lowering treatment. The plasma levels of interleukin-6 ($P < .0001$), tumor necrosis factor-α ($P < .0001$), neopterin ($P < .0001$), and high-sensitivity C-reactive protein ($P = .002$) at admission for critical limb ischemia were all significantly lower in the survivors, whereas there was no difference concerning CD40 ligand. In logistic regression adjusted for age, sex, lipid-lowering therapy, active treatment, gangrene, leukocyte count, creatinine, and serum HDL cholesterol, the inflammatory mediators tumor necrosis factor-α ($P = .0084$), neopterin ($P = .0035$), but not interleukin-6 ($P = .585$) or high-sensitivity C-reactive protein ($P = .314$) were independent risk variables of death within 1 year.

Conclusions.—Increased age, leukocyte count, creatinine, and inflammatory mediators, together with gangrene, were associated with 1-year mortality despite intervention in critical limb ischemia. For tumor necrosis factor-α and neopterin in plasma, this association was independent of the other parameters.

▶ It is becoming increasingly clear that patients with critical limb ischemia are substantially different from those with claudication or asymptomatic disease. Short-term mortality rate is significantly higher and functional outcome is worse, even with successful lower extremity arterial repair. Additionally, these poor outcomes are only partially explained by comorbidities. As demonstrated in this report, critical limb ischemia appears to be a manifestation of a systemic, inflammatory process. Some benefit in limiting mortality and limb loss is gained from the use of statins, which have an antiinflammatory effect and should be given to all these patients. However, until the systemic nature of critical limb ischemia is better understood, improving mortality rate and outcome in patients with end-stage peripheral vascular disease will remain difficult.

J. M. Seeger, MD

Rapid Foot and Calf Compression Increases Walking Distance in Patients With Intermittent Claudication: Results of Randomized Study

Ramaswami G, D'Ayala M, Hollier LH, et al (New York Methodist Hosp; LSU School of Medicine, New Orleans; Univ of California, San Diego; et al)
J Vasc Surg 41:794-801, 2005 12–20

Objective.—The aim of our pilot study was to determine the usefulness of rapid, high-pressure, intermittent pneumatic calf and foot compression (IPCFC) in patients with stable intermittent claudication, with reference to the end points of improvement in initial claudication distance (ICD) (distance at which patient feels pain or discomfort in the legs), and improvement in absolute claudication distance (ACD) (distance at which patient stops walking because the pain or discomfort becomes severe).

Methods.—Thirty male patients presenting with stable, intermittent claudication (ACD between 50 and 150 meters on treadmill testing at 3.8 km/h, 10° gradient) were recruited into this pilot study from a single center. Fifteen patients were randomized to treatment with IPCFC (applied for 1 hour twice daily in the sitting position) and were also advised to have daily exercise, and 15 patients served as controls, who were advised exercise alone. All patients received aspirin and had resting and postexercise ankle/brachial index (ABI) measured at enrollment along with ICD and ACD on treadmill testing (3.8 km/h, 10° gradient). The mean age, baseline ICD, and ACD of the treatment and control groups were 70.4 ± 7 years and 70.7 ± 9 years, 55.8 ± 15 meters and 68.4 ± 17 meters, and 86.7 ± 19 meters and 103.9 ± 27 meters, respectively. Both groups were equally matched for risk factors, including smoking, type II diabetes mellitus, and hypercholesterolemia. IPCFC was applied. The study protocol included follow-up visits at 1, 2, 3, 4, 6, and 12 months with the ABI, ICD and ACD being measured at every visit.

Results.—The percent change from baseline for ICD and ACD for each patient visit and the mean ± standard deviation (SD), standard error (SE), and median were calculated for the control and treatment groups. The percent change from baseline measurements (mean ± SD) for ICD and ACD in the control group at 4, 6, and 12 months were 2.2 ± 18 and 2.3 ± 18, 2.9 ± 17 and 5.2 ± 20, and 3.6 ± 18 and 5.8 ± 20, respectively (Fig 1). In contrast, the changes in ICD and ACD at 4, 6, and 12 months in the treatment group were 137.1 ± 128 ($P < .01$) and 84.3 ± 82 ($P < .01$), 140.6 ± 127 ($P < .01$) and 96.4 ± 106 ($P = .01$), and 150.8 ± 124 ($P < 0.01$) and 101.2 ± 104 ($P < 0.01$), respectively. Although the ABI showed a slight increase in the treatment group, these differences were not statistically significant.

Conclusions.—The results of this pilot study show that IPCFC improves walking distance in patients with stable intermittent claudication. A significant increase in ICD and ACD was seen at 4 and 6 months of treatment, respectively, and the improvement was sustained at 1 year. The combination of IPCFC with other treatment such as risk-factor modification and daily exercise may prove useful in patients with peripheral arterial occlusive disease. It may be a useful first line of therapy in patients with disabling claudication who are unfit for major reconstructive surgery. Improved walking on long-

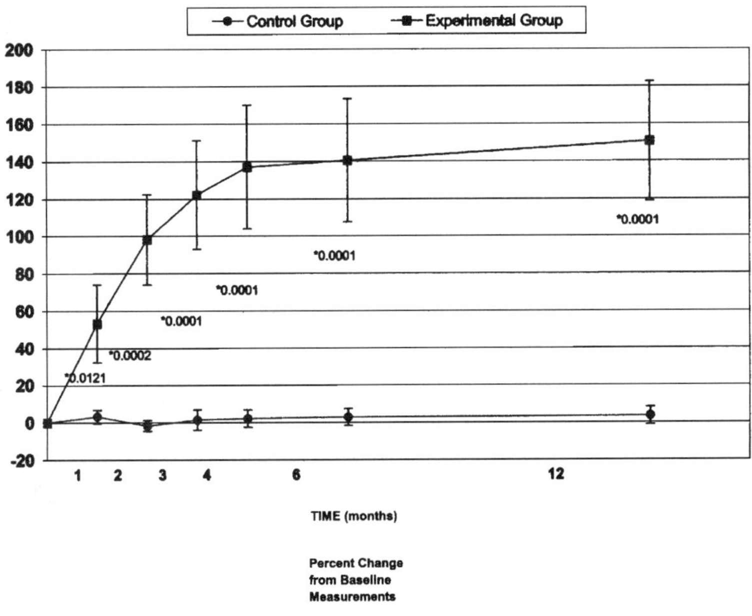

FIGURE 1.—Percent changes in the initial claudication distance in the treatment and control group (mean ± standard error of the mean) (*P value). (Courtesy of Ramaswami G, D'Ayala M, Hollier LH, et al: Rapid foot and calf compression increases walking distance in patients with intermittent claudication: Results of a randomized study. *J Vasc Surg* 41:794-801, 2005. Copyright 2005 by Elsevier.)

term follow-up and experience from different centers may establish a role for this treatment modality in the future.

► This study is seriously compromised by the small number of patients available for long-term follow-up, which severely limits any conclusions that can be drawn regarding the value of IPCFC in the treatment of patients with claudication. However, the results, though limited, are intriguing, and if further studies document the improvements in walking distance seen in this pilot study, use of this technique could provide an addition noninvasive treatment for selected patients with claudication.

J. M. Seeger, MD

Access

Autogenous Radial-Cephalic or Prosthetic Brachial-Antecubital Forearm Loop AVF in Patients With Compromised Vessels? A Randomized, Multicenter Study of the Patency of Primary Hemodialysis Access

Rooijens PPGM, Burgmans JPJ, Yo TI, et al (Med Ctr Rijnmond Zuid, The Netherlands; Diakonessenhuis, The Netherlands; Erasmus Med Ctr, The Netherlands; et al)

J Vasc Surg 42:481-487, 2005 12–21

Objective.—The construction of an autogenous radial-cephalic direct wrist arteriovenous fistula (RCAVF) is the primary and best option for vascular access for hemodialysis. However, 10%-24% of RCAVFs thrombose directly after operation or do not function adequately due to failure of maturation. In case of poor arterial and/or poor venous vessels for anastomosis, the outcome of RCAVFs may be worse and an alternative vascular access is probably indicated. A prosthetic graft implant may be a second best option. Therefore, a randomized multicenter study comparing RCAVF with prosthetic (polytetrafluoroethylene [PTFE]) graft implantation in patients with poor vessels was performed.

Methods.—A total of 383 consecutive new patients needing primary vascular access were screened for enrollment in a prospective randomized study. According to defined vessel criteria from the preoperative duplex scanning, 140 patients were allocated to primary placement of an RCAVF and 61 patients to primary prosthetic graft implantation. The remaining 182 patients were randomized to receive either an RCAVF (n = 92) or prosthetic graft implant (n = 90). Patency rate was defined as the percentage of AVFs that functioned well after implantation.

Results.—Primary and assisted primary 1-year patencies were 33% ± 5.3% vs 44% ± 6.2% (*P* = .03) and 48% ± 5.5% vs 63% ± 5.9% (*P* = .035) for the RCAVF and prosthetic AVF, respectively (Fig 2). Secondary patencies were 52% ± 5.5% vs 79% ± 5.1% (*P* = .0001) for the RCAVF and prosthetic AVF, respectively. Patients with RCAVFs developed a total of 102 (1.19/patient-year [py]) vs 122 (1.45/py; *P* = .739) complications in the prosthetic AVFs. A total of 43 (0.50/py) interventions in the RCAVF group and 79

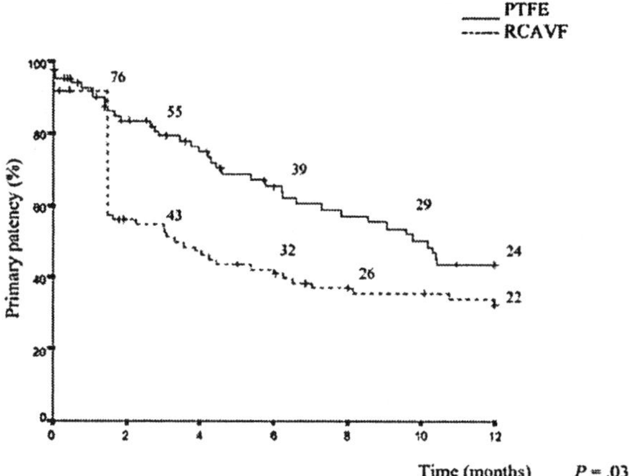

FIGURE 2.—Primary patency rates. Patency rate is shown in percentages and time in months. Number of patients is presented in the graph. *P* values calculated with the log-rank test. (Courtesy of Rooijens PPGM, Burgmans JPJ, Yo TI, et al: Autogenous radial-cephalic or prosthetic brachial-antecubital forearm loop AVF in patients with compromised vessels? A randomized, multicenter study of the patency of primary hemodialysis access. *J Vasc Surg* 42:481-487, 2005. Copyright 2005 by Elsevier.)

(0.94/py) in the prosthetic graft group were needed for access salvage (P = .077).

Conclusions.—Although there were more interventions needed for access salvage in the patients with prosthetic graft implants, we may conclude that patients with poor forearm vessels do benefit from implantation of a prosthetic graft for vascular access.

► The appropriate second choice for dialysis access construction after a RCAVF remains unclear. This study suggests that a prosthetic forearm loop arteriovenous graft may be that choice, but to achieve acceptable patency rates with such grafts, a significant number of secondary interventions were required. The question that isn't answered by this study is whether an arm procedure such as a brachiocephalic or brachiobasilic AVF would have had equal or better patency with fewer secondary interventions. Thus, this study shows that a forearm arteriovenous loop graft is a better dialysis access option than a RCAVF done by using small arteries and veins. However, the appropriate next step in access construction after RCAVF still remains unclear.

J. M. Seeger, MD

Venous

Changes in Superficial and Perforating Vein Reflux After Varicose Vein Surgery

Blomgren L, Johansson G, Dahlberg-Åkerman A, et al (Capio St Göran's Hosp, Stockholm; Univ Hosp, Uppsala, Sweden)

J Vasc Surg 42:315-320, 2005 12–22

Objectives.—This prospective duplex study was conducted to study the effect of current surgical treatment for primary varicose veins on the development of venous insufficiency ≤2 years after varicose vein surgery.

Methods.—The patients were part of a randomized controlled study where surgery for primary varicose veins was planned from a clinical examination alone or with the addition of preoperative duplex scanning. Postoperative duplex scanning was done at 2 months and 2 years.

Results.—Operations were done on 293 patients (343 legs), 74% of whom were women. The mean age was 47 years. In 126 legs, duplex scanning was done preoperatively, at 2 months and 2 years, and at 2 months and 2 years in 251 legs. Preoperative perforating vein incompetence (PVI) was present in 64 of 126 legs. Perforator ligation was not done on 42 of these; at 2 months, 23 of these legs (55%) had no PVI, and at 2 years, 25 legs (60%) had no PVI. Sixty-one legs had no PVI preoperatively, 5 (8%) had PVI at 2 months, and 11 (18%) had PVI at 2 years. In the group of 251 legs, reversal of PVI between 2 months and 2 years was found in 28 (41%) of 68 and was more common than new PVI, which occurred in 41 (22%) of 183 ($P = .003$). After 2 years, the number of legs without venous incompetence in which perforator surgery was not performed was 11 (26%) of 42 legs with preoperative PVI and 18 (30%) of 61 legs without preoperative PVI, ($P = .713$). After 2 years, new vessel formation was more common in the surgically obliterated saphenopopliteal junction (SPJ), 4 (40%) of 10, than in the saphenofemoral junction (SFJ), 17 (11%) of 151 ($P = .027$), and new incompetence in a previously normal junction was more common in the SFJ, 11 (18%) of 63, than in the SPJ, 3 (1%) of 226 ($P < 001$). Reflux in the great saphenous vein (GSV) below the knee was abolished after stripping above the knee in 17 (34%) of 50 legs at 2 months and in 22 legs (44%) after 2 years.

Conclusions.—Varicose vein surgery induces changes in the remaining venous segments of the legs that continue for several months. In most patients, perforators and the GSV below the knee can be ignored at the primary surgery. A substantial number of recurrences in the SFJ and SPJ are unavoidable with present surgical knowledge because they stem from new vessel formation and progression of disease.

► The data presented in this observational study support the concept of limiting the initial treatment of venous reflux to removal (or obliteration) of the thigh portion of the long saphenous vein. Even when PVI was present, the hemodynamic response to thigh saphenous stripping was essentially the same 2 years after treatment, whether perforators were ligated or not. Additionally, approximately 50% of the PVI resolved without vein interruption while other abnormalities, including recurrent SFJ incompetence, developed. Other reports have demonstrated that superficial venous surgery can also result in the improvement or resolution of deep venous reflux in a substantial number of patients. Thus, limiting initial therapy for venous disease to the superficial venous system is appropriate in most patients, and less invasive approaches may also be most appropriate, considering subsequent treatment of new abnormalities may be necessary.

J. M. Seeger, MD

Effectiveness of an Extracellular Matrix Graft (OASIS Wound Matrix) in the Treatment of Chronic Leg Ulcers: A Randomized Clinical Trial

Mostow EN, for the OASIS Venus Ulcer Study Group (Northeastern Ohio Univ, Akron; et al)

J Vasc Surg 41:837-843, 2005 12–23

Background.—Venous leg ulcers are a major cause of morbidity, economic loss, and decreased quality of life in affected patients. Recently, biomaterials derived from natural tissue sources have been used to stimulate wound closure. One such biomaterial obtained from porcine small-intestine submucosa (SIS) has shown promise as an effective treatment to manage full-thickness wounds. Our objective was to compare the effectiveness of SIS wound matrix with compression vs compression alone in healing chronic leg ulcers within 12 weeks.

Methods.—This was a prospective, randomized, controlled multicenter trial. Patients were 120 patients with at least 1 chronic leg ulcer. Patients were randomly assigned to receive either weekly topical treatment of SIS plus compression therapy (n = 62) or compression therapy alone (n = 58). Ulcer size was determined at enrollment and weekly throughout the treatment. Healing was assessed weekly for up to 12 weeks. Recurrence after 6 months was recorded. The primary outcome measure was the proportion of ulcers healed in each group at 12 weeks.

Results.—After 12 weeks of treatment, 55% of the wounds in the SIS group were healed, as compared with 34% in the standard-care group ($P = .0196$) (Fig 2). None of the healed patients treated with SIS wound matrix and seen for the 6-month follow-up experienced ulcer recurrence.

Conclusions.—The SIS wound matrix, as an adjunct therapy, significantly improves healing of chronic leg ulcers over compression therapy alone.

▶ Venous ulcers are common and improvements in wound management that would hasten healing of these ulcers would obviously be of value. This randomized trial demonstrates such an improvement with the use of a porcine small intestine submucosa-based dressing. It also appeared that the increased cost of the dressing was offset by fewer dressing changes and more rapid wound healing. While confirmation of these results will obviously vali-

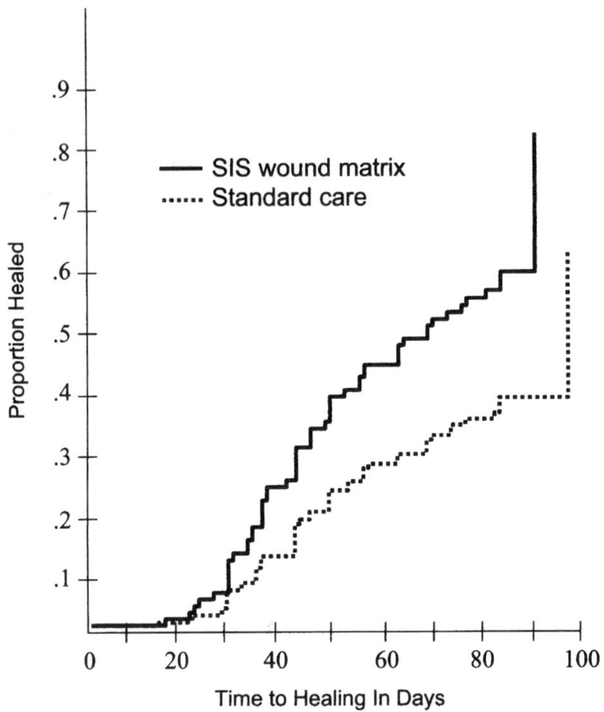

FIGURE 2.—Survival plot analysis for the small-intestine submucosa (*SIS*) wound matrix group and the standard-care group. Success was defined as 100% healing. Patients treated with SIS wound matrix were more likely to heal by 12 weeks than those in the standard-care group ($P = .0226$). (Courtesy of Mostow EN, for the OASIS Venus Ulcer Study Group: Effectiveness of an extracellular matrix graft (OASIS Wound Matrix) in the treatment of chronic leg ulcers: A randomized clinical trial. *J Vasc Surg* 41:837-843, 2005. Copyright 2005 by Elsevier.)

date this conclusion, this appears to strong evidence of the value of this wound dressing in the management of venous ulcers.

J. M. Seeger, MD

Five-Year Outcome Study of Deep Vein Thrombosis in the Lower Limbs

Asbeutah AM, Riha AZ, Cameron JD, et al (Monash Univ, Melbourne; Wesley Vascular Centre, Brisbane, Australia)

J Vasc Surg 40:1181-1189, 2004 12–24

Objective.—Venous disease was evaluated in relation to post-thrombotic syndrome 5 years after deep venous thrombosis (DVT) in patients treated with a regimen of low-molecular-weight heparin (LMWH) and warfarin in a Hospital-in-the-Home program.

Methods.—The presence of flow, reflux and compressibility in 51 patients (102 limbs, 54 with DVT and 48 without DVT) was assessed by duplex ultrasound scanning. Blood tests were carried out for prothrombotic screening. Venous disease was related to pathologic severity of post-thrombotic syndrome, characterized by the CEAP (clinical, etiologic, anatomic, pathophysiologic) classification on a scale of 0 to 6.

Results.—In the 102 limbs studied, 30 patients (59%) had an underlying thrombophilic disorder. The most common cause of DVT was postoperation and prolonged immobilization not related to postoperation. The most common thrombophilic abnormalities were anticardiolipin antibody and a deficiency of protein C or S, or both. Twenty-six limbs (48%) had proximal involvement (proximal and proximal plus distal DVT); resolution (recanalization or normal vein) in these limbs was seen in 85% at 6 months and 96% at 5 years. After 5 years, 25 of these proximal DVT limbs (96%) developed reflux and there were 4 limbs in CEAP class 0, 8 in classes 1 to 3, and 14 in classes 4 to 6. All of the 28 limbs (52%) with distal DVT showed DVT resolution by 6 months. After 5 years, 10 limbs (36%) developed reflux, and 13 limbs were in class 0, 12 in classes 1 to 3, and 3 limbs in classes 4 to 6. No DVT was detected in the 48 contralateral limbs, but reflux was detected in 25 limbs (52%), predominately in the superficial veins (16 limbs, 64%).

Conclusions.—The resolution of thrombus was more rapid and complete in patients with distal DVT than in those with proximal DVT. Patients with proximal DVT developed a more severe form of post-thrombotic syndrome that was likely related to the development of deep venous reflux. An important finding of this study was an unexpectedly high incidence of venous reflux in the apparently unaffected limb. Although these non-DVT limbs were not investigated at presentation, our data is consistent with the hypothesis that DVT may result in a more systemic disorder of venous function.

► The long-term outcome after lower extremity DVT remains relatively undefined. This interesting study confirms previous reports that distal (below the popliteal vein) DVT resolves more quickly and completely than proximal DVT and that proximal DVT is more commonly associated with venous reflux long term. Surprisingly, the study also suggests that unilateral DVT may be associated with a higher likelihood of the development of venous reflux in the contralateral "normal" extremity, although as examination of that extremity at the time of the DVT was not done, this cannot be conclusively demonstrated. It is of course possible that asymptomatic DVT also occurred in that extremity or preexisting venous abnormalities existed in both legs which predisposed the patients to DVT. Regardless, understanding the natural history of DVT is necessary to both guide subsequent follow-up and treatment as well as for comparison of DVT treatments other than anticoagulation.

J. M. Seeger, MD

Miscellaneous

Physician Supply, Treatment, and Amputation Rates for Peripheral Arterial Disease

Ho V, Wirthlin D, Yun H, et al (Rice Univ, Houston; Intermountain Health Care, Salt Lake City, Utah; Univ of Alabama Birmingham)
J Vasc Surg 42:81-87, 2005 12–25

Objective.—To test whether the availability of vascular surgeons and interventional radiologists in a region affects revascularization and amputation rates for patients with peripheral arterial disease (PAD).

Methods.—We identified all patients with PAD in the Medicare claims database in 1994 and tracked their claims through 1999. We aggregated risk-adjusted data on the 143,202 patients who survived through 1999 by Hospital Referral Region and merged this data with information on local physician supply and other regional characteristics. Instrumental variables analysis was used to account for unobserved illness severity. Main outcome measures were risk-adjusted rates of lower extremity bypass surgery, angioplasty, and amputation by region.

Results.—Increasing vascular surgeon supply in a region by approximately one standard deviation (.30/10,000 Medicare beneficiaries) is associated with a 0.9 percentage point increase in bypass surgery rates and a 1.6 percentage point reduction in amputation rates. We find weaker evidence that greater availability of interventional radiologists increases angioplasty rates and reduces amputation rates. Factors reflecting regional attractiveness, such as the rating of a region based on climate, recreation, crime, and other attributes, were strong independent predictors of the number of vascular surgeons and interventional radiologists in an area.

Conclusions.—Availability of specialists affects outcomes for PAD patients. Regional variability in specialists who treat PAD is influenced by factors other than regional medical needs. Policies aimed at increasing the supply of vascular surgeons and interventional radiologists and their provision of bypass surgery in underserved areas may help to reduce regional disparities in amputation.

► Like all population-based studies using data from administrative databases, the conclusions from this study must be taken with a large grain of salt. Additionally, many of the observations reported in this study are based on statistical modeling rather than actual outcomes. Despite this, the results of the study are intriguing. Variation in amputation rates across the country is not surprising, as similar variations in health care outcomes have previously been observed. In contrast, the favorable influence of the availability of vascular surgeons, and to a lesser degree interventional radiologists and cardiologists, on amputation rates has not been previously documented. Additionally, while the relationship between these specialties and their primary procedures (bypass, angioplasty, medical therapy) is to be expected, this finding supports the idea that a "vascular specialist" who provides all types of vascular care might provide the best treatment for a patient with peripheral vascular disease. Regardless, this observed variation in amputation rates will likely persist as the distribution of specialists in our health care system is not based on need (as also documented in this study).

J. M. Seeger, MD

13 General Thoracic Surgery

Introduction

I am honored once again to present to you, as part of the 2006 YEAR BOOK, the section on General Thoracic Surgery. The issue of lung cancer was thrust into the public limelight this past year with the death of an American icon, television anchorman Peter Jennings. He died of metastatic non–small cell lung cancer. This at least temporarily heightened the public's awareness of lung cancer. Unfortunately, it was short-lived. The issue of smoking still receives little public attention, few federal dollars, and little to no public support. Movies continue to show young leading stars and starlets smoking cigarettes. The promotion of smoking to our young continues unabated, despite its obvious irresponsibility to the future health of our society. I wonder how many executives and/or CEOs of tobacco companies encourage their children or grandchildren to smoke?

Lung cancer represents a pan-epidemic. It is the number one cancer killer in the world. It is the number one cause of cancer deaths in the United States, and in fact, lung cancer kills more men then the second, third, and fourth most common organ killers **combined**. This includes cancers of the colon, prostate, and pancreas. Similarly, lung cancer will take the lives of more women in the year 2005 than the second, third, and fourth most common solid organ tumors in women combined. This includes deaths from cancer of the breast, ovary, and colon **combined**. Thirty percent of all cancer deaths are from lung cancer, and cigarette smoking will take the lives prematurely of more than 50% of those who smoke. Yet the amount of money spent on public education to help prevent smoking is dwarfed in terms of other cancers. For this reason, the YEAR BOOK OF SURGERY will once again focus on lung cancer. We will continue to focus on this problem until we are finally able to make a dent in this pan-epidemic. The number of deaths from lung cancer is equivalent to a jumbo jet-liner crashing every day, day after day, with no survivors. The overall 5-year survival of patients with lung cancer remains a dismal 15%, and this pales in comparison to every other solid organ tumor. Perhaps the only silver lining in the death of Peter Jennings may be the increased awareness of lung cancer and the fatal risks that smokers take on a daily basis.

We have divided this section of the YEAR BOOK into 5 categories. The first consists of 2 articles about preoperative factors in patients with non–small cell lung cancer. The second category delivers 6 articles on staging patients with lung cancer. We will present new articles that evaluate the role of endoscopic ultrasound with fine-needle aspirate of mediastinal lymph nodes. We will then look at the role of PET scanning and demonstrate the lack of concordance of clinical staging compared with the actual pathologic stage of patients with non–small cell lung cancer. The third section concerns 6 articles on intraoperative staging. The concept of lymph node dissection instead of sampling will be reviewed. This section also includes articles that review the role of surgery after neoadjuvant chemotherapy in patients with non–small cell lung cancer. Our fourth category will be a miscellaneous section that evaluates other important articles in the field of general thoracic surgery. This includes an article on metasectomy for tumors that travel hematogenously to the lungs, a common part of our practice. It also features an article on the dreaded problems of stents placed for benign airway problems. The fifth and final category will once again be on lung transplantation. We hope you enjoy and find this year's version of general thoracic surgery in the YEAR BOOK to be informative.

Robert J. Cerfolio, MD

Preoperative Evaluation

Surgeon Specialty and Operative Mortality With Lung Resection

Goodney PP, Lucas FL, Stukel TA, et al (Dept of Veterans Affairs Med Ctr, White River Junction, Vt; Dartmouth-Hitchcock Med Ctr, Lebanon, NH; Dartmouth Med School, Hanover, NH; et al)

Ann Surg 241:179-184, 2005 13–1

Objective.—We sought to examine the effect of subspecialty training on operative mortality following lung resection.

Summary Background Data.—While several different surgical subspecialists perform lung resection for cancer, many believe that this procedure is best performed by board-certified thoracic surgeons.

Methods.—Using the national Medicare database 1998 to 1999, we identified patients undergoing lung resection (lobectomy or pneumonectomy) for lung cancer. Operating surgeons were identified by unique physician identifier codes contained in the discharge abstract. We used the American Board of Thoracic Surgery database, as well as physician practice patterns, to designate surgeons as general surgeons, cardiothoracic surgeons, or noncardiac thoracic surgeons. Using logistic regression models, we compared operative mortality across surgeon subspecialties, adjusting for patient, surgeon, and hospital characteristics.

Results.—Overall, 25,545 Medicare patients underwent lung resection, 36% by general surgeons, 39% by cardiothoracic surgeons, and 25% by noncardiac thoracic surgeons. Patient characteristics did not differ substantially by surgeon specialty. Adjusted operative mortality rates were lowest for cardiothoracic and noncardiac thoracic surgeons (7.6% general surgeons, 5.6% cardiothoracic surgeons, 5.8% noncardiac thoracic surgeons, $P = 0.001$). In analyses restricted to high-volume surgeons (>20 lung resections/y), mortality rates were lowest for noncardiac thoracic surgeons (5.1% noncardiac thoracic, 5.2% cardiothoracic, and 6.1% general surgeons) ($P < 0.01$ for difference between general surgeons and thoracic surgeons). In analyses restricted to high-volume hospitals (>45 lung resections/y), mortality rates were again lowest for noncardiac thoracic surgeons (5.0% noncardiac thoracic, 5.3% cardiothoracic, and 6.1% general surgeons) ($P < 0.01$ for differences between all 3 groups).

Conclusions.—Operative mortality with lung resection varies by surgeon specialty. Some, but not all, of this variation in operative mortality is attributable to hospital and surgeon volume.

▶ Although there are obvious problems in the methodology of this article, which uses a very large Medicare database, the results are interesting. This study, like so many before it, drives home the fact that operative mortality varies by the surgeon's specialty. This article shows this theory to be true with pulmonary resection. The volume of the hospital and the volume of the surgeon clearly play a role in the outcome of the patient. This is no surprise. However, large numbers are needed, as provided by this article, to prove statistically what seems like an obvious conclusion—if one has a team that performs a large number of a particular procedure day after day, that team is more likely to obtain better results than a team that performs the same procedure rarely. The basic import of this large study may affect who is reimbursed for performing pulmonary resection in the future. Further data are being compiled by insurance companies and the government to answer these difficult questions. These questions are politically volatile, difficult to answer, and more controversial than the study's findings.

R. J. Cerfolio, MD

Smoking and Timing of Cessation: Impact on Pulmonary Complications After Thoracotomy

Barrera R, Shi W, Amar D, et al (Mem Sloan-Kettering Cancer Ctr, New York)
Chest 127:1977-1983, 2005 13–2

Study Objective.—The benefit of smoking cessation just prior to surgery in preventing postoperative pulmonary complications has not been proven. Some studies actually show a paradoxical increase in complications in those quitting smoking only a few weeks or days prior to surgery. We studied the effect of smoking and the timing of smoking cessation on postoperative pulmonary complications in patients undergoing thoracotomy.

Design and Setting.—Prospective study conducted in a tertiary care cancer center in 300 consecutive patients with primary lung cancer or metastatic cancer to the lung who were undergoing anatomical lung resection.

Results.—The groups studied were nonsmokers (21%), past quitters of > 2 months duration (62%), recent quitters of < 2 months duration (13%), and ongoing smokers (4%). Overall pulmonary complications occurred in 8%, 19%, 23%, and 23% of these groups, respectively, with a significant difference between nonsmokers and all smokers ($p = 0.03$) but no difference among the subgroups of smokers ($p = 0.76$). The risk of pneumonia was significantly lower in nonsmokers (3%) compared to all smokers (average, 11%; $p < 0.05$), with no difference detected among subgroups of smokers ($p = 0.17$). Comparing recent quitters and ongoing smokers, no differences in pulmonary complications or pneumonia were found ($p = 0.67$). Independent risk factors for pulmonary complications were a lower diffusing capacity of the lung for carbon monoxide (DLCO) (odds ratio [OR] per 10% decrement, 1.41; 95% confidence interval [CI], 1.17 to 1.70; $p = 0.01$) and primary lung cancer rather than metastatic disease (OR, 3.94; 95% CI, 1.34 to 11.59; $p = 0.003$). Among smokers, a lower DLCO percent predicted (OR per 10% decrement, 1.42; 95% CI, 1.16 to 1.75; $p = 0.008$) and a smoking history of > 60 pack-years (OR, 2.54; 95% CI, 1.28 to 5.04; $p = 0.0008$) were independently associated with overall pulmonary complications.

Conclusions.—In patients undergoing thoracotomy for primary or secondary lung tumors, there is no evidence of a paradoxical increase in pulmonary complications among those who quit smoking within 2 months of undergoing surgery. Smoking cessation can safely be encouraged prior to surgery.

▶ In this interesting article, Dr Barrera and colleagues find that there is no increased risk of pulmonary complications in patients who quit smoking within 2 months of elective lung resection. This finding refutes the popular claim that patients who are lifelong smokers should not be advised to quit just before surgery. Some believe there is a paradoxic increase in pulmonary complications in patients who stop smoking just before surgery. This study divided patients into 4 distinct groups: those who never smoked, those who quit smoking more than 2 months before surgery, those who quit within 2 months before surgery, and those who continued to smoke up to the day of thoracotomy and pulmonary resection. The latter group had the highest incidence of complications. These data support the fact that surgeons along with pulmonologists should continue to encourage patients to stop smoking before undergoing elective pulmonary resection.

R. J. Cerfolio, MD

Staging of Patients with Non-Small Cell Lung Cancer

Endoscopic Ultrasound-Guided Fine Needle Aspiration of Mediastinal Lymph Node in Patients With Suspected Lung Cancer After Positron Emission Tomography and Computed Tomography Scans

Eloubeidi MA, Cerfolio RJ, Chen VK, et al (Univ of Alabama at Birmingham)
Ann Thorac Surg 79:263-268, 2005 13–3

Background.—The treatment of patients with non-small cell lung cancer (NSCLC) depends on the stage. Positron emission and computed tomography (CT) scans can identify suspicious lymph nodes that require biopsy. We prospectively evaluated the yield and accuracy of endoscopic ultrasound-guided fine needle aspiration (EUS-FNA) in sampling mediastinal lymph nodes and compared its accuracy to that of 18F-fluorodeoxyglucose positron emission tomography (FDG-PET) and CT in staging NSCLC.

Methods.—A consecutive series of patients with suspicious nodes on PET or CT scan in the posterior mediastinal lymph node stations (#5, 7, 8, or 9) were prospectively evaluated by EUS-FNA. The reference standard included thoracotomy with complete lymphadenectomy in patients with lung cancer or if EUS-FNA was benign, repeat clinical imaging, or long-term follow-up.

Results.—There were 104 patients (63 men) with 125 lesions (117 lymph nodes, 8 left adrenal glands) who underwent EUS-FNA. The sensitivity, specificity, positive predictive value, negative predictive value, and accuracy of EUS-FNA were 92.5%, 100%, 100%, 94%, and 97%, respectively. EUS-FNA was more accurate and had a higher positive predictive value than the PET or CT ($p < 0.001$) scan in confirming cancer in the posterior mediastinal lymph nodes (Table 4). EUS-FNA documented metastatic cancer to the left adrenal in all 4 patients with advanced disease. No deaths resulted from EUS-FNA. One patient experienced self-limited stridor.

Conclusions.—EUS-FNA is a safe, accurate, and minimally invasive technique that improves the staging of patients with NSCLC. It is more accurate and has a higher predictive value than either the PET scan or CT scan for posterior mediastinal lymph nodes.

▶ The role of EUS-FNA for the general thoracic surgeon continues to be better defined. This article is another in a series of EUS-FNA articles that again shows the safety, accuracy, and minimally invasive nature of EUS-FNA. EUS-FNA provides accurate and safe noninvasive staging of patients with NSCLC. As displayed in Table 4, EUS-FNA has a higher predictive value then PET scan, which is of no surprise, since PET only provides clinical suspicion whereas EUS-FNA provides pathologic proof.

R. J. Cerfolio, MD

TABLE 4.—Operating Characteristics of CT, PET, EUS and EUS-FNA in Detecting Malignancy in Suspicious Mediastinal Lymph Nodes

TEST	Sensitivity (95% CI) *p*-value	Specificity (95% CI) *p*-value	PPV (95% CI) *p*-value	NPV (95% CI) *p*-value	Accuracy (95% CI) *p*-value	LR Positive
CT	—	—	39.2% (26.7–49.4)	—	40.3% (30.9–50.5)	1.03 (0.98–1.08)
PET	—	—	40.3% (29.1–55.1)	—	50.0% (37.2–61.4)	1.30 (1.11–1.53)
EUS[a]	80.0% (64.4–90.1)	62.5% (49.5–74.3)	57.2% (43.2–70.3)	83.3% (69.8–92.5)	69.2% (59.4–77.9)	2.13 (1.50–3.03)
EUS-FNA[b]	92.5% (79.6–98.4)	100% (94.3–100)	100% (90.5–100)	95.5% (87.5–99.1)	97.1% (91.8–99.4)	118.9 (7.5–1883)

[a]EUS imaging with any 2 or more lymph node features present.
[b]*p* value (0.001) for both accuracy and PPV of EUS-FNA compared with CT and FDG-PET.
Abbreviations: CI, Confidence interval; *CT,* computed tomography; *EUS,* endoscopic ultrasound; *EUS-FNA,* endoscopic ultrasound fine-needle aspiration; *FDG,* ^{18}F-fluorodeoxyglucose; *LR,* likelihood ratio; *NPV,* negative predictive value; *PET,* positron emission tomography; *PPV,* positive predictive value.
(Courtesy of Eloubeidi MA, Cerfolio RJ, Chen VK, et al: Endoscopic ultrasound-guided fine needle aspiration of mediastinal lymph node in patients with suspected lung cancer after positron emission tomography and computed tomography scans. *Ann Thorac Surg* 79:263-268, 2005. Reprinted with permission from the Society of Thoracic Surgeons.)

Endoscopic Ultrasound Added to Mediastinoscopy for Preoperative Staging of Patients With Lung Cancer

Annema JT, Versteegh MI, Veseliç M, et al (Leiden Univ, The Netherlands; Krankenhaus Grosshansdorf, Germany)

JAMA 294:931-936, 2005 13–4

Context.—Up to 40% of thoracotomies performed for non–small cell lung cancer are unnecessary, predominantly due to inaccurate preoperative detection of lymph node metastases and mediastinal tumor invasion (T4). Mediastinoscopy and the novel, minimally invasive technique of transesophageal ultrasound–guided fine-needle aspiration (EUS-FNA) target different mediastinal lymph node stations. In addition, EUS can identify tumor invasion in neighboring organs if tumors are located adjacent to the esophagus.

Objective.—To investigate the additional value of EUS-FNA to mediastinoscopy in the preoperative staging of patients with non–small cell lung cancer.

Design, Setting, and Patients.—Prospective, nonrandomized multicenter trial performed in 1 referral and 5 general hospitals in the Netherlands. During a 3-year period (2000-2003), 107 consecutive patients with potential resectable non–small cell lung cancer underwent preoperative staging by both EUS-FNA and mediastinoscopy. Patients underwent thoracotomy with tumor resection if mediastinoscopy was negative. Surgical-pathological staging was compared with preoperative findings and the added benefit of the combined strategy was assessed.

Intervention.—The EUS-FNA examination was performed as an additional staging test to mediastinoscopy in all patients.

Main Outcome Measure.—Detection of mediastinal tumor invasion (T4) and lymph node metastases (N2/N3) comparing the combined staging by both EUS-FNA and mediastinoscopy with staging by mediastinoscopy alone.

Results.—The combination of EUS-FNA and mediastinoscopy identified more patients with tumor invasion or lymph node metastases (36%; 95% confidence interval [CI], 27%-46%) compared with either mediastinoscopy alone (20%; 95% CI, 13%-29%) or EUS-FNA (28%; 95% CI, 19%-38%) alone. This indicated that 16% of thoracotomies could have been avoided by using EUS-FNA in addition to mediastinoscopy. However, 2% of the EUS-FNA findings were false-positive.

Conclusion.—These preliminary findings suggest that EUS-FNA, when added to mediastinoscopy, improves the preoperative staging of lung cancer due to the complementary reach of EUS-FNA in detecting mediastinal lymph node metastases and the ability to assess mediastinal tumor invasion.

► This article, by Dr Annema and colleagues, that appeared in the *Journal of the American Medical Association* brought the modality of EUS-FNA to national attention. Anytime an article appears in *The New England Journal of Medicine* or *JAMA*, it deserves special attention because of the high readership that these crossover journals comprise. These articles if on a general thoracic topic will appear in the *Year Book of Surgery* even if they are not done well. There were several articles in the lay press about this particular study that was performed in the Netherlands. Although the study only had 107 patients and took 3 years to complete, it was prospective and multi-institutional, and it was performed outside the United States. These latter factors, as opposed to the quality of the science, are the main appeal to *JAMA* and *The New England Journal of Medicine*. This study showed that EUS-FNA when added to mediastinoscopy improves preoperative staging of patients with lung cancer. This is obviously not new information to general thoracic surgeons since mediastinoscopy assesses the anterior/superior nodal stations (2R, 4R, 2L, 4L, and the top of 7), whereas EUS-FNA assesses the posterior/inferior nodal stations (5, 7, 8, and 9). I do not believe that EUS-FNA can assess the 5 station, but rather the low 4L. Thus, the 2 tests are complementary as we show in the next article (Abstract 13–5).

R. J. Cerfolio, MD

Endoscopic Ultrasound-Guided Fine-Needle Aspiration in Patients With Non-Small Cell Lung Cancer and Prior Negative Mediastinoscopy

Eloubeidi MA, Tamhane A, Chen VK, et al (Univ of Alabama at Birmingham)

Ann Thorac Surg 80:1231-1240, 2005 13–5

Background.—Mediastinoscopy and endoscopic ultrasound-guided fine-needle aspiration biopsy (EUS-FNA) are complementary for staging non-small cell lung cancer (NSCLC) patients. We assessed (1) the yield of EUS-FNA of malignant lymph nodes in NSCLC patients with combined anterior and posterior lymph nodes that had already undergone mediastinoscopy and (2) the cost implications associated with alternative initial strategies.

Methods.—All patients underwent chest computed tomography (CT) and/or positron emission tomography (PET), and mediastinoscopy. Then, the posterior mediastinal stations (7, 8, and 9) or station 5 were targeted with EUS-FNA. The reference standard included thoracotomy with complete thoracic lymphadenectomy, repeat clinical imaging, or long-term clinical follow-up. A Monte Carlo cost-analysis model evaluated the expected costs and outcomes associated with staging of NSCLC.

Results.—Thirty-five NSCLC patients met inclusion criteria (median age 65 years; 80% men). Endoscopic ultrasound-guided FNA was performed in 53 lymph nodes in various stations, the subcarinal station (7) being the most common (47.3%). Of the 35 patients who had a prior negative mediastinoscopy, 13 patients (37.1%) had malignant N2 or N3 lymph nodes. Accuracy of EUS-FNA (98.1%) was significantly higher than that of CT (41.5%; $p < 0.001$) and PET (40%; $p < 0.001$). Initial EUS-FNA resulted in average costs per patient of \$1,867 (SD ± \$4,308) while initial mediastinoscopy cost \$12,900 (SD ± \$4,164.40). If initial EUS-FNA is utilized rather than initial mediastinoscopy, an average cost saving of \$11,033 per patient would result.

Conclusions.—In patients with NSCLC and combined anterior and posterior lymph nodes, starting with EUS-FNA would preclude mediastinoscopy in more than one third of the patients. Endoscopic ultrasound-guided FNA is a safe outpatient procedure that is less invasive and less costly than mediastinoscopy.

► In this article from our institution, Dr Eloubeidi and colleagues have shown that EUS-FNA may be a more cost-effective technique to use initially rather than mediastinoscopy. This may only apply to patients with both anterior and posterior mediastinal lymph nodes that are suspected to be involved with metastatic cancer.

R. J. Cerfolio, MD

The Maximum Standardized Uptake Values on Positron Emission Tomography of a Non–Small Cell Lung Cancer Predict Stage, Recurrence, and Survival

Cerfolio RJ, Bryant AS, Ohja B, et al (Univ of Alabama, Birmingham; Birmingham VA Hosp, Ala)

J Thorac Cardiovasc Surg 130:151-159, 2005 13–6

Objective.—We sought to assess whether the standard uptake value of a pulmonary nodule is an independent predictor of biologic aggressiveness.

Methods.—This is a retrospective review of a prospective database of patients with non–small cell lung cancer. Patients had dedicated positron emission tomography scanning with F-18 fluorodeoxyglucose, with the maxi-

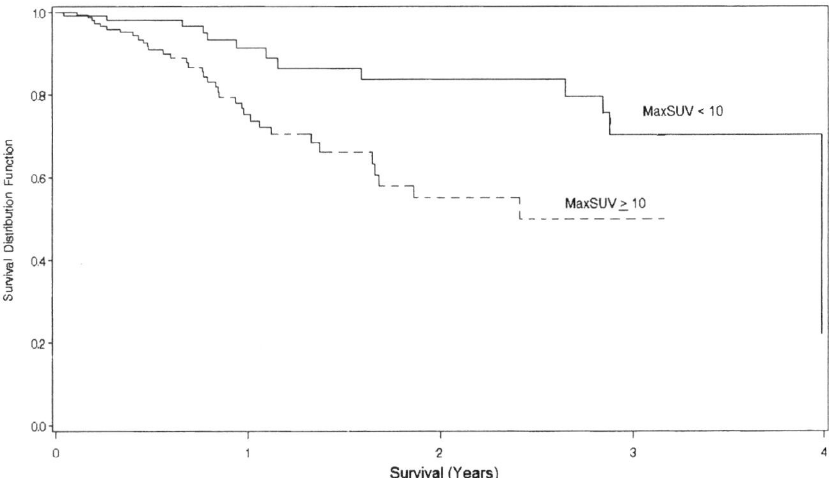

FIGURE 2.—Cox proportional hazard survival curve for all 315 patients stratified by maximum SUV. *Abbreviation: SUV,* Standardized uptake value. (Courtesy of Cerfolio RJ, Bryant AS, Ohja B, et al: The maximum standardized uptake values on positron emission tomography of a non–small cell lung cancer predict stage, recurrence, and survival. *J Thorac Cardiovasc Surg* 130:151-159, 2005. Copyright 2005 with permission from The American Association for Thoracic Surgery.)

mum standard uptake value measured. All suspicious nodal and systemic locations on computed tomographic and positron emission tomographic scanning underwent biopsy, and when indicated, resection with complete lymphadenectomy was performed.

Results.—There were 315 patients. Multivariate analysis showed patients with a high maximum standard uptake value (≥10) were more likely to have poorly differentiated tumors (risk ratio, 1.5; *P* = .005) and advanced stage (risk ratio, 1.9; *P* = .010) and were less likely to have their disease completely resected (risk ratio, 3.7; *P* = .004) (Fig 2). Maximum standard uptake value was the best predictor of disease-free survival (hazard ratio, 2.5; *P* = .039) and survival (hazard ratio, 2.8; *P* = .001). Stage-specific analysis showed that patients with stage IB and stage II disease with a maximum standard uptake value of greater than the median for their respective stages had a lower disease-free survival at 4 years (*P* = .005 and .044) (Fig 1). The ac-

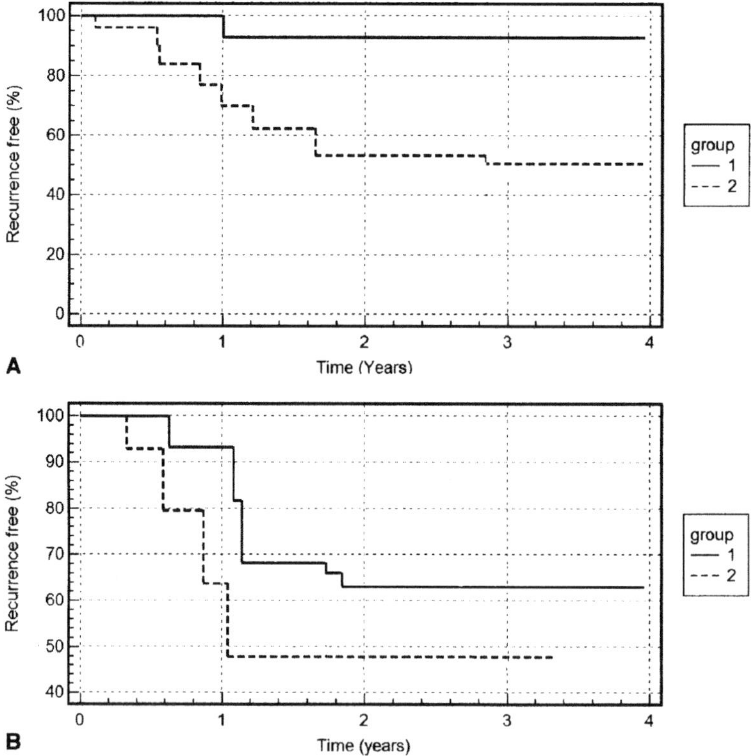

FIGURE 1.—Kaplan-Meier curves depicting disease-free survival of NSCLC comparing patients with a low maximum SUV with those with a high maximum SUV by stage. *Group 1,* Patients with a maximum SUV lower than the median maximum SUV in that stage (low maximum SUV group). *Group 2,* Patients with a maximum SUV greater than or equal to the median maximum SUV in that stage (high maximum SUV group). **A**, Stage IB NSCLC (*P* = .005); **B**, stage II NSCLC (*P* = .044). *Abbreviations: NSCLC,* Non–small cell lung cancer; *SUV,* standardized uptake value. (Courtesy of Cerfolio RJ, Bryant AS, Ohja B, et al: The maximum standardized uptake values on positron emission tomography of a non–small cell lung cancer predict stage, recurrence, and survival. *J Thorac Cardiovasc Surg* 130:151-159, 2005. Copyright 2005 with permission from The American Association for Thoracic Surgery.)

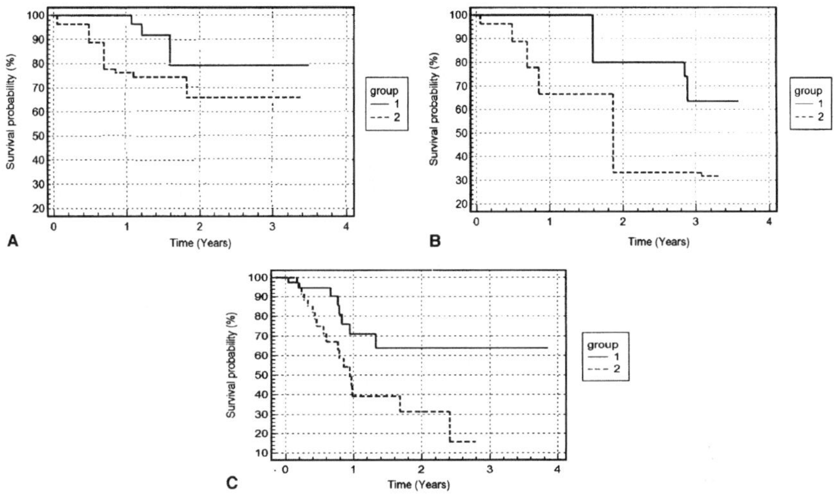

FIGURE 3.—Kaplan-Meier curves depicting the actual survival for patients with a low maximum SUV compared with those with a high maximum SUV stratified by stage. *Group 1,* Patients with a maximum SUV lower than the median maximum SUV in that stage (low maximum SUV group). *Group 2,* Patients with a maximum SUV greater than or equal to the median maximum SUV in that stage (high maximum SUV group). **A,** Stage Ib NSCLC (P = .048); **B,** stage II NSCLC (P = .028); **C,** stage IIIA (P = .0120). *Abbreviations: SUV,* Standardized uptake value; *NSCLC,* non–small cell lung cancer. (Courtesy of Cerfolio RJ, Bryant AS, Ohja B, et al: The maximum standardized uptake values on positron emission tomography of a non–small cell lung cancer predict stage, recurrence, and survival. *J Thorac Cardiovasc Surg* 130:151-159, 2005. Copyright 2005 with permission from The American Association for Thoracic Surgery.)

tual 4-year survival for patients with stage Ib non–small cell lung cancer was 80% versus 66% (P = .048), for stage II disease it was 64% versus 32% (P = .028), and for stage IIIa disease it was 64% versus 16% (P = .012) for the low and high maximum standard uptake value groups, respectively (Fig 3).

Conclusions.—The maximum standard uptake value of a non–small cell lung cancer nodule on dedicated positron emission tomography is an independent predictor of stage and tumor characteristics. It is a more powerful independent predictor than the TNM stage for recurrence and survival for patients with early-stage resected cancer. This information might help guide treatment strategies.

▶ This article, which received significant television and press coverage, shows the importance of the maximum standardized uptake value (maxSUV). The maxSUV is calculated by the software contained in an integrated positron emission tomography (PET)/CT scan or in a dedicated PET scan. It quantifies the biologic aggressiveness of a tumor in a particular host. It also determines certain pathologic characteristics of a solid organ tumor. It is a remarkable and powerful finding that the maxSUV was found to be a better and more powerful independent predictor than the current TNM staging system for recurrence and survival in patients with early resected non–small cell lung cancer. Figures 1 through 3 display the predictive power of the maxSUV.

This is not the first series to show this important finding, but it may be the largest and most carefully done. It features an electronic prospective database, which is much more accurate than a retrospective chart review. It has careful, meticulous clinical and pathologic staging, and the latter has been shown to be much more accurate than the former. It also has careful follow-up. This study shows that perhaps the biology of a tumor in a host may be more important than just its anatomic location or characteristics (ie, its size, spread to nodes, etc). This corroborates those studies that examine cellular and genetic factors that make tumors "bad actors." The maxSUV as calculated during a PET scan quantifies that concept for us and does it in a particular host. Further studies are underway to evaluate the importance of the maxSUV, not only in lung cancer but also in other solid organ tumors such as esophageal malignancy.

R. J. Cerfolio, MD

Comparison Between Clinical and Pathologic Staging in 2,994 Cases of Lung Cancer

López-Encuentra A, for the Bronchogenic Carcinoma Cooperative Group of the Spanish Society of Pneumology and Thoracic Surgery (Hosp Universitario 12 de Octubre, Madrid; et al)

Ann Thorac Surg 79:974-979, 2005 13–7

Background.—The accuracy of clinical staging in lung cancer may be evaluated by comparing it against the gold standard of pathologic staging. The objective of this paper is to compare these two staging methods in a series of 2,994 lung cancer cases operated on consecutively in Spain between 1993 and 1997.

Methods.—The raw frequency of agreement was used to compare clinical against pathologic staging and to assess the agreement. Kappa's index was used to determine the random effect of agreement.

Results.—Ninety-three percent of the entire population were men, with a mean age of 64 years (median, 66; SD, 9.6). The majority of cases were classified as squamous tumors (1,774; 59%), with complete resection (2,410; 80%), and with lobectomy or bilobectomy (1,490; 55%). The most frequently found pathologic stage was pIB (997; 37%), followed by pIIIA (524; 19%). Considering the 2,377 cases with clinical and pathologic staging data, a classification coincidence was observed in 1,108 cases (47%; Kappa's index 0.248 for stages IA through IIIB). Considering the pathologic staging as the gold standard, the agreement was 75% for stages IA-IB (Kappa's index 0.56). In general, downstaging is more frequent than upstaging.

Conclusions.—This recent series of lung cancer showed the low diagnostic accuracy of the clinical staging as compared with the pathologic staging. Diagnostic accuracy was found to be much higher in the initial IA-IB stages, as illustrated by Kappa's index.

▶ In this article, Dr López-Encuentra and colleagues show the low diagnostic accuracy of the predictive clinical stage when compared with the actual pathologic stage. In fact, the authors found that when a patient is clinically staged as IA or IB, it is only correct 75% of the time. Interestingly, downstaging was more frequently found than upstaging. This once again should make physicians use caution when treating patients based on an assumed clinical stage. We and especially our medical oncologic colleagues should not use the clinical stage as determined by CT or PET/CT to treat patients, but rather obtain biopsy specimens from suspicious sites using minimally invasive techniques if possible, to ensure these sites are not falsely positive. Too many patients are denied pulmonary resection or incorrectly given neoadjuvant therapy because of assumed metastatic disease in sites that are suspicious on PET but never proven as malignant with biopsies.

R. J. Cerfolio, MD

Improving the Inaccuracies of Clinical Staging of Patients With NSCLC: A Prospective Trial

Cerfolio RJ, Bryant AS, Ojha B, et al (Univ of Alabama at Birmingham)
Ann Thorac Surg 80:1207-1214, 2005 13–8

Background.—Clinical stage affects the care of patients with nonsmall cell lung cancer.

Methods.—This is a prospective trial on patients with suspected resectable nonsmall cell lung cancer. All patients underwent integrated positron emission tomographic scanning and computed tomographic scanning, and all suspicious metastatic sites were investigated. A, T, N, and M status was assigned. If N2, N3 and M1 were negative, patients underwent thoracotomy and complete thoracic lymphadenectomy.

Results.—There were 383 patients. The accuracy of clinical staging using positron emission tomographic scanning and computed tomographic scanning was 68% and 66% for stage I, 84% and 82% for stage II, 74% and 69% for stage III, and 93% and 92% for stage IV, respectively. N2 disease was discovered in 115 patients (30%) and was most common in the subcarinal lymph node (30%). Unsuspected N2 disease occurred in 28 patients (14%) and was most common in the posterior mediastinal lymph nodes (subcarinal, 38%; posterior aortopulmonary, 15%). It was found in 9% of patients who were clinically staged I (58% in the posterior mediastinal lymph nodes) and in 26% of patients clinically staged II (86% in posterior mediastinal lymph nodes).

Conclusions.—Despite integrated positron emission tomographic scanning and computed tomographic scanning, clinical staging remains relatively inaccurate for patients with nonsmall cell lung cancer. Recent studies suggest adjuvant therapy for stage Ib and II nonsmall cell lung cancer; thus the impact on preoperative care is to find unsuspected N2 disease. Unsuspected N2 disease is most common in posterior mediastinal lymph nodes inaccessible by mediastinoscopy. Thus one should consider endoscopic ultrasound fine-needle aspiration, especially for patients clinically staged as I and

II, even if the nodes are negative on positron emission tomographic scanning and computed tomographic scanning.

▶ This article, which was presented at the annual meeting of The Society of Thoracic Surgeons in January 2005, also shows the inaccuracies of clinical staging when compared with pathologic staging. It again found significant inaccuracies in patients with stage I, stage II, and stage III non–small cell lung cancer. It is a carefully designed and performed prospective study and again emphasizes the need for caution that patients should be pathologically and not clinically staged. Treatment decisions should not be based on suspected nodal or metastatic sites but rather on sites that have undergone definitive biopsies that prove or disprove cancer. It probably is more important for us to deliver this message to our colleagues, the medical oncologists and the radiation therapists, than it is to general and thoracic surgeons.

R. J. Cerfolio, MD

Intra-Operative Concerns

Morbidity, Survival, and Site of Recurrence After Mediastinal Lymph-Node Dissection Versus Systematic Sampling After Complete Resection for Non-Small Cell Lung Cancer

Lardinois D, Suter H, Hakki H, et al (Univ Hosp, Zurich, Switzerland; Univ Hosp, Bern, Switzerland; Univ of Zurich, Switzerland; et al)

Ann Thorac Surg 80:268-275, 2005 13–9

Background.—Mediastinal lymph-node dissection was compared to systematic mediastinal lymph-node sampling in patients undergoing complete resection for non-small cell lung cancer with respect to morbidity, duration of chest tube drainage and hospitalization, survival, disease-free survival, and site of recurrence.

Methods.—A consecutive series of one hundred patients with non-small-cell lung cancer, clinical stage T1-3 N0-1 after standardized staging, was divided into two groups of 50 patients each, according to the technique of intraoperative mediastinal lymph-node assessment (dissection versus sampling). Mediastinal lymph-node dissection consisted of removal of all lymphatic tissues within defined anatomic landmarks of stations 2-4 and 7-9 on the right side, and stations 4-9 on the left side according to the classification of the American Thoracic Society. Systematic mediastinal lymph-node sampling consisted of harvesting of one or more representative lymph nodes from stations 2-4 and 7-9 on the right side, and stations 4-9 on the left side.

Results.—All patients had complete resection. A mean follow-up time of 89 months was achieved in 92 patients. The two groups of patients were comparable with respect to age, gender, performance status, tumor stage, histology, extent of lung resection, and follow-up time. No significant difference was found between both groups regarding the duration of chest tube drainage, hospitalization, and morbidity. However, dissection required a longer operation time than sampling (179 ± 38 min versus 149 ± 37 min, $p < 0.001$). There was no significant difference in overall survival between the two groups; however, patients with stage I disease had a significantly longer disease-free survival after dissection than after sampling (60.2 ± 7 versus 44.8 ± 8 months, $p < 0.03$). Local recurrence was significantly higher after sampling than after dissection in patients with stage I tumor (12.5% versus 45%, $p = 0.02$) and in patients with nodal tumor negative mediastinum (N0/N1 disease) (46% versus 13%, $p = 0.004$).

Conclusion.—Our results suggest that mediastinal lymph-node dissection may provide a longer disease-free survival in stage I non-small cell lung cancer and, most importantly, a better local tumor control than mediastinal lymph-node sampling after complete resection for N0/N1 disease without leading to increased morbidity.

▶ Dr Lardinois and colleagues from Switzerland have presented a very important study that evaluated a consecutive series of 100 patients who have non–small cell lung cancer. The patients were divided into 2 groups. Unfortunately, they were not randomized. The authors found that those patients with stage I cancer had improved survival if a complete thoracic mediastinal lymph node dissection was performed, compared with those patients who underwent lymph node sampling. They also found improved local control for patients who were N1 as well as those who were pathologic N0. This is an extremely important study. Although there are flaws in the methodology, the article is important, and it give credence as to why the standard of care for lung cancer surgery should be to perform complete thoracic lymphadenectomy in all patients with non–small cell lung cancer. We continue to wait for the results of the large ACOSOG multi-institutional study that examined this same question in a different way.

Finally, some argue that it should be required to have documentation of lymph node removal or biopsy in order to receive surgeon reimbursement. Perhaps a pathology report that shows nodes have at least been sampled from several stations on the right (stations: 2R, 4R, 7, 8, and 9) and on the left (stations: 5, 6, 7, 8, and 9 and maybe 4L) should be necessary before submitting a bill to the insurance company for surgeon reimbursement.

R. J. Cerfolio, MD

Comparison of Morbidity, 30-Day Mortality, and Long-term Survival After Pneumonectomy and Sleeve Lobectomy for Non–Small Cell Lung Carcinoma

Ludwig C, Stoelben E, Olschewski M, et al (Univ of Freiburg, Germany)
Ann Thorac Surg 79:968-973, 2005 13–10

Background.—The advantage of sleeve lobectomy as an alternative to pneumonectomy for preserving lung function is obvious and among other arguments allows operating on patients with lung cancer who would not tolerate pneumonectomy. The purpose of this retrospective, nonrandomized study is to compare the early (30-day mortality) and late (5-year survival) outcomes of both procedures.

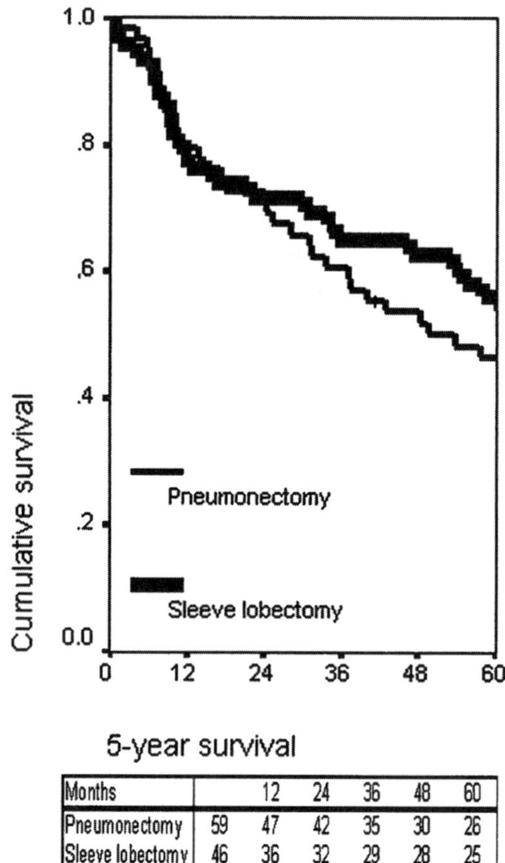

Months		12	24	36	48	60
Pneumonectomy	59	47	42	35	30	26
Sleeve lobectomy	46	36	32	29	28	25

FIGURE 2.—Survival after sleeve lobectomy or pneumonectomy with N0 nodal status. (Courtesy of Ludwig C, Stoelben E, Olschewski M, et al: Comparison of morbidity, 30-day mortality, and long-term survival after pneumonectomy and sleeve lobectomy for non–small cell lung carcinoma. *Ann Thorac Surg* 79:968-973, 2005. Reprinted with permission from the Society of Thoracic Surgeons.)

Methods.—The charts of 310 patients who underwent either pneumonectomy or sleeve lobectomy for lung cancer stages I to IIIA from 1987 to 1997 were reviewed. One hundred ninety-four patients underwent pneumonectomy, and 116 patients underwent sleeve lobectomy. Specific operative complications, i.e., anastomotic leakage versus stump dehiscence, perioperative complications, 30-day or in-hospital mortality, and 5-year survival were registered for comparison of the immediate risk of the respective procedures.

Results.—In the bronchial sleeve lobectomy group, the incidence of anastomotic leakage was 6.9% (8 of 116 patients) and the operative mortality was 4.3%. The incidence of bronchial stump fistulas after pneumonectomy was 3.6% (7 of 194 patients), and early mortality was 4.6%. All but 6 patients (98%) had a complete resection. Overall 5-year survival after sleeve lobectomy was 39% and after pneumonectomy, 27%. The distribution of

5-year survival stage by stage in either group is presented (Fig 2). Sleeve lobectomy, age younger than 65 years, pN0, and stage I are positive prognostic factors for long-term survival. In the multivariate analysis, pneumonectomy is a negative prognostic factor.

Conclusions.—The indication for pneumonectomy versus sleeve lobectomy depends on the localization of the primary tumor on the one hand, and on cardiorespiratory function, which might be more often distinctly impaired in the sleeve group, on the other hand. This could explain why the mortality in the sleeve lobectomy group was identical with that in the pneumonectomy group. However, both techniques are appropriate treatment modalities of advanced lung cancer or patients with critical functional reserve. Therefore, whenever possible, sleeve lobectomy should be performed.

▶ This retrospective review from Freiburg, Germany, from Dr Ludwig and associates compares 194 patients who had pneumonectomy with 116 who underwent sleeve lobectomy. The authors report similar survival between the 2 groups, and they found pneumonectomy to be a negative prognostic factor. This study is obviously flawed by the fact that it's retrospective, some patients could not undergo sleeve lobectomy, etc, and it has other serious methodological problems. However, it elucidates the low local recurrence rates with sleeve lobectomy if negative margins are achieved. Sleeve lobectomy continues to be the standard of care if complete R0 resection can be achieved, even if the patient could tolerate pneumonectomy. As shown in Figure 2, it is especially appealing in patients who are node negative.

R. J. Cerfolio, MD

Border Between N1 and N2 Stations in Lung Carcinoma: Lessons From Lymph Node Metastatic Patterns of Lower Lobe Tumors

Okada M, Sakamoto T, Yuki T, et al (Hyogo Med Ctr for Adults, Akashi City, Japan)

J Thorac Cardiovasc Surg 129:825-830, 2005 13–11

Objective.—Distinction of lymph node stations is one of the most crucial topics still not entirely resolved by many lung cancer surgeons. The nodes around the junction of the hilum and mediastinum are key points at issue. We examined the spread pattern of lymph node metastases, investigated the prognosis according to the level of the involved nodes, and conclusively analyzed the border between N1 and N2 stations.

Methods.—We reviewed the records of 604 consecutive patients who underwent complete resection for non–small cell lung carcinoma of the lower lobe.

Results.—There were 390 patients (64.6%) with N0 disease, 127 (21.0%) with N1, and 87 (14.4%) with N2. Whereas 11.3% of patients with right N2 disease had skip metastases limited to the subcarinal nodes, 32.6% of patients with left N2 disease had skip metastases, of which 64.2% had involvement of N2 station nodes, except the subcarinal ones. The overall 5-year survivals of patients with N0, N1, and N2 disease were 71.0%, 50.8%, and 16.7%, respectively (N0 vs N1 $P = .0001$, N1 vs N2, $P < .0001$). Although there were no significant differences in survival according to the side of the tumor among patients with N0 or N1 disease, patients with a left N2 tumor had a worse prognosis than those with a right N2 tumor ($P = .0387$). The overall 5-year survivals of patients with N0, intralobar N1, hilar N1, lower mediastinal N2, and upper mediastinal N2 disease were 71.0%, 60.1%, 38.8%, 24.8%, and 0%, respectively (Fig 3, A). Significant differ-

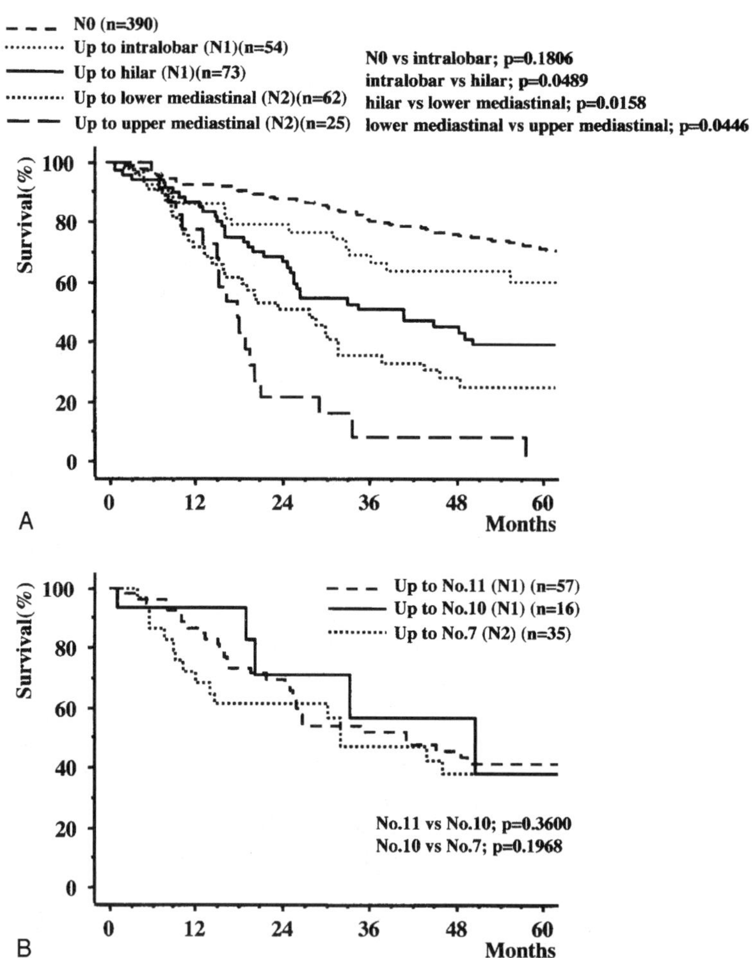

FIGURE 3.—Overall survival curves of patients subjected to complete resection for non–small cell lung cancer according to pathologic nodal status. **A**, Disease was classified as N0 disease, intralobar N1 disease, hilar N1 disease, lower mediastinal N2 disease, and upper mediastinal N2 disease. **B**, Disease was further classified as tumor involving up to either interlobar (station 11), main bronchus (station 10), or subcarinal (station 7) nodes. (Courtesy of Okada M, Sakamoto T, Yuki T, et al: Border between N1 and N2 stations in lung carcinoma: Lessons from lymph node metastatic patterns of lower lobe tumors. *J Thorac Cardiovasc Surg* 129:825-830, 2005. Copyright 2005 with permission from The American Association for Thoracic Surgery.)

ences were observed between intralobar N1 and hilar N1 disease (P = .0489), hilar N1 and lower mediastinal N2 disease (P = .0158), and lower and upper mediastinal N2 disease (P = .0446). Also, the 5-year survivals of patients with involvement up to station 11, up to station 10, and up to station 7 were 41.4%, 37.9% and 37.7%, respectively (difference not significant) (Fig 3, B).

Conclusions.—N1 and N2 diseases appeared as a combination of subgroups: intralobar N1 disease, hilar N1 disease, lower mediastinal N2 disease, and upper mediastinal N2 disease. Interestingly, the survivals of patients with involvement up to interlobar nodes (station 11), main bronchus nodes (station 10), and subcarinal nodes (station 7) were identical. These data constitute the basis for a larger investigation to develop a lymph node map in lung cancer.

▶ This article from Dr Okada and associates from Japan reviewed the records of 604 consecutive patients who underwent complete resection of non–small cell lung cancer. They assessed 390 patients who had N0 disease, 127 with N1, and 87 who had N2. The authors divided the N1 disease into interlobar and hilar N1 disease. They divided N2 disease into lower mediastinal and upper mediastinal N2 disease. This subdivision is unusual, and there are few previous data on this concept. Their findings were interesting. The survival of patients who had involvement of the interlobar or #11 station along with the 10R, or what they call the "main bronchus lymph node," along with the N2 subcarinal stations was identical. These data are shown in Figure 3. These provocative data are different from other reports, which show that metastatic involvement of the subcarinal #7 lymph node is a worse prognostic sign than any N1 node. This finding may mean that the #10 or hilar node should be treated more as an N2 node, and perhaps those patients would benefit from neoadjuvant therapy. These are important and provocative data, and further studies are needed. The Japanese continue to thoroughly investigate the role of radical lymph node dissection in the survival of many solid organ cancers, and this report echoes their significant contribution to the field of general thoracic surgery in this regard.

R. J. Cerfolio, MD

One Hundred Consecutive Pneumonectomies After Induction Therapy for Non–Small Cell Lung Cancer: An Uncertain Balance Between Risks and Benefits

Doddoli C, Barlesi F, Trousse D, et al (Université de la Méditerranée, Marseille, France; IFR Jean Roche, Marseille, France)

J Thorac Cardiovasc Surg 130:416-425, 2005 13–12

Objective.—We sought to assess postoperative outcome after pneumonectomy after neoadjuvant therapy in patients with non–small cell lung cancer.

Methods.—This retrospective study included 100 patients treated from January 1989 through December 2003 for a primary lung cancer in whom pneumonectomy had been performed after an induction treatment. Surgical intervention had not been considered initially for the following reasons: N2 disease (stage IIIA, n = 79), doubtful resectability (stage IIIB [T4, N0], n = 19), and M1 disease (stage IV [T2, N0, M1, solitary brain metastasis], n = 2). All patients received a 2-drug platinum-based regimen with a median of 2.5 cycles (range, 2-4 cycles), and 30 had associated radiotherapy (30-45 Gy).

Results.—There were 55 right and 45 left resections. Overall 30-day and 90-day mortality rates were 12% and 21%, respectively. At multivariate analysis, one independent prognostic factor entered the model to predict 30-day mortality: postoperative cardiovascular event (relative risk, 45.7; 95% confidence interval, 3.7-226.7; P = .001). Four variables predicted 90-day mortality: age of more than 60 years (relative risk, 5.06; 95% confidence interval, 1.47-17.48; P = .01), male sex (relative risk, 8.25; 95% confidence interval, 1.01-67.34; P = .049), postoperative respiratory event (relative risk, 3.64; 95% confidence interval, 1.14-9.37; P = .007), and postoperative cardiovascular event (relative risk, 7.84; 95% confidence interval, 3.12-19.71; P < .001). Estimated overall survivals in 90-day survivors were 35% (range, 29%-41%) and 25% (range, 19.3%-30.7%) at 3 and 5 years, respectively. At multivariate analysis, one independent prognostic factor entered the model: pathologic stage III-IV residual disease (relative risk, 1.89; 95% confidence interval, 1.09-3.26; P = .022).

Conclusions.—Pneumonectomy after induction therapy is a high-risk procedure, the survival benefit of which appears uncertain.

▶ This article from Dr Doddoli and colleagues from France retrospectively studied 100 patients over a 14-year period and found that pneumonectomy, after induction therapy, is a high-risk procedure. The authors reported a 30-day operative mortality of 12%. However, the staggering number is the reported 90-day mortality of 21%. It is interesting that they even report 90-day mortality, and the increase in deaths over 2 months is high. I think the 90-day mortality figure, which is rarely reported, is an important statistic. Our prospective database and others are showing that when patients are carefully followed up for more than just 1 month after surgery, there's a much higher incidence of recidivism and other complications that occur after hospital discharge. The surgical dictum of death before discharge or before 30 days may not need to change, but the concept of reporting a 90-day mortality and/or the quality of life and recidivism rate may provide even more information on the true impact of surgical procedures.

R. J. Cerfolio, MD

Preoperative Chemotherapy Does Not Increase Complications After Nonsmall Cell Lung Cancer Resection

Perrot E, Guibert B, Mulsant P, et al (Centre Hospitalier Lyon Sud, Pierre-Benite, France)

Ann Thorac Surg 80:423-427, 2005 13–13

Background.—Neoadjuvant chemotherapy before resection of nonsmall cell lung cancer seems to increase survival, mainly in the early stage. Risks of postoperative complications after chemotherapy and surgery remain controversial. Here we review our experience with patients treated in one thoracic surgery center.

Methods.—Patients undergoing resection for nonsmall cell lung cancer after induction chemotherapy between January 1993 and March 2002 were reviewed. Data collected included age, sex, preoperative forced expiratory volume in 1 second (FEV_1), hemoglobin, and arterial oxygen pressure tension (PaO_2), postoperative complications, and global survival. The main objectives were postoperative mortality and morbidity. Postoperative mortality and morbidity were defined as complications or deaths occurring within 30 days after surgery. Predictive morbidity factors were identified by univariate and multivariate analysis and overall survival by the Kaplan-Meier method.

Results.—In all, 114 patients were reviewed. Different induction chemotherapies were used, mainly cisplatin with vinorelbine or gemicitabine. Postoperative mortality was 2 of 114, 1 of 27 after pneumonectomy, and there were no deaths after lobectomy. Complications occurred in 29% of patients (33 of 114), usually infectious pneumonia and anemia requiring transfusion. Preoperative FEV_1, hemoglobin, and PaO_2 are not associated with morbidity in univariate or multivariate analysis.

Conclusions.—Preoperative chemotherapy does not increase postoperative mortality and morbidity after nonsmall cell lung cancer surgery, performed exclusively by thoracic surgeons (Table 5).

▶ This article by Dr Perrot and coauthors, also from France, has the exact opposite finding from the previous French study (Abstract 13–12). In this study of 114 patients, the authors reported only a 29% complication rate, and they had only 2 deaths. There were 27 patients who underwent pneumonectomy, and only 1 patient died. However, we are not told about the 90-day survival or late complication rate. I intentionally placed these 2 articles back to back. They are both from the same country, cover similar topics, have similar designs, and yet yield almost opposite conclusions. This illustrates the controversial nature of this topic in the field of general thoracic surgery. Table 5 presents a nice review of the literature on this topic.

R. J. Cerfolio, MD

TABLE 5.—Postoperative Mortality and Morbidity Rates in 10 Retrospective Studies Without Neoadjuvant Therapy

Author, Reference	Year	Number of Patients	Stage	Overall Mortality	Mortality After Pneumonectomy	Mortality After Lobectomy	Morbidity
Ginsberg et al [11]	1983	2,200	All stages	3.7%	6.2%	2.9%	Not specified
Deslaurier et al [12]	1994	783	All stages	3.8%			27%
Shah et al [13}	1996	313	Stage I and II	3.2%	1.6%	4.03%	6.7%
Duque et al [14]	1997	605	All stages	6.6%	13.4%	4.4%	32.4%
Wada et al [15]	1998	7,099	All stages	1.3%	3.2%	1.2%	Not specified
Joo et al [16]	2001	105	Only pneumonectomy		10.5%		
Myrdal et al [17]	2001	616	All stages	2.9%	5.7%	0.6%	30.8%
Bernard et al [18]	2001	639	Only pneumonectomy		7%		38.3%
Alexiou et al [19]	2001	206	Only pneumonectomy		6.8%		39%
Licker et al [20]	2002	193	Only pneumonectomy		9.3%		47%

(Courtesy of Perrot E, Guibert B, Mulsant P, et al: Preoperative chemotherapy does not increase complications after nonsmall cell lung cancer resection. *Ann Thorac Surg* 80:423-427, 2005. Reprinted with permission from the Society of Thoracic Surgeons.)

Visceral Pleural Invasion Is an Invasive and Aggressive Indicator of Non–Small Cell Lung Cancer

Shimizu K, Yoshida J, Nagai K, et al (Natl Cancer Ctr Hosp East, Chiba, Japan; Gunma Univ, Japan; Natl Cancer Ctr Research Inst East, Chiba, Japan)
J Thorac Cardiovasc Surg 130:160-165, 2005 13–14

Objective.—Although visceral pleural invasion by non–small cell lung cancer is considered a poor-prognostic factor, further information is lacking, especially in relation to other clinicopathologic prognostic factors. We assessed the relationship between visceral pleural invasion and other clinicopathologic characteristics and evaluated its significance as a prognostic factor.

Methods.—We reviewed 1074 patients with surgically resected T1/2 non–small cell lung cancer for their clinicopathologic characteristics and prognoses. The patients were divided into 2 groups according to visceral pleural invasion status (visceral pleural invasion group and non–visceral pleural invasion group). Both groups were compared with regard to age, sex, histology, tumor size, tumor differentiation, lymph node involvement, lymphatic invasion, vascular invasion, scar grade, nuclear atypia, mitotic index, serum carcinoembryonic antigen level, and survival. Univariate and multivariate analyses were conducted.

Results.—Visceral pleural invasion was identified in 288 (26.8%) of the resected specimens. Survival was 76.0% at 5 years and 53.2% at 10 years in the non–visceral pleural invasion group and was 49.8% at 5 years and 37.0% at 10 years in the visceral pleural invasion group (Fig 1). The difference between groups was highly significant ($P < .0001$). Visceral pleural in-

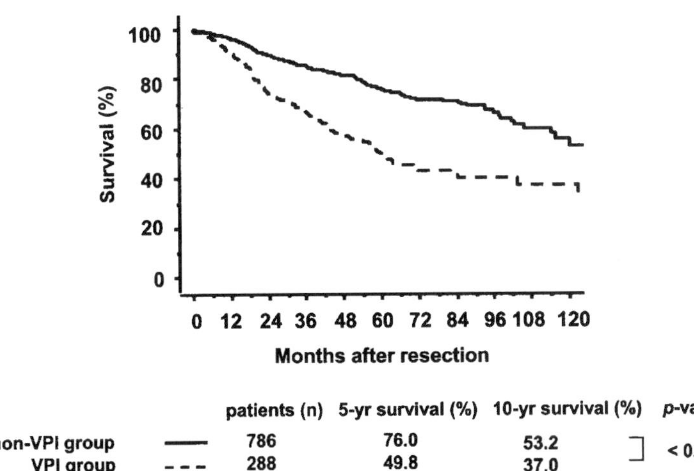

FIGURE 1.—Survival curves and overall 5- and 10-year survival for non-VPI and VPI groups. *Asterisk, P* value by log-rank test. *Abbreviation: VPI,* Visceral pleural invasion. (Courtesy of Shimizu K, Yoshida J, Nagai K, et al: Visceral pleural invasion is an invasive and aggressive indicator of non–small cell lung cancer. *J Thorac Cardiovasc Surg* 130:160-165, 2005. Copyright 2005 with permission from The American Association for Thoracic Surgery.)

vasion was also significantly associated with a higher frequency of lymph node involvement. However, regardless of N status (N0 or N1/2), there was a significant difference in survival when the visceral pleura was invaded. Visceral pleural invasion was observed significantly more frequently in tumors with factors indicative of tumor aggressiveness/invasiveness: moderate/poor differentiation, lymphatic invasion, vascular invasion, high scar grade, high nuclear atypia grade, high mitotic index, and high serum carcinoembryonic antigen level. By multivariate analysis, visceral pleural invasion proved to be a significant independent predictor of poor prognosis in non–small-cell lung cancer patients with or without lymph node involvement.

Conclusions.—Visceral pleural invasion is a significant poor-prognostic factor, regardless of N status. Our analyses indicated that visceral pleural invasion is an independent indicator of non–small cell lung cancer invasiveness and aggressiveness.

▶ Dr Shimizu and associates from Japan have evaluated the charts of 1074 patients and identified visceral pleural invasion (a non–small cell lung cancer tumor that has grown through the pulmonary parenchyma) as a poor prognostic indicator. There is a dramatic difference in the 5-year survival between a T2 and a T1 lesion as shown in Figure 1. The authors report a 76% 5-year survival for T1 lesions compared with only 50% for T2. Interestingly, this dramatic difference of a 26% drop off in survival rates continued when the 10-year survival was calculated. It was 53% compared with 37%, again favoring the T1 lesions. They concluded that visceral pleural invasion is a significant poor prognostic factor. This information, coupled with data concerning the maximum standardized values as calculated via positron emission tomography (PET) scanning, shows that T2 lesions are quite virulent, especially when compared with T1 lesions. If one could predict a lesion as invading the visceral pleura preoperatively, perhaps one should consider neoadjuvant therapy, even if it was less then 3 cm in its greatest diameter. Of course, this is not the current standard of care, and data from prospective studies that show a survival advantage for this strategy are needed.

R. J. Cerfolio, MD

Miscellaneous

Repeat Pulmonary Resection for Isolated Recurrent Lung Metastases Yields Results Comparable to Those After First Pulmonary Resection in Colorectal Cancer

Ogata Y, Matono K, Hayashi A, et al (Kurume Univ, Fukuoka, Japan)
World J Surg 29:363-368, 2005 13–15

Introduction.—Pulmonary resection for colorectal metastases is well accepted. However, the main cause of death after pulmonary resection is recurrence in the lung. The aim of this study was to clarify whether a repeat pulmonary resection was warranted in patients with recurrent lung metastases. The records of 76 patients undergoing initial pulmonary resection, including 14 patients undergoing a repeat operation for lung metastases, were reviewed for survival, operative morbidity, and mortality. Overall, pulmonary resection was performed 96 times in this group of patients. The operative mortality was 0%, morbidity involved only one case of major postoperative hemorrhage associated with the first operation. The cumulative 5-year survival rate for the 76 patients was 32%. After the second pulmonary operation, recurrence was identified in 79% (11 of 14) of the patients. In 10 patients with isolated lung recurrence after a first pulmonary resection, who showed no extrapulmonary disease before or at the time of first thoracotomy, the 3-year, and 5-year-survival rate after the second pulmonary resection was 67%, and 33%, respectively, comparing favorably with the survival rate in those who underwent primary pulmonary resection. In contrast, all 4 patients with extrapulmonary disease before or at the time of thoracotomy had poor prognosis. Repeat pulmonary operation for isolated recurrent colorectal metastases to the lung yielded results comparable to those after the first pulmonary resection in terms of operative mortality and survival in the absence of hilar/mediastinal lymph node or extrathoracic involvement.

▶ This article from Dr Ogata and colleagues from Japan examined the records of 76 patients undergoing initial pulmonary metastasectomy for colorectal carcinoma and the charts of 14 patients who underwent a repeat operation. Although these numbers are very small, this article was selected because it drives home a very important and common clinical dilemma. That is, how many times does one perform a metastasectomy on a patient who has hematogenous disease that has spread to the lungs? These authors found that patients with extrapulmonary disease before the time of thoracotomy had a worse prognosis, but that repeat pulmonary operations had similar results to the first. These data, although of course only on patients with colorectal cancer, are applicable to patients with other solid organ tumors as demonstrated in many other small institutional trials. The take-home message continues to be if the primary is under control, if the pulmonary disease can be completely resected, and if the patient's operative risks are low, metastasectomy makes sense, irrespective of the number of previous resections or the number of pulmonary nodules.

R. J. Cerfolio, MD

Lung Volume Reduction Surgery vs Medical Treatment: For Patients With Advanced Emphysema

Miller JD, Berger RL, Malthaner RA, et al (McMaster Univ, Hamilton, Ont, Canada; Harvard Med School, Boston; Univ of Western Ontario, London, Canada; et al)
Chest 127:1166-1177, 2005 13–16

Objective.—To contribute to the knowledge on the therapeutic value of lung volume reduction surgery (LVRS).

Design.—Two similar, independently conceived and conducted, multicenter, randomized clinical trials.

TABLE 5.—Outcome Differences Between Surgical and Medical Arms 6 Months After Randomization*

Outcome	CLVR Study		OBEST		Combined			
	LVRS vs Medical	p Value	LVRS vs Medical Therapy	p Value	Weighted Mean Difference	Lower 95% CI	Upper 95% CI	p Value
FEV_1, mL	246	0.036	113	0.2327	167	29	304	0.017
TLC, ml	− 959	0.010	− 1,111	0.0019	− 1,044	− 1,483	− 605	< 0.001
RV, mL	− 1,379	0.0027	− 1,316	0.0012	− 1,342	− 1,844	− 840	< 0.001
P_{CO_2}, mm Hg	− 4.80	0.030	− 4.82	0.5936	− 3.7183	− 6.960	− 0.477	0.025
D_{LCO}, mL/min/mm Hg	1.615	0.067	− 0.2137	0.8535	0.9810	− 0.334	2.296	0.144
6MWD, feet	170.0	0.066	125.5	0.190	148.8	24.3	273.2	0.019

*Values were adjusted for blocking.

Abbreviations: CLVR, Canadian Lung Volume Reduction; *OBEST,* Overholt-Blue Cross Emphysema Surgery Trial; *LVRS,* lung volume reduction surgery; *CI,* confidence interval; FEV_1, forced expiratory volume in 1 second; *TLC,* total lung capacity; *RV,* residual volume; $P_{CO}2$, partial pressure of carbon dioxide; D_{LCO}, diffusing capacity of lung for carbon monoxide; *6MWD,* 6-minute walk distance.

(Courtesy of Miller JD, Berger RL, Malthaner RA, et al: Lung volume reduction surgery vs medical treatment: For patients with advanced emphysema. *Chest* 127:1166-1177, 2005.)

Setting.—The Canadian Lung Volume Reduction (CLVR) study and the Overholt-Blue Cross Emphysema Surgery Trial (OBEST).

Methods.—Using a fixed-effects meta-analysis, the 6-month results produced by the addition of LVRS to optimal medical therapy were compared to those obtained from optimal medical therapy alone. Patients were required to have severe emphysema, marked airflow limitation (*ie*, FEV_1, 15 to 40% predicted), hyperinflation (total lung capacity [TLC], > 120% predicted), CO_2, < 55 mm Hg, and measurable dyspnea (chronic respiratory disease questionnaire [CRDQ] scores ≤ 4 for the CLVR study, or Medical Research Council dyspnea scale ≥ 1 for the OBEST). Optimal medical therapy included pulmonary rehabilitation in both arms of both studies.

Results.—The CLVR study randomized 58 patients and the OBEST randomized 35 patients for a total of 93 patients. Of these, 54 patients were randomized to undergo surgery, and 39 patients were randomized to receive medical treatment. The 6-month mortality rate (including operative mortality) in the surgical and medical cohorts was similar (5.6% vs 5.1%, respectively). A comparison of the medical and surgical arms of the combined CLVR study/OBEST population showed that LVRS was associated with a higher FEV_1 (167 mL or 24% predicted; 95% confidence interval [CI], 29 to 304; $p = 0.017$), lower residual volume (−1,342 mL or 24.5% predicted; 95% CI, −1,844 to −840; $p < 0.001$), lower TLC (−1,044 mL or 13% predicted; 95% CI, −1483 to −605; $p < 0.001$), and higher 6-min walk distance (148.8 feet; 95% CI, 24.3 to 273.2; $p = 0.019$) (Table 5). Each domain of the CRDQ showed statistically significant improvement in the surgical arm of the study, but not in the medical arm. The summary physical component scale of the Medical Outcomes Study 36-item short form (SF-36) was also more favorable in the LVRS cohort (6.9; 95% CI, 2.86 to 10.90; $p < 0.001$). The summary mental component scale of the SF-36 did not show a statistically significant difference between the two groups.

Conclusion.—Six months after randomization, LVRS produced better palliation than optimal medical therapy in patients with advanced emphysema.

▶ This extremely important article from Dr John D. Miller and associates from Canada examines a very carefully constructed and performed multicentered, randomized clinical trial on LVRS. Once again, these authors found that LVRS produced better quality of life than optimal medical therapy in patients with advanced emphysema. These results are best illustrated in Table 5. These authors show that in tightly designed, clinically constructed, and difficult-to-perform studies, LVRS beats medical therapy in properly selected patients with emphysema. The keys to surgical success are careful patient selection, meticulous intraoperative technique, and an experienced postoperative team.

R. J. Cerfolio, MD

Surgically Induced Accelerated Local and Distant Tumor Growth Is Significantly Attenuated by Selective COX-2 Inhibition

Qadri SSA, Wang J-H, Coffey JC, et al (Cork Univ, Republic of Ireland)
Ann Thorac Surg 79:990-995, 2005 13–17

Background.—Even after apparently curative resection, lung cancer recurrence continues to lead to high mortality levels. The aim of this study was to assess the effects of cyclooxygenase-2 (COX-2) inhibitor on local and systemic recurrent tumor growth.

Methods.—C57BL/6 mice underwent mammary fat pad inoculation with 3LL cells. After two weeks growth, flank tumors were resected completely and followed for recurrent tumor growth. Postresection mice were randomized to receive placebo alone (group 1) or the selective COX-2 inhibitor, rofecoxib (group 2), daily for two weeks by tube feeding. Recurrent tumor growth kinetics were compared for both groups. Two weeks following primary tumor excision animals were sacrificed, after which lungs were resected and pulmonary metastatic burden was assessed using the lung-body weight ratio. Apoptotic and mitotic indices were established for recurrent tumors and lungs, using hematoxylin and eosin histology.

Results.—Two weeks postexcision of the primary tumor, recurrent tumors in the placebo group were significantly greater than the treatment group ($p = 0.002$). While primary tumors were typically encapsulated and not adherent, recurrent tumors in the placebo group were invasive, adherent to the chest wall and the overlying wound. In contrast, recurrent tumors in the treatment group were nonadherent to the chest wall. Moreover, postoperative pulmonary metastatic burden was significantly reduced in treated animals. Histologic examination revealed increased apoptosis as well as an increase in the apoptosis-mitosis ratio in treated animals.

Conclusions.—Primary tumor excision was associated with accelerated local and systemic tumor recurrence. However, these effects were significantly attenuated using selective COX-2 inhibition. The COX-2-inhibition was associated with increased levels of apoptosis. These findings endorse a role for COX-2 inhibition in the secondary prevention of lung cancer recurrence at both local and systemic levels.

▶ We selected this interesting article (even though it is on a basic science topic as opposed to a clinical study) because it shows the positive effect that COX-2 inhibitors have for apoptosis of tumors cells. This may play a critical role in the prevention of both the local and systemic spread of non–small cell lung cancer. Although drugs that are COX-2 inhibitors have taken an unfortunate public hit recently with the lawsuits against Merck and Pfizer secondary to their possible link to deaths in isolated patients from stroke, the positive effects of these agents are undeniable. We believe over time these agents will make their use back into the clinical arena with public support, especially in patients who have adenocarcinoma. They will play an important role in preventing further cancer recurrence.

R. J. Cerfolio, MD

Outcomes of Tracheobronchial Stents in Patients With Malignant Airway Disease

Lemaire A, Burfeind WR, Toloza E, et al (Duke Univ, Durham, NC)
Ann Thorac Surg 80:434-438, 2005 13–18

Background.—Malignant central airway obstruction is difficult to manage and is associated with poor outcome. We sought to identify the short (<30 days) and intermediate (>30 days) benefits and risks of tracheobronchial stents in patients with malignant airway disease.

Methods.—Two hundred and twenty-five tracheobronchial stents were placed in 172 patients for benign (n = 32) and malignant (n = 140) disease from January 1, 1997, to May 31, 2003. The records of the patients with malignant disease were retrospectively analyzed to determine complication rate, reintervention rate, and survival. The malignant diagnoses included nonsmall cell cancer, small cell cancer, esophageal cancer, and metastatic disease.

Results.—There were 172 stents placed in 140 patients with malignant disease, with no intraoperative mortality. The mean follow-up period was 142 ± 12 days. There were 23 complications, including tumor ingrowth (n = 9), excessive granulation tissue (n = 7), stent migration (n = 5), and restenosis (n = 2). Five of the complications occurred during the short-term period (<30 days) with the remaining complications (n = 18) occurring after 30 days. The complications required interventions including laser debridement (n = 14), dilation (n = 4), and stent removal (n = 5).

Conclusions.—Tracheobronchial stents offer minimally invasive palliative therapy for patients with unresectable malignant central airway obstruction. The benefit of airway stents is particularly seen in the short-term period where they provide symptomatic improvement and have low complication risk. The major impediment is excessive granulation tissue and tumor ingrowth, which occur primarily after 30 days.

► This article by Dr Lemaire and his colleagues was presented at the annual meeting of the Southern Thoracic Surgical Association. It drives home the message that permanent wire stents should not be placed in patients with benign disease. The records of 172 patients who had 225 stents placed were examined. The most important finding was in the 32 patients who had benign disease. The authors found excessive granulation tissue at the ends of the stents to be a significant problem. This is a problem we deal with on almost a weekly basis in our practice as well. The use of permanent wire stents should be condemned in patients with benign disease in most situations.

R. J. Cerfolio, MD

Tracheoplasty for Expiratory Collapse of Central Airways

Wright CD, Grillo HC, Hammoud ZT, et al (Harvard Med School, Boston)
Ann Thorac Surg 80:259-267, 2005 13–19

Background.—Severe central airway obstruction due to expiratory collapse occurs with malacia of intrathoracic trachea and main bronchi, often with chronic obstructive pulmonary disease. Bronchoscopically observed, it is confirmed by inspiratory-expiratory computerized tomographic chest scans. Prior attempts at surgical stabilization have not given dependable results.

Methods.—Posterior tracheobronchial splinting with polypropylene mesh (Marlex) holds cartilages in more normal configuration, and fixes redundant membranous walls (Fig 5). Fourteen consecutive patients were so treated for severe dyspnea. Prior trials of various autologous and exogenous splints failed.

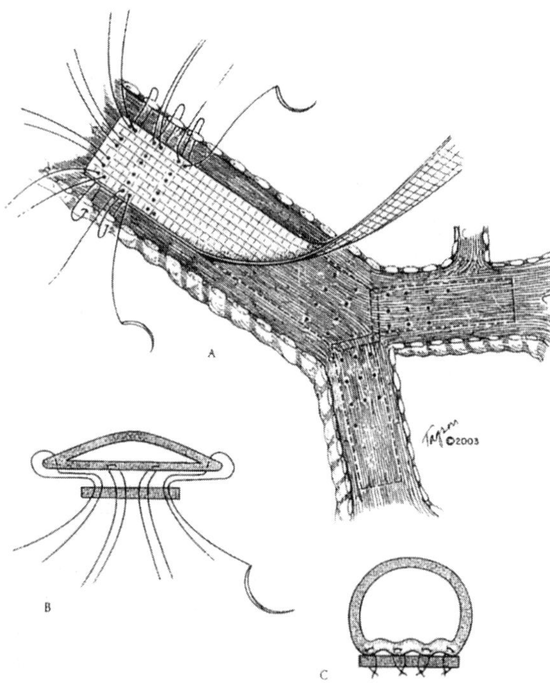

FIGURE 5.—Diagrams of posterior splinting procedure for expiratory tracheobronchial collapse. **A**, Marlex strip of appropriate width is sutured to the posterior membranous tracheal wall from the apex of the thorax to the carina. Successive rows of sutures are placed as described in the text. *Dots* indicate general placement of sutures. *Dashed lines* indicate placement of Marlex strips. **B**, Cross-sectional diagram showing placement and spacing of sutures. C, When tied, sutures pull the cartilage into more nearly normal C configurations and quilt the widened membranous wall to the Marlex. (Reproduced with permission of the artist, courtesy of Grillo HC: *Surgery of the Trachea and Bronchi*. Hamilton, Ont, Canada, BC Decker, 2004, p 647. From Wright CD, Grillo HC, Hammoud ZT, et al: Tracheoplasty for expiratory collapse of central airways. *Ann Thorac Surg* 80:259-267, 2005. Reprinted with permission from the Society of Thoracic Surgeons.)

Results.—All felt subjectively improved early, with decreased dyspnea, cough, and secretion retention, and with increased activities. Mean forced expiratory volume in 1 second rose from 51% predicted to 73% ($p = 0.009$), and peak expiratory flow rate from 49% to 70% ($p < 0.00001$). One patient was lost to follow-up (1 year), 1 died of unrelated cause (5 years), 1 died of chronic obstructive pulmonary disease (3 years), and 1 had decreased respiratory function over 5 years. Ten patients were available for long-term follow-up: 6 were judged to have an excellent result, 2 were good, and 2 were poor due to collapse of unsplinted main bronchi.

Conclusions.—Complete splinting of all malacic central airways with Marlex restores anatomic configuration and permanently prevents expiratory collapse, with relief of extreme dyspnea, cough, and secretion retention.

► Dr Wright and his associates from Boston have given an interesting alternative to the placement of stents for benign disease. As shown in the previous article (Abstract 13–18), these types of permanent expandable wire stents should almost never be used in patients with benign disease. Yet these patients suffer from respiratory distress from airways that collapse on themselves. Silicon stents, however, that can be removed and do not become ingratiated into the tracheal wall are viable options. However, they too can develop some granulation tissue and thus have long-term problems. This article, which only covers 14 patients, carefully secures the diagnosis of tracheobronchial malacia. The authors performed a right thoracotomy and a posterior splinting procedure using a Marlex strip as shown in Figure 5. This is an ingenious idea to help patients with malacia, and the authors' results are outstanding.

R. J. Cerfolio, MD

Thoracoscopic Sympathectomy for Axillary Hyperhidrosis: The Influence of T4

Licht PB, Jørgensen OD, Ladegaard L, et al (Aarhus Univ, Denmark; Odense Univ, Denmark)

Ann Thorac Surg 80:455-460, 2005 13–20

Background.—Recent data suggest that severe compensatory sweating after sympathectomy for hyperhidrosis is more common than previously reported. In particular, T2-T4 sympathectomy for axillary hyperhidrosis leads to significantly more disabling sweating compared with T2-T3 sympathectomy for palmar hyperhidrosis. However, it is not known whether this is a result of the additional transection of the T4 segment or if patients with primary axillary hyperhidrosis are more prone to experience disabling compensatory sweating.

Methods.—A follow-up study by questionnaire was made of 100 consecutive patients who underwent thoracoscopic sympathectomy for axillary hyperhidrosis at two university hospitals. Patients underwent T2-T3 sympathectomy (n = 35) or T2-T4 sympathectomy (n = 65) depending on the surgeon's preference.

Results.—The questionnaire was returned by 91% of patients after a median of 31 months. Compensatory sweating occurred in 90% of patients and was so severe in 61% that they often had to change clothes during the day. There were no significant differences in occurrence or severity of compensatory sweating between the two extents of sympathectomy. Surgical outcome, however, was significantly better after T2-T4 sympathectomy.

Conclusions.—In contrast with previous reports, the incidence of compensatory sweating was not significantly related to the extent of sympathectomy for axillary hyperhidrosis. This result suggests that patients with primary axillary hyperhidrosis are more prone to experience compensatory sweating. Although the majority of patients with axillary hyperhidrosis were satisfied after thoracoscopic sympathectomy, many regret the operation. Patients should undergo surgery only if medical treatments fail; and provided there is an indication, we recommend T2-T4 sympathectomy.

► In this article from Denmark, Dr Licht and colleagues examine the results of 100 consecutive patients who underwent thoracoscopic sympathectomy for axillary hyperhidrosis. It has been purported that patients with axillary hyperhidrosis alone who undergo VATS sympathotomy or sympathectomy have much higher rates of compensatory hyperhidrosis. The initial theory was that this was secondary to the fact that the sympathetic chain had been cut at the level of T4. However, further studies seem to show that the level of the interruption may not be the problem. Rather, patients who have axillary hyperhidrosis are more prone to get compensatory hyperhidrosis, irrespective of where the sympathetic chain is interrupted. These authors interestingly found that compensatory hyperhidrosis occurred in 90% of patients and was so severe that many patients had to change clothes during the day. Interestingly, they found no difference in the extent of compensatory sweating between those patients who had T2 to T3 sympathotomy when compared with patients who underwent division of the chain at T2 to T4. The important point of this study is the 90% compensatory hyperhidrosis rate and the fact that 61% have severe compensatory hyperhidrosis. The authors (probably correctly at least from their own data and experience) conclude that surgery shouldn't be performed in this group of patients. Patients with primary axillary hyperhidrosis are more prone to experience compensatory sweating and therefore probably should not undergo sympathectomy. An alternative therapy for these unhappy patients is to find a plastic surgeon who performs axillary liposuction. Although the data for the results of this procedure are pending, it has in our limited experience been relatively successful. Most importantly, if it fails, the patient is no worse off than before the medical intervention. This is a better situation than having the irreversible (or difficult to treat) problem of severe compensatory hyperhidrosis after sympathotomy.

R. J. Cerfolio, MD

Surgical Salvage Therapy for Malignant Intrathoracic Metastases From Nonseminomatous Germ Cell Cancer of Testicular Origin: Analysis of a Single-Institution Experience

Kesler KA, Wilson JL, Cosgrove JA, et al (Indiana Univ, Indianapolis)

J Thorac Cardiovasc Surg 130:408-415, 2005 13–21

Background.—Cisplatin-based chemotherapy followed by surgical extirpation of residual benign disease represents the usual sequence of curative therapy for metastatic nonseminomatous germ cell cancer of testicular origin. Occasionally, residual disease is malignant in the form of either a persistent nonseminomatous germ cell cancer tumor or degeneration into non–germ cell cancer. We reviewed our institution's experience with patients undergoing salvage operations to remove malignant intrathoracic metastases.

Methods.—From 1981 through 2001, 438 patients with nonseminomatous germ cell cancer had operations to remove residual intrathoracic disease after cisplatin-based chemotherapy at Indiana University Hospital. A subset of 134 patients who underwent 186 surgical procedures to remove malignant metastases is the basis of this review. Fifty-nine patients had removal of pulmonary metastases, 49 had removal of mediastinal metastases, and 26 had removal of both pulmonary and mediastinal metastases. Surgical pathology demonstrated 84 patients with persistent nonseminomatous germ cell cancer tumors, 38 with degeneration into non–germ cell cancer, and 12 with both malignant pathologic categories.

Results.—There were 4 (3.7%) operative deaths. The overall median survival was 5.6 years, with 55 (42.3%) patients alive and well after a mean follow-up of 5.1 years. Seventeen variables were analyzed by using Cox regression. Of these, older age, pulmonary metastases (vs mediastinal metastases), and 4 or more (vs 1) total intrathoracic metastases were significantly ($P \leq .01$) predictive of inferior long-term survival.

Conclusions.—Salvage thoracic surgery to remove malignant metastases from nonseminomatous germ cell cancer tumors of testicular origin can result in long-term survival in select patients. We identified variables that influence survival in this subset.

▶ Drs Kesler and Einhorn from Indiana, recognized world leaders in nonseminomatous germ cell tumors, once again present their vast experience in the surgical care of these unique patients. It is clear that this group has probably the world's largest experience in this particular area. The authors reviewed their experience with 438 patients with nonseminomatous germ cell tumors who had thoracic procedures to remove residual intrathoracic disease after cisplatin-based chemotherapy. They examined a subset of these 438 patients, specifically 134 patients who underwent repeat procedures to remove these metastases. They conclude that this technique can result in long-term survival in selected patients. This study shows that once again, repeat resection is indicated in selected patients.

R. J. Cerfolio, MD

Outcomes of COPD Lung Transplant Recipients After Lung Volume Reduction Surgery

Nathan SD, Edwards LB, Barnett SD, et al (Inova Heart and Lung Transplant Ctr, Falls Church, Va; United Network for Organ Sharing, Richmond, Va)

Chest 126:1569-1574, 2004 13–22

Study Objectives.—We sought to assess the outcomes of COPD lung transplant recipients who had previously undergone lung volume reduction surgery (LVRS), and to compare these patients to those COPD lung recipients who had not previously undergone LVRS.

Design.—Retrospective analysis of the United Network for Organ Sharing transplant database over the period between October 25, 1999, and December 31, 2002.

Patients.—All COPD patients who were listed and underwent transplantation during the time period were analyzed and categorized according to who did and did not have a history of LVRS. The two groups were compared for demographics, severity of illness, and various measures of outcomes after transplantation, including survival.

Results.—There were 791 COPD patients who underwent transplantation, of whom 50 had a history of LVRS. The two groups had similar demographics and severity of disease. There was no difference in the need for reoperation, hospital length of stay, or survival between the groups.

Conclusion.—A history of LVRS does not impact on outcomes after lung transplantation and should not influence a patient's candidacy for transplantation. Similarly, a patient's potential need for lung transplantation should not impact on the decision-making process for undergoing LVRS.

▶ Dr Nathan and colleagues from the United States have shown that LVRS does not impact on the outcome after lung transplantation and is not a contraindication to lung transplantation.

R. J. Cerfolio, MD

Lung Transplantation

Primary Graft Dysfunction and Other Selected Complications of Lung Transplantation: A Single-Center Experience of 983 Patients

Meyers BF, de la Morena M, Sweet SC, et al (Washington Univ, St Louis; Barnes-Jewish Hosp, St Louis)

J Thorac Cardiovasc Surg 129:1421-1429, 2005 13–23

Objectives.—We sought to review the incidence and outcome of lung transplantation complications observed over 15 years at a single center.

Methods.—We performed a retrospective review from our databases, tracking outcomes after adult and pediatric lung transplantation. The 983 operations between July 1988 and September 2003 included 277 pediatric and 706 adult recipients. Bilateral (74%), unilateral (19%), and living lobar

TABLE 1.—Recipients Stratified by Pediatric Versus Adult Classification

	Pediatric (n = 277)	Adult (n = 706)	*P* Value
Age (y)	10.7 ± 6.4; 12.1 (IQR, 5.4-15.8)	47.6 ± 12.2; 50.5 (IQR, 38.9-57.6)	
Sex (F)	156 (56.3%)	357 (50.6%)	.118
Diagnosis			<.001
Emphysema	0 (0%)	399 (56.5%)	
Cystic fibrosis	138 (49.8%)	118 (16.7%)	
Pulmonary vascular disease	71 (25.6%)	63 (8.9%)	
Other pulmonary disease	68 (24.6%)	126 (17.8%)	
Time on the waiting list (d)	176 (IQR, 42-465)	488 (IQR, 281-665)	<.001
Type of transplantation performed			<.001
Bilateral	204 (73.6%)	526 (74.5%)	
Single	8 (2.9%)	176 (24.9%)	
Heart-lung	16 (5.8%)	4 (0.6%)	
Bilateral lobar (living)	39 (14.1%)	0 (0%)	
Bilateral lobar (cadaveric)	4 (1.4%)	0 (0%)	
Single lobe	1 (0.4%)	0 (0%)	
Bilateral-liver	5 (1.8%)	0 (0%)	
Length of mechanical ventilation (d)	5 (IQR, 2-14)	2 (IQR, 1-4)	<.001
Length of stay in ICU (d)	7 (IQR, 4-17)	3 (IQR, 2-5)	<.001
Length of stay in hospital (d)	19 (IQR, 13-33)	17 (IQR, 12-24)	<.001
Required ECMO support after transplantation	27 (9.7%)	20 (2.8%)	<.001
Primary graft dysfunction*	62 (22.4%)	160 (22.7%)	1.000
Hospital mortality	46 (16.6%)	50 (7.1%)	<.001
Treated for airway complication	30 (10.8%)	66 (9.3%)	.476
Diagnosed with posttransplantation lymphoproliferative disease	32 (11.6%)	42 (5.9%)	.004

*Adults: arterial partial pressure of oxygen/fraction of inspired oxygen of 150 or less on initial or 24-hour arterial blood gas; Peds: mechanical ventilation >7 days, retransplantation <7 days of initial transplant, chest radiograph consistent with reperfusion injury, biopsy.

Abbreviations: IQR, Interquartile range; *ECMO*, extracorporeal membrane oxygenation.

(Courtesy of Meyers BF, de la Morena M, Sweet SC, et al: Primary graft dysfunction and other selected complications of lung transplantation: A single-center experience of 983 patients. *J Thorac Cardiovasc Surg* 129:1421-1429, 2005. Copyright 2005 with permission from The American Association for Thoracic Surgery.)

transplants (4%) comprised the bulk of this experience. Retransplantations accounted for 44 (4.5%) of the operations.

Results.—The groups differed by indication for transplantation. The adults included 57% with emphysema and 17% with cystic fibrosis, and the children included no patients with emphysema and 50% with cystic fibrosis (Table 1). Hospital mortality was 96 (9.8%) of 983, including 46 (17%) of 277 of the children and 50 (7%) of 706 of the adults. The overall survival curves did not differ between adults and children ($P = .56$). Freedom from bronchiolitis obliterans syndrome at 5 and 10 years was 45% and 18% for adults and 48% and 30% for children, respectively ($P = .53$). The causes of death for adults included bronchiolitis obliterans syndrome (40%), respiratory failure (17%), and infection (14%), whereas the causes of death in children included bronchiolitis obliterans syndrome (35%), infection (28%), and respiratory failure (21%) ($P < .01$). Posttransplantation lymphoproliferative disease occurred in 12% of pediatric recipients and 6% of adults ($P < .01$). The frequency of treated airway complications did not differ between adults and children (9% vs 11%, $P = .48$). The frequency of primary graft dysfunction did not differ between children (22%) and adults (23%), despite disparity in the use of cardiopulmonary bypass.

Conclusion.—These results highlight major complications after lung transplantation. Despite differences in underlying diagnoses and operative techniques, the 2 cohorts of patients experienced remarkably similar outcomes.

► This article from Dr Meyers and colleagues at Washington University is a retrospective review of 983 operations over a 15-year period. Although it is obviously a mixed bag of patients with a wide array of thoracic diseases, as shown in Table 1, it shows the significant morbidity of lung transplantation in adults as compared with children. Despite different indications for transplantation and the obviously different age groups, the results are quite similar.

R. J. Cerfolio, MD

► The heterogeneity of issues pertaining to success after transplantation is highly dependent upon the organ transplanted. Issues relating to success of kidney transplantation differ from those for liver, heart, and pancreas transplantation. The current article describes a single-center experience with lung transplantation. The authors describe their experience with delayed graft function and the associated morbidity. Although many variables are associated with primary graft dysfunction including ischemia time, mode of death, etc, one of the interesting observations made was the relative sparing of patients who were transplanted for emphysema as compared with individuals who underwent transplantation for pulmonary hypertension. The complication of graft dysfunction is enormous in that the mortality rate for patients with primary graft dysfunction was almost 30% compared with less than 5% for those without the condition. As this complication occurs in up to 20% of cases, addressing its cause and rectifying its complications is critical. If one can survive early primary graft dysfunction, the next major long-term complication is that of bronchiolitis obliterans. Whether the advent of new immunosuppressives will markedly alter the incidence of this complication remains to be seen. At present, bronchiolitis obliterans accounts for roughly 40% of all deaths in the adult population and 35% of all deaths in the pediatric population.

T. L. Pruett, MD

Lung Transplantation With Lungs From Donors Fifty Years of Age and Older

Fischer S, Gohrbandt B, Struckmeier P, et al (Hannover Med School, Germany)
J Thorac Cardiovasc Surg 129:919-925, 2005 13–24

Background.—A shortage of donors has led to the progressive expansion of criteria for donor selection in lung transplantation. The outcome of recipients of lungs from donors aged 50 years or older is analyzed systematically.

Methods.—From March 1998 to June 2003, 49 recipients received lungs from donors aged 50 years or older (range 50-64 years, mean 54 ± 3 years). This group of recipients was compared with 244 patients receiving lungs from donors aged less than 50 years (range 7-49 years, mean 32 ± 11 years). This study was undertaken on all 293 patients at our institution who received Perfadex-preserved lungs (Vitrolife, Göteborg, Sweden).

TABLE 4.—Outcome After Lung Transplantation by Different Age Subgroups in the Elderly Donor Cohort (Do > 50)

	Do 50-54 y (n = 31)	Do 55-59 y (n = 12)	Do > 59 y (n = 6)
Length of post-LTx ventilation (hr)	364 ± 450	307 ± 452	303 ± 221
Length of ICU stay (d)	18 ± 20	14 ± 19	7 ± 9
Survival (%)			
30 d	90 ± 2	82 ± 3	75 ± 3
3 mo	81 ± 2	73 ± 2	75 ± 3
6 mo	71 ± 1	73 ± 2	75 ± 3
12 mo	71 ± 1	73 ± 2	75 ± 3
First PaO_2/FIO_2 on the ICU	282 ± 138	261 ± 151	262 ± 113
Best FEV_1 (% of predicted FEV_1)	73 ± 22	80 ± 18	87 ± 32
Cause of death after LTx (n)	10 (32%)	4 (36%)	1 (25%)
Acute graft failure	1 (11% of deaths)	1 (25% of deaths)	0
Chronic graft failure	1 (11%)	0	0
Sepsis/multiorgan failure	4 (44%)	3 (75%)	0
Bronchial complications	1 (11%)	0	0
Cardiac/hemodynamic complications	1 (11%)	0	0
Neurologic complications	1 (11%)	0	1 (100%)
Gastroenterologic complications	0	0	0
Neoplasia	0	0	0
Unknown	1 (11%)	0	0

$P < .05$.

Abbreviations: Do > 50, Donors aged 50 years or more; *LTx*, lung transplantation; Pao_2/Fio_2, ratio of partial pressure of oxygen in arterial blood to the fraction of inspired oxygen; FEV_1, forced expiratory volume in 1 second.

Results.—Recipient age, sex, and indications for transplant did not differ significantly between groups. Also, the percentage of the different types of transplants (bilateral or single lung transplantation) performed was equal in both cohorts. Donor PaO_2/FIO_2 ratios before lung retrieval (415 ± 91 vs 439 ± 113, respectively) and length of ischemic time (347 ± 67 minutes vs 351 ± 84 minutes, respectively) did not differ significantly between the older and younger donor groups. The following posttransplant parameters were also not statistically different: first PaO_2/FIO_2 at intensive care unit arrival (274 ± 125 in the older donor group vs 253 ± 119 in the younger donor group, respectively), mechanical ventilation time (328 ± 427 hours vs 269 ± 425 hours, respectively), and length of stay in the intensive care unit (16 ± 18 days vs 14 ± 18 days, respectively). Recipient survival in the older and younger donor groups at 30 days, 3, 6, 12, 24, and 60 months was 77% ± 6%, 75% ± 6%, 73% ± 7%, 73% ± 7%, 68% ± 5%, and 68% ± 4% versus 86% ± 2%, 83% ± 3%, 80% ± 3%, 78% ± 3%, 71% ± 4%, and 66% ± 4%, respectively.

Conclusions.—Lung grafts from elderly donors have been considered as marginal organs for transplantation. However, this study indicates that transplantation of lungs from carefully selected donors aged 50 years or more may lead to similar short- and long-term outcomes compared with lungs from younger donors. The use of lungs from elderly donors may help to increase the number of donor organs in lung transplantation (Table 4).

► Dr Fischer and colleagues from Hannover, Germany, have presented a provocative report on 49 recipients who received lungs from donors that were 50 years or older. Because of the great shortage of organs and the fact that so many patients die while waiting for heart and lung transplants, articles such as these are timely and important. The bar needs to be lowered and tested at this reduced height. This article shows that in carefully selected donors who are 50 or older, the short and perhaps intermediate results are similar to patients who receive lungs from younger donors. These results are shown in Table 4. It is this type of data that will help impact on the devastating number of deaths of patients who remain on the transplant list who don't live long enough to receive an organ. These data may be applicable to other types of solid organs.

R. J. Cerfolio, MD

Subject Index

A

B

C

D

F

G

H

I

K

L

M

N

O

Q

R

S

Author Index

A

B

C

D

E

F

G

H

T

U

V

W

X

Y

Z